Updates in Neurourology

Editor

JOHN T. STOFFEL

UROLOGIC CLINICS OF NORTH AMERICA

www.urologic.theclinics.com

Consulting Editor
KEVIN R. LOUGHLIN

May 2024 • Volume 51 • Number 2

ELSEVIER

1600 John F. Kennedy Boulevard • Suite 1800 • Philadelphia, Pennsylvania, 19103-2899

http://www.theclinics.com

UROLOGIC CLINICS OF NORTH AMERICA Volume 51, Number 2
May 2024 ISSN 0094-0143, ISBN-13: 978-0-443-24690-6

Editor: Kerry Holland
Developmental Editor: Nitesh Barthwal

Urologic Clinics of North America (ISSN 0094-0143) is published quarterly by Elsevier Inc., 360 Park Avenue South, New York, NY 10010-1710. Months of issue are February, May, August, and November. Business and Editorial Offices: 1600 John F. Kennedy Blvd., Suite 1800, Philadelphia, PA 19103-2899. Periodicals postage paid at New York, NY and additional mailing offices. Subscription prices are $427.00 per year (US individuals), $100.00 per year (US students and residents), $483.00 per year (Canadian individuals), $100.00 per year (Canadian students/residents), $557.00 per year (foreign individuals), and $240.00 per year (foreign students/residents). For institutional access pricing please contact Customer Service via the contact information below. Foreign air speed delivery is included in all *Clinics* subscription prices. All prices are subject to change without notice. **POSTMASTER:** Send address changes to *Urologic Clinics of North America*, Elsevier Health Sciences Division, Subscription Customer Service, 3251 Riverport Lane, Maryland Heights, MO 63043. **Customer Service: 1-800-654-2452 (US). From outside the United States, call 1-314-447-8871. Fax: 1-314-447-8029. E-mail: JournalsCustomerServiceusa@elsevier.com (for print support)** and **JournalsOnlineSupport-usa@elsevier.com (for online support)**.

Reprints. For copies of 100 or more, of articles in this publication, please contact the Commercial Reprints Department, Elsevier Inc., 360 Park Avenue South, New York, New York 10010-1710. Tel.: 212-633-3874; Fax: 212-633-3820; E-mail: reprints@elsevier.com.

Urologic Clinics of North America is covered in MEDLINE/PubMed (*Index Medicus*), *Excerpta Medica, Current Contents/Clinical Medicine, Science Citation Index,* and *ISI/BIOMED*.

Contributors

EDITOR-IN-CHIEF

KEVIN R. LOUGHLIN, MD, MBA
Emeritus Professor of Surgery (Urology),
Harvard Medical School, Visiting Scientist,
Vascular Biology Research Program, Boston
Children's Hospital, Boston, Massachusetts,
USA

EDITOR

JOHN T. STOFFEL, MD
Member, Neurogenic Bladder Research
Group, Lapides Family Research Professor,
Chief, Neurourology and Pelvic Reconstruction
Division, Department of Urology, University of
Michigan, Ann Arbor, Michigan, USA

AUTHORS

ANDREW S. AFYOUNI, BS
Medical Student, Division of Neurourology and
Reconstructive Pelvic Surgery, Department of
Urology, University of California Irvine, Irvine,
California, USA

HUMPHREY O. ATIEMO, MD
Clinical Associate Professor, University of
Toledo, Promedica Health System, Toledo,
Ohio, USA

ULYSSES G.J. BALIS, MD
Professor, Division of Pathology Informatics,
Department of Pathology, University of
Michigan Medical School, Ann Arbor,
Michigan, USA

BRANDEE BRANCHE, MD
Urology Resident PGY-3, University of
Michigan Medical School, Ann Arbor,
Michigan, USA

ANNE P. CAMERON, MD
Professor, Department of Urology, University
of Michigan, Ann Arbor, Michigan, USA

SHANICE COX, MS
Medical Student, Burnett School of Medicine at
TCU, Fort Worth, Texas, USA

IRENE CRESCENZE, MD
Clinical Assistant Professor, Department of
Urology, Ohio State University, Columbus,
Ohio, USA

JOHN DELANCEY, MD
Norman F. Miller Professor of Gynecology,
Department of Obstetrics and Gynecology,
University of Michigan Medical School,
Michigan, Ann Arbor, USA

TAIWO DODO-WILLIAMS, BS
Medical Student, UC San Diego School of
Medicine, La Jolla, California, USA

CHRISTOPHER S. ELLIOTT, MD, PhD
Division of Urology, Attending Physician,
Department of Urology, Stanford University
Medical Center, Santa Clara Valley Medical
Center, Valley Specialties Center, San Jose,
California, USA

MARC A. FURRER, MD, FEBU
Head Physician, Department of Urology,
Solothurner Spitäler AG, Kantonsspital Olten,
Olten, Switzerland; Bürgerspital Solothurn,
Solothurn, Switzerland, Department of Uro-
Neurology, National Hospital for Neurology and
Neurosurgery and UCL Institute of Neurology,

London, United Kingdom; Department of Urology Inselspital, University of Bern, Bern, Switzerland

NATALIA GARCÍA-PEÑALOZA, MD
Urology Resident PGY-1, UC San Diego School of Medicine, La Jolla, California, USA

KELLY T. HARRIS, MD
Pediatric Urologist, Division of Urology, Children's Hospital Colorado, Aurora, Colorado, USA

LATANYA LOFTON HOGUE, MD
Clinical Assistant Professor, Department of Orthopedic Surgery, Wake Forest School of Medicine, Atrium Health, Carolinas Rehabilitation, Charlotte, North Carolina, USA

CATALINA K. HWANG, MD
Fellow, Division of Urology, Children's Hospital Colorado, Aurora, Colorado, USA

CATHERINE FRANCES INGRAM, MD
PGY-4 Resident, Department of Urology, Baylor College of Medicine, Houston, Texas, USA

GIULIA M. IPPOLITO, MD, MS
Assistant Professor, Department of Urology, University of Michigan, Ann Arbor, Michigan, USA

MICHAEL JUSZCZAK, MD
Physician, Department of Physical Medicine and Rehabilitation, Tower Health, Reading Hospital Rehabilitation at Wyomissing, Reading, Pennsylvania, USA

MICHAEL KENNELLY, MD
Clinical Professor, Department of Urology, Wake Forest School of Medicine, Atrium Health, Carolinas Rehabilitation, Charlotte, North Carolina, USA

THOMAS M. KESSLER, MD, FEBU
Head Physician, Department of Neuro-Urology, Balgrist University Hospital, University of Zürich, Zürich, Switzerland

ROSE KHAVARI, MD
Professor, Department of Urology, Houston Methodist Hospital, Houston, Texas, USA

JANE T. KURTZMAN, MD
Visiting Instructor, Division of Urology, Department of Surgery, University of Utah, Salt Lake City, Utah, USA

JOHN A. LINCOLN, MD, PhD
Associate Professor, Department of Neurology, Baylor College of Medicine, McGovern Medical School, UT Health Neurosciences Neurology, Houston, Texas, USA

MAYRA LUCAS, MD, MPH
Urology Resident PGY-1, University of California, San Francisco School of Medicine, San Francisco, California, USA

JEREMY B. MYERS, MD, FACS
Chief, Division of Urology, Professor, Department of Surgery, University of Utah, Salt Lake City, Utah, USA

JALESH N. PANICKER, MD, DM, FRCP
Consultant, Faculty of Brain Sciences, Department of Uro-Neurology, National Hospital for Neurology, UCL Queen Square Institute of Neurology, University College London, London, United Kingdom

ZHINA SADEGHI, MD
Assistant Professor, Department of Urology, Division of Neurourology and Reconstructive Pelvic Surgery, University of California Irvine, Irvine, California, USA

YAHIR SANTIAGO-LASTRA, MD
Associate Professor, Division of Urogynecology, Neuro-Urology and Reconstructive Pelvic Surgery, Department of Urology, UC San Diego School of Medicine, San Diego, California, USA

KAZUKO SHEM, MD
Chief, Department of Physical Medicine and Rehabilitation, Santa Clara Valley Medical Center, San Jose, California, USA

JOHN T. STOFFEL, MD
Member, Neurogenic Bladder Research Group, Lapides Family Research Professor, Chief, Neurourology and Pelvic Reconstruction Division, Department of Urology, University of Michigan, Ann Arbor, Michigan, USA

BLAYNE WELK, MD, MSc
Assistant Professor, Departments of Surgery, and Epidemiology and Biostatistics, Western University, London, Ontario, Canada

GLENN T. WERNEBURG, MD, PhD
Department of Urology, Glickman Urological and Kidney Institute, Cleveland Clinic Foundation, Cleveland, Ohio, USA

VIVIAN WONG, MD
Urology Resident, Department of Urology, Ohio State University, Columbus, Ohio, USA

DAN WOOD, PhD, MBBS, FRCS(Urol)
Adolescent and Reconstructive Urologist, Division of Urology, Children's Hospital Colorado, Aurora, Colorado, USA

YI XI WU, PhD
Researcher, Division of Neurourology and Reconstructive Pelvic Surgery, Department of Urology, University of California Irvine, Irvine, California, USA

LISA YU, RN
Clinical Care Coordinator, Neurourology, Incontinence, Reconstruction, University of Michigan, Michigan Medicine, Ann Arbor, Michigan, USA

YU ZHENG, MD
FPRMS Fellow, Department of Urology, University of Michigan, Ann Arbor, Michigan, USA

Contents

The Neurogenic Bladder Research Group (NBRG) was formed with the mission to optimize quality of life (QoL), surgical outcomes, and clinical care of patients with neurogenic lower urinary tract dysfunction. One of the original priorities of the organization was to support creation of the NBRG Spinal Cord Injury (SCI) Registry. The aim of this Registry was to establish a prospective database, in order to study bladder-related QoL after SCI. The study enrolled close to 1500 participants from across North America over an 18 month time-period (January 2016–July 2017).

Lower urinary tract symptoms (LUTS) are highly prevalent in individuals with multiple sclerosis (MS). However, assessment of these symptoms is often hindered by vague definitions or absence of screening in asymptomatic patients. It is crucial to exercise caution when applying the non-neurogenic definition of urinary retention in this population. For men with MS experiencing persistent and treatment-resistant LUTS, urodynamic studies should be used to identify the underlying causes of symptoms. Although numerous therapies are presently accessible for managing LUTS in MS, there is a need for further investigation into emerging treatments such as percutaneous tibial nerve, and noninvasive brain stimulation.

The health care needs children with spina bifida evolve over their lifetime; continued, regular contact with appropraitely trained, multidisciplinary providers is crucial to a patient's health and quality of life. Substantial research has been conducted to improve the transition process starting at an early age; however, there continue to be strong barriers to successful transition. This article reviews key aspects of the care of patients with spina bifida, the impact of inadequate transition to adult care, barriers to transition, and offers a potential vision for the future.

Patients with Parkinson's disease (PD) have disturbances in their bladder and sleep physiology that lead to nocturia and overactive bladder (OAB). These symptoms can be extremely bothersome and impact not only their quality of life (QoL) but also the QoL of their caretakers. We aim to highlight the changes in bladder and sleep physiology in PD and explore OAB/nocturia treatment strategies in this population.

Bladder compliance is the relationship between detrusor pressure and bladder storage volume. We discuss the definition of compliance, how it may be accurately measured, and its clinical relevance. Specifically, we discuss the association between low compliance and upper urinary tract deterioration. We discuss medical and surgical therapies that have been demonstrated to improve compliance and reduce upper tract risk. Finally, we propose a model, which not only considers compliance but also differential pressure between the bladder and ureters, and how this may also be an accurate predictor of upper tract deterioration. We call for further investigation to test this model.

Detrusor sphincter dyssynergia (DSD) is defined as a detrusor contraction concurrent with an involuntary contraction of the urethral and/or periurethral striated muscles typically occurring in a patient with a spinal cord lesion above the sacral cord. Consequently, high urethral closure pressures during the detrusor contraction leads to high intravesical voiding pressure and large postvoid residuals, which can lead to significant complications in up to 50% of patients if DSD is not treated and followed-up regularly. DSD treatment options are centered around symptomatic management rather that addressing the underlying causative mechanisms.

The evaluation of people with neurogenic lower urinary tract dysfunction (NLUTD) often involves objective parameters, however quality of life (QOL) assessments are crucial for patient-centered care. This article discusses how to measure QOL and urinary symptoms in NLUTD and highlights various questionnaires such as the Qualiveen, Neurogenic Bladder Symptom Score (NBSS), and the Incontinence Quality of Life Questionnaire (I-QOL). These questionnaires focus on bladder-related QOL or symptoms and have been validated in multiple NLUTD populations. These tools are important for advancing research and the clinical care of NLUTD patients, and have the potential to impact decision-making and improve patient outcomes.

Urethral function declines by roughly 15% per decade and profoundly contributes to the pathogenesis of urinary incontinence. Individuals with poor urethral function are more likely to fail surgical management for stress incontinence that focus on improving urethral support. The reduced number of intramuscular nerves and the morphologic changes in muscle and connective tissue collectively impact urethral function as women age. Imaging technologies like MRI and ultrasound have advanced our understanding of these changes. However, substantial knowledge gaps remain. Addressing these gaps can be crucial for developing better prevention and treatment strategies, ultimately enhancing the quality of life for aging women.

Urinary Catheters: Materials, Coatings, and Recommendations for Selection   253

John T. Stoffel and Lisa Yu

Urinary catheters have been used for more than 3000 years, although materials have changed from wood to silver to rubber. Research continues to try and find the optimal catheter materials, which improve safety and quality of life. Advantages when comparing newer catheter materials are not always obvious but catheters coated with a hydrophilic layer may reduce urethral trauma and the incidence of urinary tract infections. However, extrapolation of the data is limited by lack of end-point standardization and heterogenous populations.

The Role of Upper Extremity Motor Function in the Choice of Bladder Management in Those Unable to Volitionally Void due to Neurologic Dysfunction   263

Michael Juszczak, Kazuko Shem, and Christopher S. Elliott

It is estimated that 425,000 individuals with neurologic bladder dysfunction (spinal cordinjury, spina bifida and multiple sclerosis) are unable to volitionally void and must rely oncatheter drainage. Upper extremity (UE) motor function is one of the most important factors indetermining the type of bladder management chosen in individuals who cannot volitionally void. Novel bladder management solutions for those with impaired UE motor function and concurrent impairments involitional voiding continue to be an area of need. Those with poor UE motor function more often choose an indwelling catheter, whereas those with normal UE motor function more often choose clean intermittent catheterization.

Integrating Patient Preferences with Guideline-Based Care in Neurogenic Lower Urinary Tract Dysfunction After Spinal Cord Injury   277

Vivian Wong, Giulia M. Ippolito, and Irene Crescenze

Individual and social factors are important for clinical decision-making in patients with neurogenic bladder secondary to spinal cord injury (SCI). These factors include the availability of caregivers, social infrastructure, and personal preferences, which all can drive bladder management decisions. These elements can be overlooked in clinical decision-making; therefore, there is a need to elicit and prioritize patient preferences and values into neurogenic bladder care to facilitate personalized bladder management choices. For the purposes of this article, we review the role of guideline-based care and shared decision-making in the SCI population with neurogenic lower urinary tract dysfunction.

The systematic review and workshop recommendations by the Neurogenic Bladder Research Group offer a comprehensive framework for evaluating health disparities in adult neurogenic lower urinary tract dysfunction (NLUTD). The study acknowledges the multifaceted nature of health, highlighting that medical care, though critical, is not the sole determinant of health outcomes. Social determinants of health significantly influence the disparities seen in NLUTD. This report calls for a shift in focus from traditional urologic care to a broader, more inclusive perspective that accounts for the complex interplay of social, economic, and health care factors in managing NLUTD.

This article discusses the ideal neurogenic bladder management team for patients who have neurogenic lower urinary tract dysfunction (NLUTD). It emphasizes the importance of a diverse team, including urologists, physiatrists, neurologist and others, working collaboratively to prevent complications and enhance patient outcomes. Owing to the unique nuances of the various neurologic conditions and patterns of NLUTD dysfunction, the roles of different specialists in the interdisciplinary team are outlined. This article describes 3 team models: multidisciplinary, interdisciplinary, and transdisciplinary, highlighting the benefits of collaborative approaches.

Primary care plays an important role in caring for neurogenic bladder patients. Clinicians should assess neurogenic bladder patients for common urologic symptoms/signs and refer to urology if refractory or safety issues are identified.

UROLOGIC CLINICS OF NORTH AMERICA

SERIES OF RELATED INTEREST
Surgical Clinics of North America
https://www.surgical.theclinics.com/

Erratum

An article in the November 2023 issue of *Urologic Clinics of North America* (50:4) has an incorrect title. Please note that "Management of Urologic Complications After Genital Gender-Affirming Surgery in Transgender and Nonbinary Patients" by R. Craig Sineath, Finn Hennig, Geolani W. Dy should be correctly listed as "Current State of Urology Residency Education on Caring for Transgender and Non-Binary Patients" by R. Craig Sineath, Finn Hennig, Geolani W. Dy.

Urol Clin N Am 51 (2024) xiii
https://doi.org/10.1016/j.ucl.2024.03.002
0094-0143/24/© 2024 Published by Elsevier Inc.

Foreword

The Neurourology Journey: From Pads to Jack Lapides and Intermittent Catheterization to Multidisciplinary Management

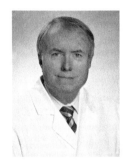

Kevin R. Loughlin, MD, MBA
Editor-in-Chief

This issue of Urologic Clinics of North America, edited by John T. Stoffel, represents the culmination of centuries of study of voiding dysfunction—its causes and treatments. Descriptions of urinary incontinence from spinal cord injury can be found as early as the second millennium BC in Egyptian manuscripts.[1,2] Claudius Galen (129–201 AD) is credited as being the first to perform physiologic experiments on the lower-urinary tract, and he concluded that micturition is achieved by contraction of the abdominal muscles. Leonardo da Vinci (1452–1519) performed human dissections of the urinary tract and completed anatomic drawings of the bladder and pelvis and concluded, "muscles which open and close the passage of the urine into the mouth of the bladder neck," was his explanation for the act of voiding.[3]

In North America, Benjamin Franklin (1706–1790) is credited with developing a silver catheter to aid in the treatment of his brother's bladder stones and then later to treat himself.[4] However, until the twentieth century, the understanding of all types of urinary dysfunction was rudimentary, and the treatment was largely empirical. It is fair to identify a landmark article by Jack Lapides, MD[5] (1914–1995) on the utility and safety of clean, intermittent catheterization in the management of urinary tract disease, as the beginning of the modern understanding of urinary tract function and treatment. It is indeed fitting that the guest editor of this issue, John T. Stoffel, is the Lapides Family Research Professor at the University of Michigan, and he carries on that institution's rich history of neurourology expertise.[6]

Urol Clin N Am 51 (2024) xv–xvi
https://doi.org/10.1016/j.ucl.2024.02.009
0094-0143/24/© 2024 Published by Elsevier Inc.

The article, "Bladder Compliance: How We Define It and Why It Is Important" particularly resonated with me because one of my teachers, Subbarao V. Yalla, had a keen interest in bladder compliance and its impact on urinary tract function.[7] He was a skilled teacher and made a difficult subject understandable.

Dr Stoffel has gathered many of the world's experts in neurourology in this single issue. The world of modern neurourology is now defined by the multidisciplinary management of urologic surgeons, neurologists, nurse practitioners, and basic scientists. I hope the readers enjoy reading this issue as much as I did.

Kevin R. Loughlin, MD, MBA
Vascular Biology Research Laboratory
Boston Children's Hospital
300 Longwood Avenue
Boston, MA 02115, USA

E-mail address:
kloughlin@partners.org

REFERENCES

1. Breasted JH. The Edwin Smith surgical papyrus: hieroglyphic transliteraturation, translation and commentary V1. Chicago: University of Chicago Oriental Institute; 1930.
2. Joachim H. Papyrus Ebers. Berlin: G. Reimer; 1890.
3. Schultheiss D, Gruenewald V, Jonas U. Urodynamic aspects in the anatomical work of Leonardo da Vinci (1452–1519). World J Urol 1999;17:137–44.
4. Catheterization: relief in a tube: catheters remain steadfast treatment for urinary disorders. Didusch Museum. Available at: https://urologichistory. museum/histories/urologictreatment/catheterization. [Accessed 20 February 2024].
5. Lapides J, Diokno AC, Silber SJ, et al. Clean, intermittent self-catheterization in the treatment of urinary tract disease. J Urol 1972;107(3):458–61.
6. Bloom DA, McGuire EJ, Lapides J. A brief history of urethral catheterization. J Urol 1994;151:317–25.
7. Sullivan MP, Yalla SV. Detrusor contractility and compliance characteristics in adult male patients with obstructive and nonobstructive voiding dysfunction. J Urol 1996;155(6):1995–2000.

Preface

Neurogenic Bladder: A Complex Puzzle with Multiple Pieces

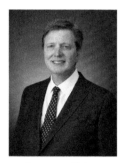

John T. Stoffel, MD
Editor

What is a neurogenic bladder? If we use a definition, neurogenic bladder is broadly defined as any bladder function that is impacted by a neurologic condition. However, this definition suffers when trying to describe a "typical" or "index" person with a neurogenic bladder. It could describe a person with multiple sclerosis–impacted urinary incontinence from neurologically derived detrusor overactivity. Or it could be a spinal cord–injured person performing intermittent catheterization for urinary retention related to detrusor underactivity. Now contrast this broad definition to oncologic malignancies. Although all have cancer, it would be foolish to group them all under a single definition. Yet this is what has happened with neurogenic bladder. The American Urological Association's recent guidelines on Neurogenic Bladder Care begin to address this broad definition problem by grouping patients as low, medium, and high risk for complications, but more work needs to be done to differentiate the nuances between neurogenic bladder patients. It the goal of this issue of *Urologic Clinics of North America* to change the conversation around neurogenic bladder and to begin to think about it in terms of a collection of subtypes with specific treatment needs rather than as a single entity.

The issue starts by highlighting urologic needs for four common neurologic conditions, Spinal Cord Injury, Spina Bifida, Multiple Sclerosis, and Parkinson Disease. As noted above, neurogenic bladder is too frequently treated as a common end point for completely different conditions. For example, whereas a spinal cord injury is an acute, focal trauma to a specific area, multiple sclerosis is an insidious chronic process that diffusely impacts broad regions of the central nervous system. Since the neurologic conditions differ by mechanism of injury and by chronicity, the overall care differs between populations in terms of expectations and schedule. **Fig. 1** highlights disparate conditions affecting the nervous system that create a "neurogenic bladder." These four articles help demonstrate how urologic care needs to adjust to the specifics of the neurologic condition to optimize safety and quality of life.

We expand on this theme further by examining how neurogenic bladder physiology tends to be viewed as dichotomous variables rather than on a spectrum of severity. When caring for neurogenic bladder patients, we frequently group physiology by urodynamic findings (**Fig. 2**), that is, low bladder compliance, detrusor sphincter dyssynergia (DSD), and stress incontinence. However, physiology is likely considerably more variable on

Urol Clin N Am 51 (2024) xvii–xix
https://doi.org/10.1016/j.ucl.2024.02.008
0094-0143/24/© 2024 Published by Elsevier Inc.

urologic.theclinics.com

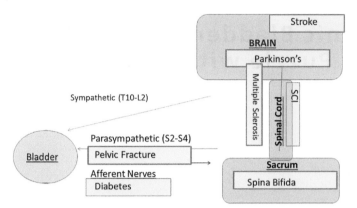

Fig. 1. Partial list of neurologic conditions causing neurogenic bladder. SCI, spinal cord injury.

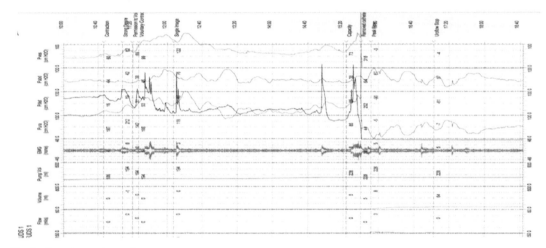

Fig. 2. Sample urodynamic trace.

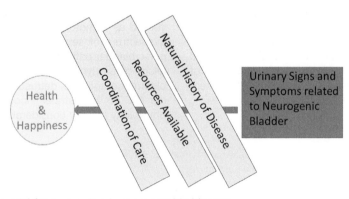

Fig. 3. Conceptual model for personalized neurogenic bladder care.

how it can impact patient care. Articles on validated neurogenic bladder quality-of-life questionnaires, bladder compliance, DSD, and urethral physiology explore potentially new opportunities to classify and define these conditions for the future.

Neurogenic bladder care is also very dependent on understanding timelines for delivering care and the tools needed to enact it. The issue examines this by highlighting the use of catheters in managing a person with a neurogenic bladder. The article on the history of catheters and technological choices in manufacturing helps set the stage for an article on why some patients struggle with performing intermittent catheterization. The article on pathways brings these limitations back into focus and demonstrates how shared decision making around care plans is crucial for long-term success.

Finally, the issue details how neurogenic bladder care requires more than just a urologist to be involved. Articles on developing a neurogenic bladder team and involving primary care for neurogenic bladder surveillance provide a blueprint for streamlining the long-term care that patients with a neurogenic bladder will require.

Neurogenic bladder care can be complex, and best care has yet to be determined for the numerous people affected by it. The Neurogenic Bladder Research Group (NBRG.org) was formed

to explore these problems in greater detail. The topics in this issue were generated through NBRG think tank discussions, and several NBRG members contributed to the individual articles exploring these in greater detail. It is the hope of NBRG that neurogenic bladder continues to advance as a model for personalized medicine in which condition, resources, and care coordination are not thought of as barriers to care (**Fig. 3**) but instead are considered necessary components of the conversation. We hope you enjoy reading our issue.

DISCLOSURES

Dr J.T. Stoffel discloses the following: Neurogenic Bladder Research Group (leadership); Flume Catheters (scientific advisor); Spine X (scientific advisor).

John T. Stoffel, MD
Department of Urology
University of Michigan
3875 Taubman Center
1500 East Medical Center Drive
Ann Arbor, MI 48109, USA

E-mail address:
jstoffel@med.umich.edu

Bladder-Related Quality of Life After Spinal Cord Injury
Findings from the Neurogenic Bladder Research Group Spinal Cord Injury Registry

Jeremy B. Myers, MD[a],*, Jane T. Kurtzman, MD[a]

KEYWORDS

- Spinal cord injury • Bladder • Urinary • Complications • Quality of life
- Patient-reported outcome measures

KEY POINTS: NEUROGENIC BLADDER RESEARCH GROUP SPINAL CORD INJURY REGISTRY

- Participants were recruited over an 18 month period and followed longitudinally over 1 year

- Inclusion criteria: >18 year old, English-speaking, acquired spinal cord injury (SCI) of any level or disability

- Variables included: demographics, injury characteristics, SCI complications, and psychosocial aspects of health-related quality of life

- Final cohort was 1479

- Participants answered extensive patient-reported outcome measure panels at enrollment and throughout the 1 year study

STUDY METHODS

The study included adult, English-speaking patients with acquired and nonprogressive spinal cord injury (SCI) (**Box 1**).[1] Study participants were recruited from clinical settings, such as urology and physical medicine and rehabilitation clinics. They were also recruited at SCI events, outreach to SCI advocate groups, and via social media—particularly via Facebook advertisements (**Fig. 1**). Stakeholders participated in all aspects of study design and implementation. Stakeholders included individuals with SCI, physical medicine and rehabilitation physicians, urologists, and SCI caregivers (**Fig. 2**).

Participants underwent an initial interview with study personnel about their medical, surgical, and injury history, as well as the management of their bladder over time. Participants then answered an extensive set of patient-reported outcome measures (PROMs), intended to study bladder-related quality of life (QoL), as well as the multifaceted experience with QoL and SCI. They were paid for their time, from enrollment to the completion of the study. The longitudinal study period was 1 year in duration, during which participants completed nonvalidated questionnaires about complications and/or changes in bladder management, as well as the same PROMs administered at the beginning of the study every 3 months. Participants underwent an exit interview at the end of the study, to confirm changes in bladder management and/or complications during the study period, as well as completing their final panel of PROMs. Participants were included in the study if they completed the study interview and the initial panel of PROMs. There was no review of medical records or physical examination as a requirement for entry into the study, and in most cases, the data were self-reported by participants.

[a] Division of Urology, Department of Surgery, University of Utah, 50 N Medical Drive, Salt Lake City, UT, 84103, USA
* Corresponding author.
E-mail address: jeremy.myers@hsc.utah.edu

Urol Clin N Am 51 (2024) 163–176
https://doi.org/10.1016/j.ucl.2024.02.004
0094-0143/24/© 2024 Elsevier Inc. All rights reserved.

Box 1
Study inclusion and exclusion criteria

Inclusion Criteria:

- Age ≥18 years
- Ability to effectively communicate in English
- Ability to provide informed consent
- Willing to participate and answer 5 sets of questionnaires over 1 year
- Acquired SCI: examples include traumatic, spinal cord stroke, malignancy (not active), surgical injury, and transverse myelitis

Exclusion Criteria:

- Congenital SCI: examples include cerebral palsy, spina bifida, myelomeningocele, caudal regression, and sacral agenesis
- Progressive SCI: examples include multiple sclerosis, active malignancy, progressive neurologic diseases leading to SCI, and myelopathies
- Not English fluent

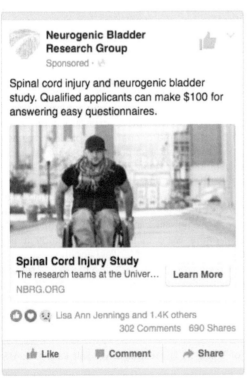

Fig. 1. Example of Facebook advertising for the NBRG SCI Registry Study. (*From* Neurogenic Bladder Research Group (NBRG.ORG).)

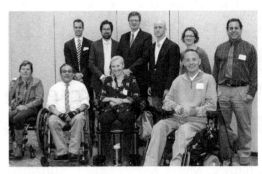

Fig. 2. Study investigators and patient and clinical stakeholders for the NBRD SCI Registry Study. Myers JB, Stoffel JT, Elliott SP, Welk B, Herrick JS, Lenherr SM. Sex Differences in Bladder Management, Symptoms, and Satisfaction After Spinal Cord Injury. J Urol. 2023 Oct;210(4):659-669. https://doi.org/10.1097/JU.0000000000003611. Epub 2023 Jul 3. PubMed PMID: 37395612.

Bladder Management

We grouped primary bladder management into 4 categories: clean intermittent catheterization (CIC), indwelling catheters (IDC: Foley catheter and suprapubic tube [SPT]), surgery (augmentation cystoplasty with or without catheterizable channel, catheterizable channel alone, conduit urinary diversion [colon conduit, ileal conduit, ileovesicostomy], and continent catheterizable pouch), and voiding (volitional voiding into a toilet, condom catheter, Credé or Valsalva voiding, leaking into pads/diapers). If participants used more than one method of bladder management, they were asked which one they considered as their primary bladder management and classified accordingly. An example of individual using mixed methods of bladder management is a participant who uses CIC during the day and a Foley catheter at night to control nocturnal polyuria. In analyses of bladder management, we used CIC as the reference category since it is often considered the gold standard for bladder management due to the lower medical complication rates compared to IDC.[2]

Primary and Secondary Outcomes

The primary outcome for most of the studies was the *Neurogenic Bladder Symptom Score* (*NBSS*). The *NBSS* has been validated in SCI and is primarily focused on bladder symptoms.[3,4] The overall *NBSS* ranges from 0 to 74 with lower scores indicating better function and less symptom burden. In addition, in some of the studies, we reported the Spinal Cord Injury Measurement System (SCI-QoL) *Bladder Difficulties* item bank. The SCI-QoL consists of many different item banks validated in individuals with SCI, which assess multiple aspects of the health and psychosocial impact of SCI.[5] Specifically, the SCI-QoL *Bladder Difficulties* item bank assesses the ability to perform a bladder program, incontinence concerns, and bladder-related impacts on daily life.[6] Some studies also used the SCI-QoL *Independence* and the SCI-QoL *Positive Affect and Well-Being (Positive Affect)* item banks to measure psychosocial aspects of health-related QoL. SCI-*QoL Independence* assesses perceptions of personal independence, ability to communicate needs with others, and a sense of control over one's life.[5,7,8] SCI-QoL *Positive Affect* assesses sense of well-being, life satisfaction, and purpose.[8–10]

The SCI-QoL questionnaire concentrates on feelings about bladder function and symptoms, while the NBSS characterizes the magnitude of symptoms. SCI-QoL questionnaires rely on item response theory and computer-adaptive testing, which enables the questionnaires to adapt to participant answers. SCI-QoL item banks have a mean score of 50 and a range of 0 to 100, with lower scores indicating less difficulty.

Secondary outcomes, in many of the studies, included the scores in the 3 subdomains of the *NBSS*: (1) *Incontinence* (range 0–29), which assesses the severity and impact of incontinence, (2) *Storage and Voiding* (range 0–22), which assesses urgency, ability to store urine effectively, and problems with bladder emptying (which are applicable whether a catheter is used or not), and (3) *Consequences* (range 0–23), which assesses the severity and frequency of urinary tract infections (UTIs), bladder and kidney stones, and medication use for bladder management. In addition to the 3 subdomains of the NBSS, there is a final question about bladder-related satisfaction; *Satisfaction* (range 0–4) is an independently scored QoL question, which asks about satisfaction with urinary function.[3] This QoL question is phrased: "If you had to live the rest of your life with how your bladder (or urinary reservoir) currently works, how would you feel?"

Statistical Analysis

The majority of data about bladder-related QoL were analyzed utilizing cross-sectional data from the study initial interview and PROMs. If there were missing data from the PROMs, the next set of PROMs was used to substitute the missing data. Other missing data were dealt with by multiple imputation. Baseline and follow-up factors, beyond the variables being analyzed, were incorporated into the imputation model to account for dependence of the missing data mechanism on other measured factors.

In the vast majority of studies, multiple linear regression models were used to test the association between study covariates and primary and secondary outcomes. For covariates in the models, estimated beta coefficients were reported, which measure the magnitude of change associated with that variable. Beta coefficients were reported with 95% confidence intervals and *P*-values. Negative change in beta coefficients of our outcomes all signified improved QoL or decreased bladder symptoms. Statistical analyses were conducted in R v. 3.4.1[11]; significance was assessed at the 0.05 level, and all tests were two-tailed.

Covariates

The covariates, in most of the analyses, were grouped by (1) primary bladder management, (2) demographics, (3) injury characteristics, (4) SCI complications, and (5) psychosocial aspects of health-related QoL (**Table 1**).

NEUROGENIC BLADDER RESEARCH GROUP SPINAL CORD INJURY REGISTRY PARTICIPANT COHORT

Over an 18 month period, 1479 participants were recruited to the study and completed baseline PROMS and the study enrollment interview (**Fig. 3**). Bladder management was very similar to other large series reported in the literature, and the key characteristics are summarized in **Table 2**. Bladder management consisted of CIC in 51%, IDC in 18%, surgery in 13%, and voiding in 18%.[2] The vast majority of patients managed with surgery had undergone augmentation cystoplasty; less frequently, patients had conduit urinary diversion. The cohort of participants was similar to many other SCI studies: male predominant (60%), level in the majority was paraplegia (57%), median age of 45 year old (IQR 34.1, 54.1), and median time from injury of 11 years (IQR 5.1, 22.4). Given that for many patients, the time since injury was greater than 10 years, participants were quite experienced about their bladder management and many had tried different bladder management strategies or had urinary complications over their history with SCI.

WHAT OUR RESEARCH SHOWED ABOUT BLADDER-RELATED QUALITY OF LIFE
Bladder Management and Quality of Life

Our main study results divided participants by level (paraplegia vs tetraplegia) and analyzed how bladder management was associated with bladder-related symptoms and QoL.[12] We analyzed participants with tetraplegia and

Table 1
Covariates separated by bladder management, demographics, injury characteristics, spinal cord injury complications, and psychosocial aspects of health-related quality of life

Variable	Definition
Bladder Management	
Primary bladder management, those using more than one method asked, which management they considered their main bladder management method	
CIC	
IDC	Foley urethral catheter, SPT
Surgery	Bladder augmentation with or without catheterizable channel, catheterizable channel alone, urinary diversion (conduit or continent catheterizable pouch)
Voiding	Condom catheter, involuntary leaking, volitional voiding
Demographics	
Age	
Sex	Self-reported by participants
Obese	BMI $\geq$ 30 kg/m^2
Education	Bachelor's degree or higher
Employed for wages	
Injury Characteristics	
Level	Tetraplegia (cervical level 1–8) vs paraplegia (thoracic level 1 and below, including sacral levels and cauda equina)
Years since injury	
Complete injury	AIS "A" or if unknown participants asked if they had a complete or incomplete injury
SCI Complications	
Chronic pain	Asked: "do you experience chronic pain?"
Number of UTIs	Categorical: 0, 1–3, $\geq$4, self-reported by participants
Severe bowel dysfunction	Neurogenic Bowel Dysfunction Score > 14
Psychosocial Measures	
SCI-QoL Independence	
SCI-QoL Positive Affect	

Abbreviations: AIS, American Spinal Injury Association Impairment Scale; BMI, body mass index; CIC, clean intermittent catheterization; IDC, indwelling catheter; UTI, urinary tract infection; severe bowel dysfunction—Neurogenic Bowel Dysfunction Score $\geq$ 14.

Missing values: Obese (BMI $\geq$ 30 kg/m^2) (346), Education (1), Employment (1), Complete injury (65), Chronic pain (2), Number of UTIs (1), Hospitalization for UTI (1).

paraplegia separately because the considerations for bladder management differ significantly between these cohorts. In addition, statistical analysis of the interaction of level (paraplegia vs tetraplegia) and outcome measures found significant differences in the overall *NBSS*, as well as many of the subdomains of *NBSS*, based upon level. Level was defined as tetraplegia (cervical level 1–8) or paraplegia (thoracic level 1 and below, including sacral levels and cauda equina).

Overall, we found that participants managed with surgery and IDCs had significantly less associated bladder symptoms, assessed via the *NBSS*, than those managed with CIC. This applied to both paraplegic and tetraplegic participants. Participants who managed their bladders with voiding had substantially worse associated bladder symptoms than CIC. The results of the SCI-QoL *Bladder Difficulties* item bank also revealed a similar hierarchy, especially in tetraplegia. The magnitude of the change; however, was much less in this measure compared to the *NBSS*. In the *NBSS* subdomains (*Incontinence, Storage and Voiding, Consequences,* and *Satisfaction*), both surgery and IDC were associated with significantly lessened incontinence symptoms in paraplegia and with IDC in tetraplegia, compared to participants performing CIC. Similarly, in *Storage and Voiding* participants fared much better with surgery or IDC compared to CIC. However, in *Satisfaction* only surgery was associated with better

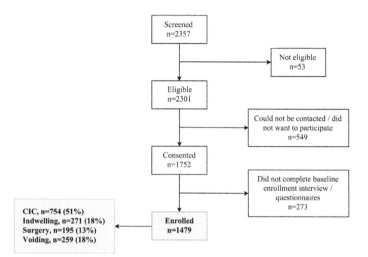

Fig. 3. Study consort diagram.

satisfaction compared to CIC. There were many other relationships established in this study between patient and injury characteristics and bladder symptoms, which were explored in further studies from the Neurogenic Bladder Research Group (NBRG) SCI Registry.

The finding that participants, regardless of level, had less bladder symptoms associated with IDCs compared to CIC challenged the axiomatic view that CIC is the best bladder management method or "gold standard" for individuals with SCI. An observation from a seminal paper from Cameron and colleagues also supports this very confounding finding.[13] In this study, the authors used the Model Systems Database to analyze bladder management over time in individuals with SCI. They found that in the patients discharged from rehabilitation doing CIC, 70% of the patients stopped CIC over the subsequent years of follow-up. Most of this change occurred in the first 5-year period; however, there was a steady decline in utilization over time, and the patients who stopped CIC mainly elected to transition to a chronic IDC. This observation exposed a disconnect between providers' recommendation for CIC as the gold standard for bladder management and the actual choices that patients make for their bladder management after SCI. We suspected that this patient-driven transition from CIC to IDC could be explained by a lower burden of bladder symptoms for IDC compared to CIC and our findings subsequently support this hypothesis.

In order to better characterize the frequent transition in individuals with SCI from CIC to IDC, we looked at a subset of participants in the PCORI study who had utilized CIC in the past but had moved to IDC for their bladder management.[14] As part of the study enrollment interview, participants were asked if they had utilized CIC in the past and why they switched to a chronic IDC. There were a total of 176 participants who had started CIC but stopped and were utilizing IDCs, almost exclusively an SPT. Differences in this participant group, included 62% of 176 participants, were tetraplegic, compared to the overall cohort, which was 43% tetraplegic. This difference is intuitive, since a major indication for IDC use can be limited hand function and inability to perform CIC. In the overall participant group, the leading reasons for stopping CIC were (1) inconvenience, (2) incontinence, and (3) too many infections associated with CIC. Following these 3 reasons was, "not wanting to be dependent upon others," which was of higher concern in those participants with tetraplegia. The data support our experience with talking to individuals with SCI, in clinic, where often the theme of convenience is of primary concern surrounding the choice to switch from CIC to an SPT. For example, one can imagine the challenges of an individual with tetraplegia who takes 15 to 30 minutes to catheterize, while balancing attendance in college classes. In this circumstance, an individual transitioning to an SPT may minimize embarrassing leakage episodes, time away from important responsibilities (such as college courses), dangerous autonomic dysreflexia, and increased UTI risk (due to poor adherence to timely catheterization).

The Association Between Surgery and Bladder-Related Quality of Life

In our initial study of the association between different bladder managements and bladder-related QoL, surgery was associated with less bladder symptoms and higher bladder-related satisfaction in comparison to CIC. The vast majority

Table 2
Characteristics of 1479 participants grouped by level (paraplegia vs tetraplegia)

Variable	All Patients	Paraplegia	Tetraplegia	P-Value
Number of participants	1479	843 (57%)	636 (43%)	
Bladder Management				
CIC	754 (51%)	525 (62%)	229 (36%)	<.001
IDC	271 (18%)	83 (10%)	188 (30%)	
Surgery	195 (13%)	101 (12%)	94 (15%)	
Voiding	259 (18%)	134 (16%)	125 (20%)	
IDC Types (n = 271)				
Foley	81 (30%)	32 (39%)	49 (26%)	.038
SPT	190 (70%)	51 (61%)	139 (74%)	
Surgery Types (n = 195)				
Conduit	35 (18%)	12 (12%)	23 (24%)	.15
Continent pouch	7 (3%)	4 (4%)	3 (3%)	
Augmentation cystoplasty - catheterizable channel + catheterizable channel	126 (65%) 79 47	70 (70%)	56 (60%)	
Catheterizable channel alone	27 (14%)	15 (15%)	12 (13%)	
Voiding Specifics (n = 259)				
Condom catheter	59 (23%)	16 (12%)	43 (34%)	.003
Spontaneous voiding	200 (77%)	118 (88%)	82 (66%)	<.001
Type of Voiding (n = 259)				
Volitional (toilet)	77 (30%)	32 (24%)	45 (36%)	<.001
Leak (diapers/condom catheter)	71 (27%)	26 (19%)	45 (36%)	
Maneuvers (Valsalva/Credé)	97 (37%)	67 (50%)	30 (24%)	
Unspecified	14 (5%)	9 (7%)	5 (4%)	
Demographics				
Age: median (IQR)	44.9 (34.4, 54.1)	45.5 (35.1, 54.4)	44.7 (33.3, 53.3)	.049
Range	(18, 86)	(18, 83.3)	(18.4, 86)	
Sex: male	894 (60%)	469 (56%)	424 (67%)	<.001
Obese (BMI > 30 kg/m^2)	351 (25%)	227 (28%)	124 (20%)	<.001
Education	603 (41%)	331 (39%)	272 (43%)	.18
Employment	863 (59%)	514 (61%)	349 (55%)	.021
Injury Characteristics				
Chronic pain	1024 (69%)	605 (72%)	419 (66%)	.019
Years since injury: median (IQR)	11 (5.1, 22.4)	10.6 (5, 21.9)	11.7 (5.3, 23.1)	.33
- Range	(0, 54.8)	(0, 53.7)	(0.1, 54.8)	
Complete injury	564 (38%)	379 (45%)	185 (29%)	<.001
SCI Complications				
Number of UTIs				
0	388 (26%)	226 (27%)	162 (26%)	.43
1–3	677 (46%)	374 (44%)	303 (48%)	

(continued on next page)

Table 2 *(continued)*				
Variable	All Patients	Paraplegia	Tetraplegia	P-Value
≥ 4	413 (28%)	243 (29%)	170 (27%)	
Hospitalization for UTI	177 (12%)	85 (10%)	92 (15%)	.009
Severe bowel dysfunction	569 (42%)	309 (40%)	260 (44%)	.14

Missing values: Obese (BMI > 30 kg/m²) (21), Education (1), Employment (1), Complete injury (6), Chronic pain (2), Number of UTIs (1), Hospitalization for UTI (1).

Abbreviations: BMI, body mass index; bladder augmentation, enterocystoplasty with or without a catheterizable channel; catheterizable channel, a separate catheterizable channel without augmentation or catheterizable pouch; chronic pain, participants asked "do you experience chronic pain?"; CIC, clean intermittent catheterization; complete injury, American Spinal Injury Association Impairment Scale (ASI) "A" or if ASI grade unknown participants asked if they are complete or incomplete; conduit, colon or ileal conduit, ileovesicostomy; continent pouch, right colon or other continent catheterizable pouch; education, having achieved a bachelor's degree or higher; employment, making wages (including self-employment); IDC, indwelling catheter; UTI, urinary tract infection; number of UTIs and hospitalization in last year, severe bowel dysfunction—Neurogenic Bowel Dysfunction Score ≥ 14.

of participants having had surgery and had bladder augmentation, with very few undergoing urinary diversion (see **Table 2**). In an effort to explore the role of surgery and specifically augmentation cystoplasty, we studied QoL between 3 groups performing CIC.[15] These groups included participants who (1) performed CIC, (2) utilized onabotulinum toxin and CIC (CIC-BTX), and (3) had augmentation cystoplasty and used CIC (CIC-AUG). In this study, we hypothesized that participants utilizing onabotulinum toxin and having undergone bladder augmentation surgery would have better bladder-related QoL compared to those doing CIC alone.

In total, 879 patients performed CIC, when those having had augmentation cystoplasty were included. The percent of participants in each group consisted of: 67% CIC, 19% CIC-BTX, and 15% CIC-AUG. Gratifying for urologic surgeons, we found that CIC-AUG patients had substantially associated improved QoL measures compared to both other groups. CIC-AUG participants had less bladder symptoms (*NBSS Total*) compared to both other groups, as well as improved feelings about bladder function (*SCI-QoL Bladder Difficulties*). Specifically, participants who had undergone augmentation cystoplasty had an associated better *Incontinence* and *Satisfaction* subdomain scores compared to both other groups. The overall findings supported the important role of surgery for individuals seeking to continue CIC. Surgery can be particularly impactful for patients who have problems with catheterizing effectively (inconvenience), and/or detrusor overactivity incontinence (incontinence), both of which were themes identified by participants of the NBRG SCI Registry as the leading reason for discontinuation of CIC. In addition to addressing inconvenience and incontinence, surgery with concomitant creation of a catheterizable channel at the time of augmentation cystoplasty

can address a leading concern in individuals with tetraplegia, which is increased independence and not wanting to be dependent upon others for bladder management.

Surgery, however, is associated with high morbidity, including high perioperative complications and a significant risk of reoperation and/or revision surgery in the future.[16] In addition, our data from the NBRG SCI Registry showed that participants who had surgery were more likely to have worse neurogenic bowel dysfunction compared to other bladder management groups. This may be because patients who have worse neurogenic bowel dysfunction are more likely to have worse bladder-related QoL,[12] and as a result, may be more likely to pursue surgery. However, it may also be that surgery itself induces worsened bowel function in individuals with SCI. In patient–clinician shared decision-making, these are very important negative QoL consequences that need to be contrasted to the improvements in bladder-related QoL associated with surgery.

KEY FINDINGS: BLADDER MANAGEMENT STRATEGIES AND QUALITY OF LIFE

- IDC has less associated bladder symptoms than CIC, even after adjusting for numerous variables including demographics, injury characteristics, and SCI complications.
- IDC, however, has well-established worse medical morbidity than CIC.
- Surgery, mostly augmentation cystoplasty, also has less associated bladder symptoms than those performing CIC and in addition has higher associated bladder satisfaction.
- Individuals with SCI stopping CIC and switching to IDC do so because of inconvenience, incontinence, and a perceived higher UTI rate.

PARTICIPANT FACTORS AND HOW THEY AFFECT BLADDER-RELATED QUALITY OF LIFE
Sex

A very consistent finding, in our studies of the NBRG SCI Registry, is that women have an associated higher burden of bladder symptoms and worse bladder-related satisfaction.[12] This relationship was explored further in a study focused upon the differences in QoL between men and women.[17] In this study, there were significant differences between women and men regarding their bladder management. Women were less likely to use CIC (43% vs 57%, $P < .001$) and much more likely to utilize surgery (23% vs 7%, $P < .001$; **Table 3**). There was no difference in participants with urinary conduits or continent catheterizable pouches between sexes; however, augmentation cystoplasty with or without catheterizable channel or catheterizable channel alone was surgeries performed at a much higher rate in women (19% vs 4%, $P<.001$). The observed higher rates of catheterizable channel creation make sense since women have unique anatomic challenges compared to men, when catheterizing in the sitting position. In another survey study, we looked at the time it took to catheterize and found women who were obese took two times as long to catheterize as nonobese women.[18] Sex was not in itself associated with increased catheterization times, in this study; however, there was also a very high rate of catheterizable channel creation in the cohort of women. Having a high rate of catheterizable channel creation may have moderated differences in time and burden of catheterization between women and men within the study.

The NBRG SCI Registry study also explored why bladder symptom burden and satisfaction were worse in women. In an unadjusted analysis, women had worse overall bladder symptoms, as demonstrated by the total *NBSS*, which was 16% worse than for men. This difference was also evident within every subdomain of the *NBSS*, including *Satisfaction*. In the adjusted analysis, bladder management methods that have been well demonstrated to decrease bladder symptoms (IDC and surgery) had greater effect in women and men. There was decreased symptom burden in women with IDC (-11.8 in women vs -6.7 in men, $P = .001$), as well as surgery (-5.3 vs -2.6, respectively, $P = .001$).

We hypothesized at the beginning of the study that worse bladder-related QoL would be explained by worse incontinence in women. Scores in the subdomain *Incontinence* were in fact better (lower) in both women and men with IDCs and with surgery; however, this was also true of scores in *Storage and Voiding* as well as *Satisfaction*. Thus, the overall worsened bladder-related QoL in women appeared to be spread across different domains of bladder function and satisfaction.

We also noted a complex relationship between measures of mental health and psychosocial aspects of health-related QoL, in women, and bladder-related QoL. In an unadjusted analysis, we previously found that women with SCI had worse associated overall mental health compared to men (measured by the SCI adapted *Short-Form 12* [*SF-12*]); however, we were not able to adjust for the association of mental health with bladder symptoms.[18] In the main NBRG study of

Table 3
Sex-stratified differences in bladder management

Variable	All Patients (N = 1479)	Female (N = 585)	Male (N = 894)	P-Value
Bladder Management (%)				
Clean intermittent catheterization	754 (51.0)	249 (42.6)	505 (56.5)	<.001
Indwelling catheter	271 (18.3)	107 (18.3)	164 (18.3)	
Surgery	195 (13.2)	132 (22.6)	63 (7.0)	
Spontaneous voiding	259 (17.5)	97 (16.6)	162 (18.1)	
Surgery Types (N = 195) (%)				
Any Surgery	195 (13.2)	132 (22.6)	63 (7.0)	<.001
Conduit	35 (2.4)	15 (2.6)	20 (2.2)	<.001
Continent pouch	8 (0.5)	4 (0.7)	4 (0.4)	
Augmentation cystoplasty	79 (5.3)	49 (8.4)	30 (3.4)	
Augmentation cystoplasty + catheterizable channel	47 (3.2)	39 (6.7)	8 (0.9)	
Catheterizable channel (no augment)	26 (1.8)	25 (4.3)	1 (0.1)	

sex and bladder-related QoL, however, we were able to adjust for psychosocial aspects of health-related QoL and found that in women, measures of higher independence (SCI-QoL *Independence*) correlated to less bladder symptoms, while in men, better positive affect and well-being (SCI-QoL *Positive Affect*) correlated to less bladder symptoms. Overall, the studies show that the relationship (similar to many of the findings from the NBRG SCI Registry) between sex and bladder-related QoL is very complex and not easily explained by one simple difference, such as worse incontinence.

KEY FINDINGS: SEX AND BLADDER-RELATED QUALITY OF LIFE

- Women have more bladder symptoms and worse satisfaction than men. The reasons for this are multifactorial and evidence points to worse incontinence, as well as worse storage and voiding symptoms.
- Women utilize surgery, especially augmentation cystoplasty and catheterizable channel creation at much higher rates than men.
- There is greater benefit in overall reduction of bladder symptoms with the use of both surgery and IDCs in women compared to men, even when adjusting for many factors that affect bladder-related QoL.

Age

The age of participants had a profound association with bladder-related symptoms and satisfaction. In the main analysis of bladder management and associated QoL, age was a demographic co-variate.[12] In the assessment of overall bladder symptoms (total *NBSS*), among paraplegics participants, for every decade older there was an associated decrease in bladder symptoms. This observation was also true for many subdomains of the *NBSS*. When participants were stratified by sex, men also showed a decrease in bladder symptoms, which was significant with age.[17] The reasons for this relationship are not clear and may have to do with age being a confounder with time from injury, which also was shown to be associated with less bladder symptoms and greater satisfaction.[19]

Obesity

All analyses from the NBRG SCI Registry consistently demonstrate that there is an associated negative effect of obesity of bladder-related QoL.[12] The effect of obesity was found in tetraplegic participants for overall bladder symptoms (total *NBSS*) and noted in the subdomains of *Incontinence* and *Storage and Voiding*.

Injury Characteristics and How they Affect Bladder-related Quality of Life

Injury characteristics, which were identified a priori by the research stakeholder team, and those felt to be relevant to bladder-related QoL were injury completeness, level, and time from injury.

Level of Injury

Paraplegia and tetraplegia represent substantially different levels of physical disability, and therefore, we suspected would have differing bladder management strategies and potentially QoL outcomes as well. Therefore, injury levels were analyzed separately. Despite this, however, we found that in both groups, patients who managed their bladder with IDC or surgery had fewer bladder symptoms than CIC, while those who managed their bladders with voiding had more bladder symptoms. There were also fewer bladder management difficulties among both tetraplegic and paraplegic patients who had surgery or an IDC, when compared to CIC. Injury level also did not appear to influence the findings that surgery was associated with higher bladder satisfaction than CIC.[12]

Overall, we found that paraplegic patients more commonly utilized CIC than tetraplegic patients (62% vs 36%) and less commonly utilized IDC (10% vs 30%). Tetraplegic patients were slightly younger and more likely to be male, but less likely to be obese and less often employed than paraplegic patients. Tetraplegic participants also had significantly lower rates of chronic pain and complete SCI.

Interestingly, unadjusted analysis demonstrated that compared to paraplegic participants, tetraplegics had overall significantly fewer bladder symptoms (mean NBSS of 26 ± 10.9 vs 21.7 ± 10.1, respectively, $P <. 001$) and SCI-QoL difficulties (mean 59.3 ± 7.5 vs 56.5 ± 7.5, respectively, $P < .001$). Tetraplegic participants also had significantly better NBSS subdomain scores in *Incontinence* ($P < .001$), *Storage and Voiding* ($P < .001$), and *Satisfaction* ($P = .002$), but worse *Consequences* ($P = .019$) scores than paraplegic participants.[12] We suspected these results were related to our findings that tetraplegic participants less commonly utilized CIC and more commonly utilized IDC than paraplegic participants. Subsequent multivariable analysis in each injury group supported this hypothesis by demonstrating that CIC is independently associated with worse NBSS scores than IDC. Additionally, SCI-QoL difficulties scores were significantly better for tetraplegic participants managed with IDC than CIC. This was not the case among paraplegic participants in whom only surgery was associated with improved QoL scores compared to CIC. Since it is potentially more physically challenging and burdensome for tetraplegic patients to perform CIC than paraplegic patients, we postulated that IDCs may be more likely to improve QoL in tetraplegic patients and paraplegics.

A second NBRG SCI Registry study, which more closely examined the impact of specific SCI levels on QoL outcomes related to CIC, challenged this hypothesis.[20] In this NBRG study, participants who performed CIC (n = 753) were classified into 3 categories of injury level based on the anatomic likelihood of upper extremity (UE) function: (1) C1–C5, (2) C5–C8, and (3) T1 and below. Participants self-reported injuries as complete versus incomplete and provided data regarding fine motor function using the SCI-QoL *Fine Motor Function*. Participants were dichotomized into 2 groups: dissatisfied and neutral/satisfied based on their response to the NBSS urinary *Satisfaction* question. Those who answered "unhappy" or "mostly unsatisfied" were categorized as "dis-satisfied" with urinary QoL and everyone else as "neutral/satisfied." Interestingly, while the authors identified several variables that were associated with CIC dissatisfaction (female sex, shorter time from injury, frequent UTIs, and bowel dysfunction), neither level of SCI nor fine motor skills influenced patient dissatisfaction rates. Caregiver dependence for CIC was also not an influencing factor. This was perhaps less surprising, since we know from other NBRG work that participant decision to perform CIC, and continuing to perform CIC, is highly associated with preserved UE function.[21] Therefore, this cohort of participants who primarily perform CIC was likely biased toward participants with some degree of preserved UE function and independence. One additional important finding, however, was that patients who reported decreased physical and emotional health using the SF-12 questionnaire, were significantly more likely to be dissatisfied with CIC. This finding together with the lack of association to injury level, suggest that physical disability in-and-of-itself does not necessarily directly impact QoL, but rather that psychosocial adaptation and functioning may be a more important variable in QoL outcomes. This theory may also help explain why tetraplegic participants have overall better bladder symptom scores and QoL scores, despite having more significant physical disability than paraplegic participants. However, further work is needed to better understand these outcomes.

COMPLICATIONS OF SPINAL CORD INJURY AND HOW THEY AFFECT BLADDER-RELATED QUALITY OF LIFE

We considered the following SCI-related complications as covariates in our study: frequency of UTIs, chronic pain, and severe bowel dysfunction. In addition, we also analyzed the rates of hospitalization over the study 1 year follow-up time period.

Urinary Tract Infection

Escalation in UTI rates and management of UTIs can be one of the most common reasons that individuals with SCI seek medical care from urologists. After a short time of working with individuals with SCI, a provider realizes the impact of UTIs on daily QoL, the significant anxiety that patients have about UTIs and urosepsis, and how challenging, for patients and providers, the management of chronic UTIs can be. UTIs were very common in participants in the NBRG SCI Registry with participants reporting 1 to 3 years in 46%, 4 to 6 years in 15%, and greater than 6 years in 13%.[22] In our analyses of bladder management methods and associated bladder-related QoL, it was readily apparent that despite adjusting for other covariates, including SCI level, UTI rates were one of the most profound factors associated with greater bladder symptoms and worse satisfaction.[12] In fact, having $\geq$ 4 self-reported UTIs in the last 12 months had the most profound association with increased bladder symptoms and worse satisfaction of any of the covariates within the model (+7.24 paraplegia, +5.41, both $P < .001$).

Because of the substantial importance of UTIs on bladder-related QoL, UTI was investigated in greater depth using the data from the NBRG SCI Registry. In one study, the rates of self-reported UTI and hospitalization for UTI with different bladder management methods were studied. In this study, the authors found a progressive increase in UTI risk from the reference category of volitional voiding to use of diapers or condom catheter, to CIC, to the highest risk category IDC (**Fig. 4**).[23] In fact, those participants using IDC had a 4.3 ($P < .001$)-fold risk of UTI compared to those that were volitional voiding. The severity of UTI also followed these risk categories with 22% of participants with IDC requiring hospitalization for UTI in the last 12 month period. Other factors that were associated with increased UTI risk and severity were female sex and older participants.

In another NBRG SCI Registry study, the association between UTI rate and measures of bladder-related QoL was analyzed.[22] The authors utilized the SCI-QoL *Bladder Complications* item bank

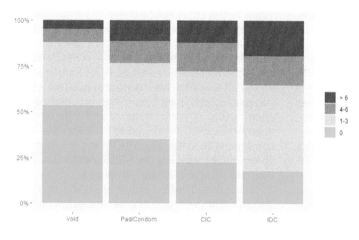

Fig. 4. Self-reported urinary tract infection rates, in the last 12 months, with different bladder managements.

and analyzed the effects of UTI rate. They found that the increased rates of UTI were associated with limiting daily activities, increased spasticity, and increased avoidance of going out. The SCI-adapted SF-12[24] was also used to analyze the effect of UTIs and the authors found that increased UTI rate was associated with worse scores in the *Physical Health* domain, but not associated with any changes in the *Mental Health* domain. Overall, these findings support the importance of UTIs to not only bladder-related QoL but also to overall health-related QoL.

In another study of hospitalization, which utilized longitudinal 1 year data from the NBRG SCI Registry, 33% of participants were seen in the emergency department or admitted during the study time period.[25] In 50% of this group, the reason for these hospital encounters was urologic with 85% of the urologic visits being related to UTI or other urologic infection. Not surprisingly, the highest odds of requiring a hospital encounter for urologic care were in participants using IDCs (OR 3.35) followed by surgery (OR 2.57) and CIC (OR 2.56) compared to spontaneous voiding (all significant $P = .003$). Although authors did not utilize PROMs extensively in this study, the *SF-12 Physical Health* domain was associated with higher risk and the *Mental Health* domain tended to be worse in those needing hospitalizations or emergency room (ER) visits for urologic problems.

Pain

Two variables were used in studies to assess pain and its association with bladder-related QoL. First, patients were asked "Do you have chronic pain?" Second, the SCI-QoL item bank called *Pain Interference*, which used similar methodology (computer-adaptive testing) as most SCI-QoL PROMs was utilized.[26] Other measures, such as a Likert scale of average pain experienced over the last week or

the use of narcotic pain medicines, had very high correlation to both of these variables. In the overall participant cohort, 1024 (69%) answered that they experienced chronic pain.[12] Chronic pain occurred at a lower rate in tetraplegic compared to paraplegic participants (66% vs 72%, $P < .019$). In adjusted models, utilizing the question "Do you have chronic pain?" there were significant associations with the subdomains of the *NBSS,* including associated worse *Storage and Voiding* in tetraplegic participants and worse *Consequences* in paraplegic participants. Also, in sex-stratified analysis, men had more associated overall bladder symptoms *(NBSS)* with chronic pain.[17]

In the second study involving pain, the PROM SCI-QoL *Pain Interference* was utilized as a variable and participants were grouped into tertiles based upon their severity of pain.[27] Participants in the highest tertile of the SCI-QoL *Pain Interference* had associated worse measures of overall bladder symptoms *(NBSS)*, feelings about their bladder (SCI-QoL *Bladder Difficulties*), and in the *Satisfaction* subdomain of the *NBSS.* This relationship was not subtle in the studies and demonstrates how pain can affect many aspects of an individual's experience after SCI.

Bowel Dysfunction

Bowel dysfunction was measured using the *Neurogenic Bowel Dysfunction (NBD) Score.* Bowel dysfunction was defined as binary in most of the studies as severe bowel dysfunction (≥ 14 points on the *NBD*) or not severe.[28] There were associations between severe bowel dysfunction and some measures of bladder symptoms and satisfaction, depending upon SCI level.[12] For example, participants with paraplegia have associated greater *Incontinence* scores and worse *Satisfaction*, while participants with tetraplegia had higher *Consequences* scores.

Bowel function was investigated in a separate NBRG study, and after excluding participants with a colostomy, 570 (42%) had severe bowel dysfunction with the remaining having mild/moderate bowel dysfunction.[29] In fact, the mean NBD score was 12 (SD 6), within the entire cohort. In a multivariable adjusted model, variables associated with severe bowel dysfunction were bladder management method and worse autonomic dysreflexia. Participants using IDCs or having had surgery had a significant odds ratio of 2.16 (P < .001) and 1.79 (P = .02), respectively, associated with severe bowel dysfunction. Autonomic dysreflexia was assessed using several questions from the nonvalidated Autonomic Dysfunction Following Spinal Cord Injury (ADFSCI) PROM,[30] and for every point increase in the ADFSCI, there was an associated 5% higher incidence of severe bowel dysfunction. These overall observations support intuitive assumptions about the interconnectedness between bladder and bowel dysfunction, as well as the link between severe bowel dysfunction and a higher burden of autonomic dysreflexia in at risk individuals. The connection between bladder management and severe bowel dysfunction is not well understood. Perhaps those with worse bladder symptoms, who fail CIC and go on to IDC or surgery have worse bowel function or it may be that there is a more direct link. For instance, in surgery, variable lengths and areas of the bowel are used for urologic reconstruction, and although data are lacking about the overall effects of urologic reconstructive surgeries and bowel function postoperatively, there is a potentially causal link. This is an area we are investigating with prospective studies before and after surgery in neurogenic bladder patients.

PSYCHOSOCIAL ASPECTS OF HEALTH-RELATED QUALITY OF LIFE AND THEIR EFFECT ON BLADDER-RELATED QUALITY OF LIFE

We hypothesized that an individual's resilience could affect their perceived bother, symptoms, and satisfaction with their bladder management after SCI. There were many measures of resilience, independence, and positive affect, which were included in the panel of PROMs participants answered over the course of the NBRG SCI Registry study. These and other variables were referred to as psychosocial aspects of health-related QoL. We realized many of these measures would have significant overlap with one another. For instance, one would expect the SF-12 Mental Health domain could have high correlation with the SCI-QoL Positive Affect. In order to address the overlap between PROMs, we first created a Pearson correlation

matrix and a priori selected PROMs that had low correlation between one another and also had face value in measuring aspects of psychosocial aspects of health-related QoL.[27] The PROMs that were used for the study were SCI-QoL Pain Interference, SCI-QoL Positive Affect, and SCI-QoL Independence. Participants were then grouped based upon tertiles of each measure and independent adjusted models were used to establish the relationship between the given PROM and 3 outcomes. These outcomes were the NBSS, NBSS Satisfaction, and SCI-QoL Bladder Difficulties.

As mentioned before, pain had significant associations with worse outcome measures, which was stepwise with each tertile of the SCI-QoL Pain Interference. The findings for participants within the middle or upper tertile (better) SCI-QoL Positive Affect had analogous results to the effects of pain, but opposite: where better positive affect was associated with less bladder symptoms. There was less effect for SCI-QoL Independence, which was only associated with less bladder symptoms (NBSS) and higher Satisfaction in the highest tertile (best) measures of independence. The reasons that better positive affect and independence associate with less bladder symptoms are not clear; there could be confounding variables that are associated with better measures or that individuals with better independence and positive affect could have less actual bladder symptoms or are not as bothered by the symptoms and tend to underreport them in PROMs.

KEY FINDINGS: PSYCHOSOCIAL ASPECTS OF HEALTH-RELATED QUALITY OF LIFE AND BLADDER SYMPTOMS AND SATISFACTION

- Three PROMs, from the SCI-QoL, were used to measure psychosocial aspects of health-related QoL.
  ○ SCI-QoL Pain Interference
  ○ SCI-QoL Independence
  ○ SCI-QoL Positive Affect
- Worse pain had significant associations with worse bladder-related QoL.
- Participants within the highest tertile (best) measures of independence and positive affect had associated less bladder symptoms and better satisfaction.

LIMITATIONS

There are many limitations to this study. One obvious limitation was inclusion bias, where those individuals with bladder problems were more likely to join the study. Another limitation is that participants' history was self-reported and may be prone to recall bias. An example of the problems with self-reporting is quantifying UTIs. We were not able to confirm participant self-reported UTIs with review of culture data or prescription of antibiotics. In fact, UTI treatment was not a part of the interview and some of these UTIs may have been self-treated with hydration. There was also heterogeneity in the bladder management groups' surgery and voiding. Participants in these groups had very different types of management (see **Table 2**). However, the intention of surgery is to improve bladder-related QoL by bypassing the bladder or expanding and defunctionalizing the bladder, so we felt that combining participants with varying surgeries was justified. Also, given that some of the surgery groups, such as conduit urinary diversion, were small, it was not practical to perform subgroup analyses. Similarly with the voiding group, the spectrum of participants included volitional voiding into a toilet to leaking into diapers, but the rational for combining these participants is none were using catheters in order to empty their bladder. Another limitation is that in some of the studies, SCI-QoL *Satisfaction* was used as an interval scale; this PROM is a 5-point scale and reviewers argued strongly within some of the studies to use this as an ordinal scale.[17] Despite these limitations, the NBRG SCI Registry is the largest study within the contemporary literature with extensive PROMs examining the multifaceted nature of bladder management and QoL after SCI.

SUMMARY

A full understanding of the multitude of factors affecting bladder-related symptoms and satisfaction will never be possible because of the uniqueness of the human experience. However, the NBRG SCI Registry Study has thoroughly explored this complex relationship and upended many of the assumptions that were commonly made about bladder-related QoL after SCI. The findings as a whole represent an excellent springboard for development of a shared decision-making tool for patients and clinicians. A shared decision-making tool is some of the current work being done by the NBRG.

CLINICS CARE POINTS

- Indwelling catheters have less associated bladder symptoms compared to individuals performing clean intermittent catheterization. This observation is important but needs to be contrasted to the well-established higher medical morbidity of indwelling catheters in shared decision-making.

- Augmentation cystoplasty plays a key role in preserving the ability to continue clean intermittent catheterization in those individuals preferring this bladder management and is associated with less bladder symptoms and high bladder satisfaction.

- Women have more bladder symptoms and worse satisfaction than men. The reasons for this are multifactorial. In addition, women utilize surgery at a much higher rate than men, especially bladder augmentation surgery.

- Bladder symptoms and satisfaction is truly multifaceted and affected by demographics, injury characteristics, spinal cord injury complications, and psychosocial aspects of health-related quality of life.

DISCLOSURE

J Myers was the primary investigator and received salary support from a Patient-Centered Outcomes Research Institute Award, which supported much of the research reported within this article. This work was (partially) supported through a Patient-Centered Outcomes Research Institute, United States (PCORI) Award (CER14092138). All statements in this report, including its findings and conclusions, are solely those of the authors and do not necessarily represent the views of PCORI.

REFERENCES

1. Patel DP, Lenherr SM, Stoffel JT, et al, Neurogenic Bladder Research Group. Neurogenic Bladder Research G: Study protocol: patient reported outcomes for bladder management strategies in spinal cord injury. BMC Urol 2017;17(1):95.
2. Cameron AP, Wallner LP, Forchheimer MB, et al. Medical and psychosocial complications associated with method of bladder management after traumatic spinal cord injury. Arch Phys Med Rehabil 2011; 92(3):449–56.
3. Welk B, Morrow S, Madarasz W, et al. The validity and reliability of the neurogenic bladder symptom score. J Urol 2014;192(2):452–7.
4. Welk B, Lenherr S, Elliott S, et al. The Neurogenic Bladder Symptom Score (NBSS): a secondary assessment of its validity, reliability among people with a spinal cord injury. Spinal Cord 2018;56(3): 259–64.
5. Tulsky DS, Kisala PA, Victorson D, et al. Overview of the Spinal Cord Injury–Quality of Life (SCI-QOL)

measurement system. J Spinal Cord Med 2015; 38(3):257–69.

6. Tulsky DS, Kisala PA, Tate DG, et al. Development and psychometric characteristics of the SCI-QOL Bladder Management Difficulties and Bowel Management Difficulties item banks and short forms and the SCI-QOL Bladder Complications scale. The journal of spinal cord medicine 2015;38(3):288–302.

7. Tulsky DS, Kisala PA, Victorson D, et al. Methodology for the development and calibration of the SCI-QOL item banks. J Spinal Cord Med 2015;38(3):270–87.

8. Labs SRA. Spinal Injuries Database. Available at: https://www.sralab.org/rehabilitation-measures.

9. Bertisch H, Kalpakjian CZ, Kisala PA, et al. Measuring positive affect and well-being after spinal cord injury: Development and psychometric characteristics of the SCI-QOL Positive Affect and Well-being bank and short form. J Spinal Cord Med 2015;38(3):356–65.

10. Tulsky DS, Kisala PA, Victorson D, et al. Developing a contemporary patient-reported outcomes measure for spinal cord injury. Arch Phys Med Rehabil 2011; 92(10 Suppl):S44–51.

11. Team R.C. A language and environment for statistical computing. Vienna, Austria: R Foundation for Statistical Computing; 2017.

12. Myers JB, Lenherr SM, Stoffel JT, et al, Neurogenic Bladder Research Group. Patient reported bladder related symptoms and quality of life after spinal cord injury with different bladder management strategies. J Urol 2019. 101097JU0000000000000270.

13. Cameron AP, Wallner LP, Tate DG, et al. Bladder management after spinal cord injury in the United States 1972 to 2005. J Urol 2010;184(1):213–7.

14. Patel DP, Herrick JS, Stoffel JT, et al, Neurogenic Bladder Research Group NBRG.org. Neurogenic Bladder Research G: Reasons for cessation of clean intermittent catheterization after spinal cord injury: Results from the Neurogenic Bladder Research Group spinal cord injury registry. Neurourol Urodyn 2020;39(1):211–9.

15. Myers JB, Lenherr SM, Stoffel JT, et al, Neurogenic Bladder Research Group NBRG. org. The effects of augmentation cystoplasty and botulinum toxin injection on patient-reported bladder function and quality of life among individuals with spinal cord injury performing clean intermittent catheterization. Neurourol Urodyn 2019;38(1):285–94.

16. Cheng PJ, Keihani S, Roth JD, et al. Contemporary multicenter outcomes of continent cutaneous ileocecocystoplasty in the adult population over a 10-year period: A Neurogenic Bladder Research Group study. Neurourol Urodyn 2020;39(6):1771–80.

17. Myers JB, Stoffel JT, Elliott SP, et al. Sex Differences in Bladder Management, Symptoms, and Satisfaction After Spinal Cord Injury. J Urol 2023;210(4):659–69.

18. Dekalo A, Myers JB, Kennelly M, et al. General and bladder-related quality of life: A focus on women living with spinal cord injury. Neurourol Urodyn 2022;41(4):980–90.

19. Moghalu O, Stoffel JT, Elliott SP, et al. Time-Related Changes in Patient Reported Bladder Symptoms and Satisfaction after Spinal Cord Injury. J Urol 2022;207(2):392–9.

20. Crescenze IM, Myers JB, Lenherr SM, et al. Predictors of low urinary quality of life in spinal cord injury patients on clean intermittent catheterization. Neurourol Urodyn 2019;38(5):1332–8.

21. Elliott CS, Stoffel JT, Myers JB, et al. Validation of Upper Extremity Motor Function as a Key Predictor of Bladder Management After Spinal Cord Injury. Arch Phys Med Rehabil 2019;100(10):1939–44.

22. Theisen KM, Mann R, Roth JD, et al. Frequency of patient-reported UTIs is associated with poor quality of life after spinal cord injury: a prospective observational study. Spinal Cord 2020;58(12):1274–81.

23. Roth JD, Pariser JJ, Stoffel JT, et al. Patient subjective assessment of urinary tract infection frequency and severity is associated with bladder management method in spinal cord injury. Spinal Cord 2019;57(8):700–7.

24. Dudley-Javoroski S, Shields RK. Assessment of physical function and secondary complications after complete spinal cord injury. Disabil Rehabil 2006; 28(2):103–10.

25. Crescenze IM, Lenherr SM, Myers JB, et al. Self-Reported Urological Hospitalizations or Emergency Room Visits in a Contemporary Spinal Cord Injury Cohort. J Urol 2021;205(2):477–82.

26. Amtmann D, Cook KF, Jensen MP, et al. Development of a PROMIS item bank to measure pain interference. Pain 2010;150(1):173–82.

27. Moghalu O, Stoffel JT, Elliott S, et al, Neurogenic Bladder Research Group. Neurogenic Bladder Research G: Psychosocial aspects of health-related quality of life and the association with patient-reported bladder symptoms and satisfaction after spinal cord injury. Spinal Cord 2021;59(9): 987–96.

28. Krogh K, Christensen P, Sabroe S, et al. Neurogenic bowel dysfunction score. Spinal Cord 2006;44(10): 625–31.

29. Stoffel JT, Barboglio-Romo P, Lenherr SM, et al. Factors impacting bowel symptoms in a contemporary spinal cord injury cohort: results from the Neurogenic Bladder Research Group Registry. Spinal Cord 2021;59(9):997–1002.

30. Hubli M, Gee CM, Krassioukov AV. Refined assessment of blood pressure instability after spinal cord injury. Am J Hypertens 2015;28(2):173–81.

Voiding Phase Dysfunction in Multiple Sclerosis

Contemporary Review of Terminology, Diagnosis, Management, and Future Directions

Catherine Frances Ingram, MD[a], John A. Lincoln, MD, PhD[b], Rose Khavari, MD[c],*

KEYWORDS

- Multiple sclerosis • Voiding dysfunction • Urodynamics • Neurogenic bladder
- Lower urinary tract symptoms

KEY POINTS

- Lower urinary tract symptoms (LUTS; storage phase or voiding phase) are common in individuals with multiple sclerosis (MS).
- Diligence should be used when applying non-neurogenic criteria of urinary retention to patients with MS. As individuals with MS often have a decreased bladder capacity, an absolute postvoid residual (PVR) value may not be meaningful without the knowledge of bladder capacity.
- Owing to the risk of development of a urinary disorder, all patients with MS, regardless of symptoms, should be screened for proper bladder emptying (voiding dysfunction) with relevant history taking in the clinic and by obtaining a baseline PVR.
- In men with MS and refractory LUTS, urodynamics should be performed. The bladder outlet obstruction index and bladder contractility index should be calculated to determine the etiology of their LUTS as neurogenic versus obstructive or both in origin.
- Numerous therapies are available for LUTS in MS, including pelvic floor muscle training, pharmacologic options, catheterization, and peripheral tibial nerve stimulation. However, to date, there is no one best option specific to voiding dysfunction.

INTRODUCTION

Multiple sclerosis (MS) is an immune-mediated demyelinating disease of the central nervous system (CNS).[1] It is also the most common debilitating disease of the CNS in young adults.[2] New research has shown that infection with Epstein-Barr virus (EBV) may trigger the onset of MS and that possessing the human leukocyte antigen HLA-DR15 may increase the likelihood of developing MS

after an EBV infection.[1,3] Despite these advances in understanding the etiology of MS, we are many years away from developing an effective method for prevention or a cure. In addition, although there are numerous disease modifying therapies shown, in the aggregate, to reduce clinical relapse and disability progression, none are used to treat symptoms of MS. Therefore, at this time, we must work to manage the symptoms of MS that,

[a] Department of Urology, Baylor College of Medicine, 1 Baylor Plaza, Houston, TX 77030, USA; [b] Department of Neurology, McGovern Medical School, UT Health Neurosciences Neurology, 6431 Fannin Street, MSB 7.222, Houston, TX 77030, USA; [c] Department of Urology, Houston Methodist Hospital, 6560 Fannin Street Suite 2100, Houston, TX 77030, USA
* Corresponding author.
E-mail address: rkhavari@houstonmethodist.org

Urol Clin N Am 51 (2024) 177–185
https://doi.org/10.1016/j.ucl.2024.01.005
0094-0143/24/© 2024 Elsevier Inc. All rights reserved.

more than often, impact the day-to-day activities of our patients.

Lower urinary tract symptoms (LUTS) are one of the most common and bothersome sequelae of MS and occur in up to 1 of 10 patients during their initial disease presentations.[4] Moreover, nearly 100% of patients will endorse LUTS within 10 years after their MS diagnosis is first made.[5] However, owing to the progressive nature of MS and its transient distribution throughout the CNS, patients' LUTS vary greatly both in character and time of onset. Therefore, the diagnosis and management of LUTS in MS is highly patient-dependent and easily confounded.

An understanding of the neuropathology behind MS is critical for effectively managing the spectrum of LUTS that can be seen. LUTS in MS could include storage and/or voiding.

- Storage phase symptoms: urinary frequency, urgency, incontinence.
- Voiding phase symptoms: hesitancy, intermittency, incomplete bladder emptying, urinary retention, or both phases (**Fig. 1**).

In MS, the origin of patient's symptoms is the demyelination of signal-carrying axons (or the destruction of white matter), which leaves behind characteristic *plaques* that are seen on diagnostic imaging. This demyelination can occur anywhere in the CNS, including the spinal cord, brain, and optic nerves.[6] The integral components of the CNS control over the micturition cycle, are spread throughout the CNS, and they rely on signals being reliably sent among themselves for proper functioning of both phases of bladder control: storage and voiding (bladder emptying).[7] Therefore, a patient with MS may present with storage or voiding complaints depending on the sites of their lesions, and their symptoms may change during the course of their disease.

The dynamic nature of LUTS associated with MS can make even the application of terminology for defining a patient's symptoms challenging. With this in mind, our goal is to (1) review the terminology for describing voiding dysfunction (VD) in MS; (2) discuss the multiple modalities available for evaluation and diagnosis of VD; and (3) examine management options, ranging from catheterization to neurostimulation. Special considerations will be provided for men with MS where bladder outlet obstruction (BOO) due to prostate pathology can contribute to VD. Finally, we will strive to speculate on future directions for the treatment of VD in MS.

TERMINOLOGY AND LIMITATIONS OF THE STATUS QUO

Most MS patients present with storage dysfunction symptoms, including urinary frequency, urgency, nocturia, and incontinence, making overactive bladder complaints the hallmark of LUTS in MS.[5] However, urodynamic (UDS) findings in several studies have shown that VD is present in up to 70% of patients with MS, including those who are asymptomatic from a LUTS standpoint.[8,9] Therefore, incomplete bladder emptying and urinary retention are similarly significant problems in MS. Not having a consensus on the definition, terminology, and diagnosis has made management challenging, especially when it comes to intervention or the need for initiation or continuation of catheterization. The combined 2021 American Urologic Association (AUA) and Society of Urodynamics, Female Pelvic Medicine and Urogenital Reconstruction guidelines regarding neurogenic lower

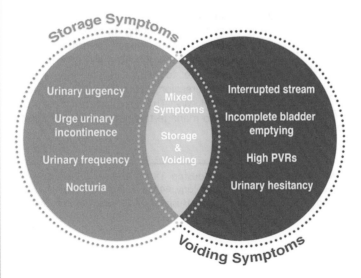

Fig. 1. Storage and voiding phase symptoms.

urinary tract dysfunction (NLUTD) do not afford any clarity to these problems.[10]

DIAGNOSIS AND EVALUATION OF VOIDING DYSFUNCTION IN MULTIPLE SCLEROSIS

The diagnosis of VD in MS is less resolute, as oftentimes patients have no urinary complaints. Therefore, should attempts at diagnosis wait until the patient becomes symptomatic or should some sort of screening occur? At what point in their disease process should patients be referred to a urologist? The European Association of Urology guidelines on neurourology vaguely state that "early diagnosis and treatment are essential," and do not specify a timeline.[11] The AUA guidelines for NLUTD assume that the patient has already been referred and has urinary symptoms secondary to their neurologic disorder.[10] MS guidelines published by the American Academy of Neurologists do not include any guidance for urinary tract surveillance or state when a urology referral is necessary. Thus, other groups have attempted to provide answers to these questions.

De Ridder and colleagues attempted to define the neurologist's role in the management of VD in MS.[12] They recommend for neurologists to perform a short evaluation of voiding function in all MS patients, regardless of symptoms, and that at minimum this evaluation should include questioning the patient about LUTS. They also outline instances when a patient should be referred to urology, including in the case of recurrent infections and a postvoid residual (PVR) greater than 100 to 150 mL. The UK consensus panel, consisting of multiple urologic groups, states that only patients with MS who complain of LUTS should be assessed for VD.[13] Nonetheless, the International Francophone Neuro-Urological Study Group, which includes urologists, neurologists, and PM&R physicians, recommend that patients with MS without urinary symptoms should be screened with at least a simple questionnaire and PVR.[14] The Multiple Sclerosis Study Group-Italian Neurology Society, composed of similar specialists as the French group, agrees with this recommendation.[15] It is also our recommendation that all patients with MS be screened for VD with questioning and by obtaining a PVR regardless of symptoms, as development of a urinary disorder should always be suspected in these patients. Two questionnaires that can be used and that have been developed specifically for the MS population are the Qualiveen questionnaire and the Neurogenic Bladder Symptom Score (NBSS).

For patients with MS who have LUTS, the urologist should begin with a thorough history and physical examination, urinalysis, and PVR, as well as uroflowmetry and voiding diary as indicated. In general, we advocate for withholding more meticulous diagnostic tests if the patient meets the following criteria: a low PVR, no spinal cord lesions, no recurrent UTIs, normal renal function, stable LUTS, and the ability to spontaneously void. However, in patients with MS who do not meet these criteria, we advocate for obtaining baseline multichannel video UDS testing and a renal ultrasound (RUS), as well as administering an MS-specific questionnaire.

Postvoid Residual

Several attempts have been made to provide patient guidance regarding PVR and complications of incomplete bladder emptying. In the non-neurogenic population, chronic urinary retention has been defined by the AUA committee for Quality Improvement and Patient Safety as 2 PVRs of at least 300 mL recorded in a time period lasting at least 6 months.[16] Diligence should be employed when applying this definition to patients with MS, as individuals with MS have a smaller bladder capacity and an absolute value of PVR may not be meaningful without the knowledge of bladder capacity.

UDS reports have shown that patients with MS often have decreased bladder capacities secondary to storage issues such as detrusor overactivity (OD) and rarely due to impaired bladder compliance.[17–20] One study of 54 female participants with MS who had UDS studies performed, showed an average bladder capacity was 287 mL.[21] Therefore, most of these patients would not have met the non-neurogenic definition of urinary retention even if they were unable to empty their bladders. Moreover, the relapsing-remitting type of MS is by far the most common, and a typical relapse will usually be symptomatic for 2 months before recovery, a significantly shorter amount of time than the 6 months required to meet the AUA's definition of chronic urinary retention.[22] Thus, the cutoff for urinary retention in non-neurogenic patients can be difficult to apply in MS.

Several treatment algorithms have defined significant urinary retention in MS as a PVR of 100 mL and recommend beginning catheterization at this value.[4,12,13,23,24] The authors suggest taking the patient's total bladder capacity, urinary flow rate, and symptoms into consideration, however, before initiating invasive bladder management based on this strict cutoff. As an example, the Italian Multiple Sclerosis Group considers residual volumes that are at least one-third of bladder capacity significant, which allows for greater PVRs to be acceptable in patients with larger intravesical volumes.[15] Moreover, for those patients whose PVRs are low but for whom emptying the bladder takes excessive time, as characterized by a decreased flow rate for voided volume on the Liverpool nomogram, clean intermittent catheterization (CIC) can be considered to decrease the amount of time expended in the bathroom. We recommend a maximum flow rate below the 10th percentile curve as the limit for CIC initiation, or according to patient preference.[25] Finally, patients' symptoms, as well as goals, should be taken into careful consideration before initiating CIC.

Urodynamics

Typically, LUTS do not correlate with UDS findings and a wide variety of patterns are seen.[26] In most reports, DO is the most common finding, followed in sequence by detrusor sphincter dyssynergia (DSD) and hypocontractility.[26,27] A recent systematic review that included 1524 patients found that DO was seen in 53% of patients, DSD in 43%, and atonic bladder in 12%.[28] Although the diagnosis of DO on UDS does not usually change management for a patient presenting with storage complaints, knowing whether a patient has DSD or atonic bladder is essential for understanding the reason for an elevated PVR, for example, in a male patient where benign prostatic hyperplasia (BPH) could be a confounding factor. Furthermore, although more rare in MS than in patients with spinal cord injury (SCI), DSD, and altered compliance can lead to deterioration of the upper and lower urinary tracts, and are important to track with UDS.[18–20] Thus, patients with these findings should undergo UDS screening.

Upper Tract Imaging

Upper tract damage and renal dysfunction are much less common sequelae from impaired voiding in MS as compared with SCI.[26,29] In one retrospective review of 249 patients with MS, only 5% had abnormal upper tract findings.[30] In another study that looked at renal function in 92 patients, mean creatinine clearance was normal and did not correlate with the severity of MS, type of MS, or UDS results; in total, only 5 patients had abnormal ultrasound findings.[31] One study that evaluated upper tract changes over time rather than in a single setting found that 5.8% of patients had abnormal upper tract findings on initial imaging; a median of 61 months later, this number had increased to 12.4%. Still, no abnormal creatinine values were observed regardless of RUS results.[29] Nonetheless, out of an abundance of caution, the AUA neurogenic bladder guidelines recommend to obtain an annual BMP and RUS for MS patients with unknown upper track risk including poor compliance, DSD, prior abnormal RUS, or below normal renal function.[10]

Questionnaires

Several questionnaires are available to assess MS patients' symptoms and bladder effects on quality of life (QoL). These are important to administer both before and after treatment to evaluate the consequences of any therapy. Which questionnaire to choose, however, is left at the provider's discretion. It is important that the chosen questionnaire be validated in the neurogenic bladder population and in the language in which it is being used. Two questionnaires that were created and validated specifically for urinary symptoms in the population with MS are the Qualiveen, and the NBSS and their respective short-forms. The Qualiveen is a QoL questionnaire which consists of 30 items that broadly address storage and voiding symptoms, as well as urinary incontinence.[32,33] The NBSS is a symptom score that includes 24 questions that likewise cover storage and voiding symptoms and continence, but it also includes questions about neurogenic bladder complications, bladder management, and QoL.[34] In addition, the Actionable Bladder Symptom Screening Tool, which was developed and validated in 2013 for following DO symptoms in patients with MS, is also available.[35] Other less neurospecific urinary symptom questionnaires, like the AUA symptom index and the standardized International Consultation on Incontinence Questionnaire (ICIQ) modules for male and female patients can likewise be used to track patient urinary symptoms over time with the ultimate goal being a metric for treatment efficacy.[36,37]

Men with Multiple Sclerosis: Special Considerations During Evaluation

MS is 2 to 3 times more common in women than men.[38] Perhaps for this reason there is a lack of literature regarding best management practices for men with MS and concomitant anatomic BOO. Because the average life expectancy for men with MS is 72 years, most of these patients will develop some degree of BPH over their lifetime.[39,40] Therefore, the provider should keep in mind that LUTS in male patients with MS can be secondary to neurogenic dysfunction, BOO, or a combination of both. UDS with pressure flow testing is the most important modality for identifying the etiology of LUT dysfunction in these patients.[11] When performing UDS, bladder outlet obstruction index (BOOI) and bladder contractility index should be calculated. A composite nomogram, such as the one produced by Abrams, can be used to place the patient in 1 of 9 categories based on bladder contractility and obstruction.[41,42] The use of cystometrogramography to determine compliance and the presence of OD, and electromyography (EMG) to determine the presence of DSD (functional obstruction), are also important to perform before a management decision is chosen. Cystoscopy should be performed in men with a BOOI indicating possible obstruction, keeping in mind that men performing CIC are at higher risk of urethral stricture development. For men with MS and BPH who are obstructed with good contractility, transrectal ultrasound sizing should be performed. Good voluntary sphincter control should be assured with UDS to decrease the risk of de novo urinary incontinence following BOO surgery.[43] Afterward, following failure with medical management, these patients should be offered BOO surgery. Currently, no data exist regarding the best surgery for BPH in this patient population.[44] Thus, we recommend transurethral resection of the prostate as the current gold standard in non-neurogenic patients.[45]

MANAGEMENT OF VOIDING DYSFUNCTION IN MULTIPLE SCLEROSIS
Pelvic Floor Muscle Training

Rehabilitation programs consisting of pelvic floor muscle training (PFMT) have been shown in multiple systematic reviews to improve patients' urinary symptom burden.[46–48] These studies have reported significant results in nocturia, urge incontinence, daytime frequency, and voided volume. According to some UDS studies, total bladder capacity can also be improved with PFMT.[48] Moreover, PFMT has been shown to be even more efficacious when combined with pelvic floor electrostimulation than when performed alone.[49] Therefore, in MS patients with significant LUTS, referral to a physiatrist for PFMT is an acceptable noninvasive first step.

Pharmacologic Therapy

No medication has been specifically designed for LUTS in patients with MS. Therefore, the provider must choose from multiple available urologic drugs and decide what to prescribe based on symptoms and UDS findings. Often, a combination of medications is required. The types of drugs available can be simply divided into alleviating either storage or voiding symptoms. Antimuscarinic drugs are typically the first-line option for patients with storage symptoms. Some of the most common are oral solifenacin, trospium, oxybutynin, and tolterodine, and all of these have shown

to be effective in the neurourological population.[50–55] However, none of these medications has been proven superior for LUTS in MS, and one should be chosen over another based on its side effect profile and mechanism of action. The provider should also consider the risk of exacerbating cognitive symptoms in older patients with dementia who receive antimuscarinics.[56] Mirabegron, a beta-3-adrenergic receptor agonist, either alone or combined with desmopressin, has been shown to improve LUTS in patients with MS.[57,58]

The medication options for storage symptoms are fewer and less proven. The cholinergic drug bethanecol should theoretically augment detrusor contractility and bladder emptying but is not typically prescribed.[59] Moreover, alpha-blockers, like tamsulosin, seem to enhance bladder emptying and decrease PVR based on limited analysis.[60]

Catheterization

For MS patients with adequate hand function who are unable to empty their bladders, CIC has long been preferred over indwelling catheters due to the decreased risk of infection.[61] More recent studies have shown that prelubricated hydrophilic catheters should be used whenever possible to decrease urinary tract infection (UTI) risk, and it is common practice that patients should catheterize themselves at a minimum of 4 times a day.[62–64] Of note, QoL should be taken into consideration when initiating catheterization. Despite the proven medical benefit of CIC, many patients prefer indwelling catheters due to convenience and comfort, and this choice should be respected. When an indwelling catheter is chosen, there are some data that support recommending a suprapubic tube (SPT) over a transurethral catheter due to an association with less discomfort and serious long-term complications, for example, urethral erosion.[65,66] Owing to the remitting nature of the most common subtype of MS, SPTs in this population may be only temporary devices for bladder emptying rather than lifelong implements.

OnabotulinumtoxinA Injections

In MS patients with storage symptoms that are refractory to oral medications, intravesical onabotulinumtoxinA (Botox) injections may be considered. Several studies, recently reviewed in a study by Kaviani and colleagues, have shown the efficacy of Botox for augmenting urinary symptoms in patients with MS for several months before having to be redone, and despite its serial nature, Botox does not seem to become less effective after multiple treatments.[67–69] Before the procedure, patients should be warned about the risk of postoperative retention and UTIs. 200 U Botox has been shown to be noninferior to 300 U, and there is no consensus regarding the injection pattern, although most physicians utilize a trigone-sparing template.[70] However, 2 recent clinical trials in patients with SCI showed evidence favoring including the trigone in Botox injections to decrease episodes of incontinence and detrusor pressures.[71,72]

Peripheral Tibial Nerve Stimulation

A recent systematic review and meta-analysis published in 2022 by Vecchio and colleagues evaluated 21 publications regarding peripheral tibial nerve stimulation (PTNS) and PFMT in the treatment of bladder dysfunction in MS.[48] The authors deemed that most of the included studies had a low risk of bias, making their quality of evidence high. Nocturia, daytime frequency, voided volume, and urge incontinence were significantly improved with PTNS. Moreover, maximum cystometric capacity was shown to improve after 3 months of PTNS. Still, many more studies are needed to confirm PTNS as a standard therapy in the treatment of MS resultant LUTS.

FUTURE DIRECTIONS

One new and exciting management option for LUTS in the MS population is noninvasive brain stimulation. Repetitive transcranial magnetic stimulation is one form of this new technology. It works by targeting specific cortical networks to excite and inhibit and has been shown to improve LUTS and pelvic pain in disparate neurologic conditions.[73,74] Patients can receive the stimulation over the course of several days to 2 weeks depending on the protocol used. Although innovative, much work remains to be done to make noninvasive brain stimulation a mainstream therapy.

SUMMARY

LUTS in MS is extremely common. However, diagnosis and evaluation can be hampered by ambiguous definitions and lack of screening in asymptomatic patients. Caution should be observed when employing the non-neurogenic definition of urinary retention in this population due to decreased bladder capacity, and low flow rate as compared with the Liverpool nomogram can be considered toward initiating catheterization. In men with MS and refractory LUTS, UDS should be utilized to determine the etiology of their symptoms. Finally, multiple therapies are currently available for the treatment of LUTS in MS, though many novel therapies, including PTNS and noninvasive brain stimulation, require additional research to determine their efficacy.

CLINICS CARE POINTS

- Clinicians should assess lower urinary tract symptoms of individuals with MS with respect to both voiding phase and storage phase abnormalities.
- It is important to note that many indiviuals with MS will have both storage and voiding symptoms.
- Post void residual value is menaing ful when it is repeated more than once and interpreted int he context of total baldder volume in the setting of MS.

FUNDING

RK is partially funded by NIDDK R01DK134340.

DISCLOSURE

The authors have nothing to disclose.

REFERENCES

1. Bjornevik K, Cortese M, Healy BC, et al. Longitudinal analysis reveals high prevalence of Epstein-Barr virus associated with multiple sclerosis. Science 2022;375(6578):296–301.
2. Ramagopalan SV, Sadovnick AD. Epidemiology of multiple sclerosis. Neurol Clin 2011;29(2):207–17.
3. Nielsen TR, Rostgaard K, Askling J, et al. Effects of infectious mononucleosis and HLA-DRB1*15 in multiple sclerosis. Mult Scler 2009;15(4):431–6.
4. Tornic J, Panicker JN. The Management of Lower Urinary Tract Dysfunction in Multiple Sclerosis. Curr Neurol Neurosci Rep 2018;18(8):54.
5. Panicker JN, Fowler CJ, Kessler TM. Lower urinary tract dysfunction in the neurological patient: clinical assessment and management. Lancet Neurol 2015; 14(7):720–32.
6. Dobson R, Giovannoni G. Multiple sclerosis - a review. Eur J Neurol 2019;26(1):27–40.
7. Alan W, Partin P, Roger R, et al. Campbell-walsh-wein urology. 12th edition. Philadelphia, PA: Elsevier; 2021.
8. Cetinel B, Tarcan T, Demirkesen O, et al. Management of lower urinary tract dysfunction in multiple sclerosis: a systematic review and Turkish consensus report. Neurourol Urodyn 2013;32(8):1047–57.
9. Jaekel AK ea, Winterhagen Fl, Zeller FL, et al. Neurogenic Lower Urinary Tract Dysfunction in Asymptomatic Patients with Multiple Sclerosis. Biomedicines

2022. https://doi.org/10.3390/biomedicines1012
3260.

10. Ginsberg DA, Boone TB, Cameron AP, et al. The
AUA/SUFU guideline on adult neurogenic lower uri-
nary tract dysfunction: diagnosis and evaluation.
J Urol 2021;206(5):1097–105.

11. Groen J, Pannek J, Castro Diaz D, et al. Summary of
European Association of Urology (EAU) Guidelines
on Neuro-Urology. Eur Urol 2016;69(2):324–33.

12. De Ridder D, Van Der Aa F, Debruyne J, et al.
Consensus guidelines on the neurologist's role in
the management of neurogenic lower urinary tract
dysfunction in multiple sclerosis. Clin Neurol Neurosurg 2013;115(10):2033–40.

13. Fowler CJ, Panicker JN, Drake M, et al. A UK
consensus on the management of the bladder in
multiple sclerosis. Postgrad Med 2009;85(1008):
552–9.

14. de Seze M, Ruffion A, Denys P, et al. The neurogenic
bladder in multiple sclerosis: review of the literature
and proposal of management guidelines. Mult Scler
2007;13(7):915–28.

15. Ghezzi A, Carone R, Del Popolo G, et al. Recommendations for the management of urinary disorders
in multiple sclerosis: a consensus of the Italian Multiple Sclerosis Study Group. Neurol Sci 2011;32(6):
1223–31.

16. Stoffel JT, Peterson AC, Sandhu JS, et al. AUA White
Paper on Nonneurogenic Chronic Urinary Retention:
Consensus Definition, Treatment Algorithm, and
Outcome End Points. J Urol 2017;198(1):153–60.

17. Moussa M, Abou Chakra M, Papatsoris AG, et al.
Perspectives on urological care in multiple sclerosis
patients. Intractable Rare Dis Res 2021;10(2):62–74.

18. Ciancio SJ, Mutchnik SE, Rivera VM, et al. Urodynamic pattern changes in multiple sclerosis. Urology
2001;57(2):239–45.

19. Cox LC, Wittman D, Papin JE, et al. Analysis of Urinary Symptoms and Urodynamic Findings in Multiple Sclerosis Patients by Gender and Disease
Subtype. J Neurol Neurobiol 2015;1(2). https://doi.
org/10.16966/2379-7150.105.

20. Litwiller SE, Frohman EM, Zimmern PE. Multiple sclerosis and the urologist. J Urol 1999;161(3):743–57.

21. Lemack GE, Frohman EM, Zimmern PE, et al. Urodynamic distinctions between idiopathic detrusor overactivity and detrusor overactivity secondary to
multiple sclerosis. Urology 2006;67(5):960–4.

22. Rolak LA. Multiple sclerosis: it's not the disease you
though it was. Clin Med Res 2002;1(1):57–60.

23. Panicker JN. Neurogenic Bladder: Epidemiology,
Diagnosis, and Management. Semin Neurol 2020;
40(5):569–79.

24. Amarenco G, Chartier-Kastler E, Denys P, et al. First-
line urological evaluation in multiple sclerosis: validation of a specific decision-making algorithm.
Mult Scler 2013;19(14):1931–7.

25. Haylen BT, Ashby D, Sutherst JR, et al. Maximum
and average urine flow rates in normal male and female populations - the Liverpool nomograms. Br J
Urol 1989;64(1):30–8.

26. Hinson JL, Boone TB. Urodynamics and multiple
sclerosis. Urol Clin North Am 1996;23(3):475–81.

27. Dillon BE, Lemack GE. Urodynamics in the evaluation of the patient with multiple sclerosis: when are
they helpful and how do we use them? Urol Clin
North Am 2014;41(3):439–44.

28. Stoffel JT. Chronic Urinary Retention in Multiple Sclerosis Patients: Physiology, Systematic Review of Urodynamic Data, and Recommendations for Care.
Urol Clin North Am 2017;44(3):429–39.

29. Fletcher SG, Dillon BE, Gilchrist AS, et al. Renal
deterioration in multiple sclerosis patients with neurovesical dysfunction. Mult Scler 2013;19(9):
1169–74.

30. Onal B ea, Siva A, Buldu I, et al. Voiding Dysfunction
due to Multiple Sclerosis - a Large Scale Retrospective Analysis. Int Braz J Urol 2009;35(3):326–33.

31. Krhut J, Hradilek P, Zapletalova O. Analysis of the
upper urinary tract function in multiple sclerosis patients. Acta Neurol Scand 2008;118(2):115–9.

32. Bonniaud V, Bryant D, Parratte B, et al. Development
and validation of the short form of a urinary quality of
life questionnaire: SF-Qualiveen. J Urol 2008;180(6):
2592–8.

33. Bonniaud V, Bryant D, Parratte B, et al. Qualiveen: a
urinary disorder-specific instrument for use in clinical trials in multiple sclerosis. Arch Phys Med Rehabil 2006;87(12):1661–3.

34. Welk B, Morrow S, Madarasz W, et al. The validity
and reliability of the neurogenic bladder symptom
score. J Urol 2014;192(2):452–7.

35. Burks J, Chancellor M, Bates D, et al. Development
and validation of the actionable bladder symptom
screening tool for multiple sclerosis patients. Int J
MS Care. Winter 2013;15(4):182–92.

36. Abrams P CL, Wagg A, Wein A. Patient-reported
outcome assessment. In: Diaz DC, et al, ed. Incontinence: 6th International Consultation on Incontinence 6th edition. 2013.

37. Barry MJ, Fowler FJ Jr, O'Leary MP, et al. The Amer-
ican Urological Association Symptom Index for
Benign Prostatic Hyperplasia. J Urol 1992;197(2S):
S189–97.

38. Howard J, Trevick S, Younger DS. Epidemiology of
Multiple Sclerosis. Neurol Clin 2016;34(4):919–39.

39. Ragonese P. Mortality studies for multiple sclerosis:
still a useful tool to analyse long-term outcome.
J Neurol Neurosurg Psychiatry 2017;88(8):617.

40. Berry Sj, Walsh PC, Ewing LL, et al. The development of human benign prostatic hyperplasia with
age. J Urol 1984;132(3):474–9.

41. Abrams P. Bladder outlet obstruction index, bladder
contractility index and bladder voiding efficiency:

three simple indices to define bladder voiding function. BJU Int 1999;84(1):14–5.

42. Victor N. Pressure Flow Urodynamic Studies - The Gold Standard for Diagnosing Bladder Outlet Obstruction. Rev Urol 2005;7 Suppl(Suppl 6):S14–21.

43. Staskin DSVY, Siroky MB, Siroky MB. Post-prostatectomy continence in the Parkinsonian patient: the significance of poor voluntary sphincter control. J Urol 1988;140(1):117–8.

44. Noordhoff TC, Groen J, Scheepe JR, et al. Surgical Management of Anatomic Bladder Outlet Obstruction in Males with Neurogenic Bladder Dysfunction: A Systematic Review. Eur Urol Focus 2019;5(5):875–86.

45. Sandhu JS, Bixler BR, Dahm P, et al. Management of lower urinary tract symptoms attributed to benign prostatic hyperplasia (BPH): AUA Guideline amendment 2023. J Urol 2023;211(1):11–9.

46. Sparaco M, Bonavita S. Pelvic Floor Dysfunctions and Their Rehabilitation in Multiple Sclerosis. J Clin Med 2022;11(7). https://doi.org/10.3390/jcm11071941.

47. Yavas I, Emuk Y, Kahraman T. Pelvic floor muscle training on urinary incontinence and sexual function in people with multiple sclerosis: A systematic review. Mult Scler Relat Disord 2022;58:103538.

48. Vecchio M, Chiaramonte R, P DIB. Management of bladder dysfunction in multiple sclerosis: a systematic review and meta-analysis of studies regarding bladder rehabilitation. Eur J Phys Rehabil Med 2022;58(3):387–96.

49. McClurg D, Ashe RG, Lowe-Strong AS. Neuromuscular electrical stimulation and the treatment of lower urinary tract dysfunction in multiple sclerosis–a double blind, placebo controlled, randomised clinical trial. Neurourol Urodyn 2008;27(3):231–7.

50. Cameron AP, Clemens JQ, Latini JM, et al. Combination drug therapy improves compliance of the neurogenic bladder. J Urol 2009;182(3):1062–7.

51. Amarenco G, Sutory M, Zachoval R, et al. Solifenacin is effective and well tolerated in patients with neurogenic detrusor overactivity: Results from the double-blind, randomized, active- and placebo-controlled SONIC urodynamic study. Neurourol Urodyn 2015;36(2):414–21.

52. Apostolidis A, et al. Neurologic Urinary and Faecal Incontinence. In: P. Abrams LC, S. Khoury & A. Wein, ed. Incontinence 6th Edition. 2017.

53. Ethans KD, Nance PW, Bard RJ, et al. Efficacy and safety of tolterodine in people with neurogenic detrusor overactivity. J Spinal Cord Med 2004;27(3):214–8.

54. Isik AT, Celik T, Bozoglu E, et al. Trospium and cognition in patients with late onset Alzheimer disease. J Nutr Health Aging 2009;13(8):672–6.

55. Madhuvrata P, Singh M, Hasafa Z, et al. Anticholinergic drugs for adult neurogenic detrusor overactivity: a systematic review and meta-analysis. Eur Urol 2012;62(5):816–30.

56. Dmochowski RR, Thai S, Iglay K, et al. Increased risk of incident dementia following use of anticholinergic agents: A systematic literature review and meta-analysis. Neurourol Urodyn 2021;40(1):28–37.

57. Welk B, Hickling D, McKibbon M, et al. A pilot randomized-controlled trial of the urodynamic efficacy of mirabegron for patients with neurogenic lower urinary tract dysfunction. Neurourol Urodyn 2018;37(8):2810–7.

58. Zachariou A, Filiponi M, Baltogiannis D, et al. Effective treatment of neurogenic detrusor overactivity in multiple sclerosis patients using desmopressin and mirabegron. Can J Urol 2017;24(6):9107–13.

59. Barendrecht MM, Oelke M, Laguna MP, et al. Is the use of parasympathomimetics for treating an underactive urinary bladder evidence-based? BJU Int 2007;99(4):749–52.

60. Tornic J, Tornic J, Sýkora R, et al. Alpha-blockers for treating neurogenic lower urinary tract dysfunction in patients with multiple sclerosis: A systematic review and meta-analysis. A report from the Neuro-Urology Promotion Committee of the International Continence Society (ICS). Neurourol Urodyn 2019;38(6):1482–91.

61. Lapides J, Diokno AC, Silber SJ, et al. Clean, intermittent self-catheterization in the treatment of urinary tract disease. J Urol 1972;107(3):458–61.

62. Giannantoni ASS, Scivoletto G, Scivoletto G, et al. Intermittent catheterization with a prelubricated catheter in spinal cord injured patients: A prospective randomized crossover study. J Urol 2001;166:130.

63. RCaT R. Intermittent catheterisation with hydrophilic and non-hydrophilic urinary catheters: Systematic literature review and meta-analyses. BMC Urol 2017.

64. Woodbury MG, Hayes KC, Askes HK. Intermittent catheterization practices following spinal cord injury: a national survey. Can J Urol 2008;15:4065.

65. Ahluwalia RSJN, Kouriefs C, Kouriefs C, et al. The surgical risk of suprapubic catheter insertion and long-term sequelae. Ann R Coll Surg Engl 2006;88:210.

66. Zimmern PEHH, Leach GE, Leach GE, et al. Transvaginal closure of the bladder neck and placement of a suprapubic catheter for destroyed urethra after long-term indwelling catheterization. J Urol 1985;134:554.

67. Ginsberg D, Gousse A, Keppenne V, et al. Phase 3 efficacy and tolerability study of onabotulinumtoxinA for urinary incontinence from neurogenic detrusor overactivity. J Urol 2012;187:2131.

68. Grosse J, Kramer G, Stöhrer M. Success of repeat detrusor injections of botulinum a toxin in patients with severe neurogenic detrusor overactivity and incontinence. Eur Urol 2005;47:653.

69. Kaviani AKR, Khavari R. Disease-specific outcomes of botulinum toxin injections for neurogenic detrusor overactivity. Urol Clin 2017;44:463–74.

70. Schurch B dSM, Denys P, Denys P, et al. Botulinum toxin type a is a safe and effective treatment for neurogenic urinary incontinence: results of a single treatment, randomized, placebo controlled 6-month study. J Urol 2005;174:196–200.

71. Hui CKX, Chonghe J, Chonghe J, et al. Combined detrusor-trigone BTX-A injections for urinary incontinence secondary to neurogenic detrusor overactivity. Spinal Cord 2016;54:46–50.

72. T A, A M. Botulinum toxin-A injections into neurogenic overactive bladder–to include or exclude the trigone? A prospective, randomized, controlled trial. J Urol 2010;184:2423–8.

73. Mazeaud CSB, Khavari R, Khavari R. Noninvasive brain stimulation in the treatment of functional urological and pelvic floor disorders: a scoping review. Neurourol Urodyn 2023.

74. Khavari R, Tran K, Helekar SA, et al. Noninvasive, individualized cortical modulation using transcranial rotating permanent magnet stimulator for voiding dysfunction in women with multiple sclerosis: a pilot trial. J Urol 2022;207(3):657–68.

Barriers to Transitional Care in Spina Bifida

Catalina K. Hwang, MD, Kelly T. Harris, MD, Dan Wood, PhD, MBBS, FRCS(Urol)*

KEYWORDS

- Spina bifida • Myelomeningocele • Transitional care • Health care transitions • Young adult
- Delivery of health care

KEY POINTS

- Key urologic goals throughout the lifetime of patients with spina bifida are preservation of renal function, continence, and prevention of complications.
- Patients who are poorly compliant with self-care tasks and routine surveillance, including outpatient visits with specialists, are at risk for hospitalization and worse outcomes related to preventable conditions.
- Barriers to transition are multifactorial, ranging from communication deficits and knowledge gaps between pediatric and adult providers, to health literacy, as well as patient preferences.
- Successful transition to adult care will require a patient-directed approach involving the input of family and caretakers, general practitioners, subspecialists outside of urology.

INTRODUCTION

Spina bifida (SB) is a congenital neural tube defect including a spectrum of severity from spina bifida occulta to myelomeningocele. An estimated 1400 new cases of SB are born each year in the United States.[1] Of these, 85% are expected to live into adulthood.[2] We should expect a continued increase in the number of affected adults. SB has a heterogeneous phenotype, affecting multiple organ systems and often does not correlate with spinal level of insult or degree of severity at that level.

Transitional care is the process of allowing an adolescent to gain appropriate independence. This article focusses on the health care setting but the principle applies in education and other areas of daily living. Primary components include educating adolescents on their past medical and surgical history, on how to make appointments, medication management, and self-advocacy. Special attention is required to bridge the gap between pediatric-centered and adult-centered practices. For those with chronic childhood diseases, failure to transition is associated with worse health outcomes, nonadherence, higher health care utilization, and decreased quality of life. The American Academy of Pediatrics (AAP), American Academy of Family Physicians (AAFP), American College of Physicians, and the American Society of Internal Medicine wrote a consensus statement in 2002 to achieve the Healthy People 2010 goal "that all young people with special health care needs will receive the services needed to make necessary transitions to all aspects of adult life, including health care, work and independent living."[3] Despite this statement's release 2 decades ago, there remain significant barriers and resistance to the transition process for many patients with SB.

This review aims to summarize 4 components of transitional care within the SB community to

1. Review the changing needs of patients with SB and importance of long-term care in patients with SB,
2. Describe the barriers in transition,
3. Highlight the impact of inadequate transition to adult care, and
4. Propose solutions and a potential vision for the future.

Division of Urology, Children's Hospital Colorado, 13123 East 16th Avenue, Box 323, Aurora, CO 80045, USA
* Corresponding author.
E-mail address: dan.wood@childrenscolorado.org

Urol Clin N Am 51 (2024) 187–196
https://doi.org/10.1016/j.ucl.2024.01.006

NEEDS OF THE ADOLESCENT AND ADULT PATIENT WITH SPINA BIFIDA

The gold standard in the pediatric care of SB is a multidisciplinary approach. Those involved may include neurosurgery, orthopedics, colorectal, urology, rehabilitation medicine, physical therapy, and psychology among others. The extent of involvement of any specialty varies on a case-by-case basis and may change with the development and growth of the child.

From a urologic standpoint, the bladder and outlet may change over the lifetime of the patient. The neurogenic bladder will continue to evolve over time, with added considerations including prostatic growth and hormonal changes of the female urethra.[4] This emphasizes the need for regular follow-up that should include, at a minimum, renal imaging and blood tests that include an assessment of renal function. Urodynamics may be indicated if there are significant changes, such as new incontinence, hydronephrosis on renal ultrasound, or urinary tract infections (UTIs).

The key urologic goals for these patients are

- Preservation of renal function
- Continence
- Prevention of other complications, for example, UTIs and skin breakdown

Patients need careful, expert evaluation and follow-up to ensure that these needs are attended to. In many cases, surgical intervention will be required to achieve some/all of these key objectives. The precise timing of surgery will depend on the degree of insult and the patient/parent decision-making. Surveillance strategies and medical considerations for this population have been described elsewhere.[5]

Continence

If continence has not already been achieved by adolescence, this needs discussion as a patient considers transitional care. It is estimated that 92.6% of older patients with SB use some form of bladder management with 76.8% performing clean intermittent catheterization (CIC).[6] Patient self-reported degree of continence is found to be predictive of bother and quality of life, and outcomes may be compounded by concurrent fecal incontinence.[7] The rate of urinary continence varies among studies, ranging between 63% continent and 66% incontinent.[6–8] This reflects differences in the clinical definitions of continence and reemphasizes the importance of counseling patients on realistic expectations following reconstructive surgeries, as well as factoring in the potential impact on a patient's quality of life, to inform these decisions. Therefore, frequent contact with health care providers is critical not only to monitor success with bladder management but also to ensure patients and their families are well apprised of their condition and options to balance medical and quality of life outcomes.

Many have found that most adolescents and adults with SB have the desire and ability to obtain a higher education, to work, to live independently, to have partnered romantic relationships, and to create families. However, the cognitive ability of patients with SB can also vary. Those with significant impairment may have diminished ability and/or motivation to achieve continence and to participate in self-care.[9] Factors including the degree of motor deficit, social support, and other socioeconomic factors may affect social participation, education, and desire for employment. These may further affect self-care needs, as well as the ability to assume mastery of these tasks.[10,11] These challenges are compounded in adolescence by the social and emotional changes inherent at this time in life.

Sexual Education

Issues regarding sex and sexuality naturally become more important as patients age and need to be recognized as part of the care for an adolescent/adult with SB. Patients with SB have normal desire to form intimate relationships but reports show that conversations regarding sex and intimacy are only initiated by physicians in one-third of cases.[12] Erectile dysfunction, ejaculatory dysfunction, and/or lack of sensation may be present depending on the level of the spinal defect. With higher spinal lesions, azoospermia in men may be more prevalent, whereas orgasm in female may be diminished.[12–15] Although objective evaluation may take time or involve some investigation, patients themselves report strong preference for these conversations with their physicians.[16,17]

Pregnancy is another issue that is important to manage with adult women with SB. Unfortunately, recent data suggest a longer length of stay and higher morbidity rate to both the mother and the infant in pregnancies of women with SB.[18] Counseling on high-dose folic acid supplements (3 months before conception and through the first trimester) and the prevalence of false-positive urine pregnancy tests, if bowel has been used in the urinary tract, must be provided.[19,20] Women with any urologic reconstruction benefit from having a urologist comfortable with such reconstruction present at their delivery. Pre-emptive discussion in early adulthood provides important information and shared care between urology and high-risk obstetrics is important throughout pregnancy.

Assessment of Chronic Conditions

Chronic diseases of adulthood add to the problem list for patients as they age. Obesity and metabolic syndrome become more prevalent in adults.[21] This may contribute to inactivity and is, in some cases, exacerbated by progressive skeletal deformities, loss of access to mobility devices or orthotics, diminished social participation, and increased morbidity such as osteoporosis, and skin break-down. Obesity contributes to an increased risk of morbidity following surgery and may impact a pa-tient's surgical candidacy. This is in addition to the potential for respiratory and cardiovascular impair-ment that may be present and need to be evalu-ated preoperatively.

This highlights the important role that primary care providers (PCPs) have in the care of adult patients as pediatric providers, especially sub-specialists, are unlikely to have the skills neces-sary to care for adult conditions such as diabetes and heart failure. This is reflected in Na-tional SB registry studies and in single-institution experiences that demonstrate that surgical clinic utilization is highest in childhood, with or-thopedic surgery and neurosurgery clinic utiliza-tion decreasing with age. Adults with SB have a higher utilization of primary care compared with children.[22,23]

Recent data suggest that young adults with SB are less likely to graduate from high school or to be employed.[24] These recent data maintain more historical trends in the United States where roughly half of graduates have a regular job, although cohorts in the United Kingdom have higher education and employment rates.[25,26] In a 2006 survey study, Young and colleagues found that although 39% of adolescents considered themselves in good health, just 5% of adults re-ported the same. More than half of adults with SB identify themselves as permanently disabled. For some, there is a lifelong dependence on care-givers.[27] Although poor mobility and impaired ex-ecutive function may add to challenges in social participation, the most important predictors of disability or unemployment status are low educa-tion and poor bowel continence.[24,27,28] Patients with SB are more likely than those without to have public insurance, and to be admitted from the emergency department, and to have higher mean monetary charges per encounter.[29]

THE IMPACT OF POOR TRANSITION TO ADULT CARE

Although some patients with SB may do well outside of health care, others may experience significant complications related to their condition. Preventable conditions are those that with self-care and routine surveillance should rarely result in hospitalization or urgent procedures. A list of such preventable conditions is provided in **Box 1**. Self-care tasks include self-catheterization, enema

---

Box 1
Potentially preventable conditions in spina bifida

Urologic
  UTIs/pyelonephritis
  Urinary tract calculus
  Renal calculi
  Renal dysfunction, end-stage renal disease
  Complications related to reconstruction (eg, bladder perforation, stomal complication, ureteric stenosis, and malabsorption)
  Sexual dysfunction
  Infertility

Colorectal
  Constipation
  Fecal incontinence

Orthopedic
  Loss of mobility
  Osteomyelitis
  Osteoporosis
  Complications relating to poorly fitting de-vice/prosthesis musculoskeletal pain

Neurosurgical
  VP shunt malfunction
  Seizure control
  Other complications associated with Chiari malformation

Integumentary
  Pressure ulcers and other skin wounds
  Graft complications

Endocrine
  Obesity and its sequelae

Respiratory
  Respiratory failure (eg, related to contractures)

Psychiatric
  Mental health concerns

Other
  Surgical complications

delivery, skin checks, and medication use. These tasks should help preserve skin integrity and ambulatory status, which tend to decline with age.[23] Reasons for failure of self-care are multifactorial, and include limited resources, health literacy, self-management, or problem-solving skills and personal motivation. Lower self-management is associated with higher rates of hospitalization.[30]

Urologic Complications

Good urologic self-care should reduce episodes of pyelonephritis and complications related to urolithiasis. The consequences of nonadherence to regimens can be severe. For example, noncompliance with CIC may result in poor bladder emptying and/or unsafe bladder pressures leading to renal failure; for a patient who has been previously augmented, bladder perforation is a dangerous risk. Other urologic complications include metabolic changes after bladder augmentation and formation of bladder stones. An estimated one-third of patients with a continent catheterizable channel mechanism will require surgical revision of the stoma.[31] Patients may also experience problems related to slow colonic transit and abnormal sphincter function. This can lead to ventriculoperitoneal shunt (VP) shunt malfunction and diminished quality of life.[32]

Increased Hospital Admissions

Patients with SB have higher health care utilization compared with patients without chronic conditions. Numerous studies have consistently demonstrated that adults with SB have a higher ED utilization compared with children, up to double the rate.[33,34] Up to 47% of hospital admissions among adults with SB were for preventable conditions. These included pressure ulcers, osteomyelitis, nephrolithiasis, and "serious urologic infections." This may result from inadequate access to primary and/or preventative care. Matta and colleagues[35] found that within the Canadian universal health care system, there was no change in the rate of PCP visits between adolescence and adulthood but there remained a modest increase in the relative risk of having an ED visit.

Dicianno and Wilson[36] also reported that preventable conditions caused one-third of hospital admissions for adults with SB. This may represent an improvement from the 47% reported by Kinsman and Doehring,[37] although their definition of a preventable condition was broader and any difference is likely also impacted by global improvements in care. A survey distributed using social media, by Lai and colleagues,[38] found that missing medical visits and having more emergency room visits for a urologic problem were independently associated with having a history of more prior urologic surgeries. This suggests that patients with prior surgeries are at risk from both potential complications and noncompliance with their own treatment regime.

COMPONENTS OF TRANSITION

Several suggestions have been offered for the intentional design of transition programs. These include flexible timing to initiate the transition process, with a long preparation period leading up to the transition. An emphasis has been placed on packaging a patient's medical/surgical histories and creating an overlap between the pediatric and preselected adult providers.

Core Elements

The 2018 Clinical Report on Health Care Transition from the AAP, AAFP, and ACP defined 6 core elements of transition: transition policy, transition tracking and monitoring, transition readiness, transition planning, transfer and/or integration into adult-centered care, and transition completion and ongoing care with adult clinician.[39] These are not exclusive to SB but are intended to represent benchmarks necessary for successful transition of patients with any chronic disease of childhood. Three separate implementation guides are available for download to suit varying practices and target patient populations (https://www.gottransition.org/six-core-elements/).

Many programs have integrated the Transition Readiness Assessment Questionnaire (TRAQ), which is a validated patient-reported questionnaire with domains of self-management and self-advocacy. Questions include medication management, keeping appointments, tracking health issues, communication with providers, and managing daily activities.[40] The TRAQ-SB supplement has a specific focus on patients with SB, with additional questions on skin damage, bowel and urinary management, VP shunt complication awareness, and equipment ordering and repair.[41]

Implementation

These together reflect a consensus for the critical components of a successful transition process. Even so, there remains no gold standard on best practice for implementation. In a 2018 survey of 34 responding SB programs via the Spina Bifida Association, most programs reported consistent patient education regarding the transition process, although patient readiness assessment was less frequently utilized.[42] Although most programs discussed education, mobility, weight, bladder, and bowel management, most did not discuss sexuality or reproductive health—issues that are clearly important to patients and within the urologist's scope of practice. There was self-reported lack of communication between adult and pediatric providers. Just 20% of clinics had an adult provider present at a transition-specific visit. Internal review of the process was also rare, perhaps reflecting inattention to the patient and overall clinic outcomes.

An in-depth review of transition programs described in the literature is outside the scope of this article and is available elsewhere.[43,44] In brief, heterogeneity in program design, reported primary outcomes, and implicit challenges in capturing long-term outcomes make interpretation of available data difficult. Even so, we expect transition programs to yield benefit with regards to independence, offering patient support, and decreasing health care utilization.[22,45,46] However, even within well-established referral systems linking pediatric and adult clinics dedicated to SB, many patients delay establishing care with an adult provider. The rate of successful transfers in some instances is less than half.[47,48]

Interestingly, a study of adult patients seen at 2 dedicated SB clinics found that one-third of patients underwent surgical intervention after their initial presentation to the clinic.[47] Roughly 10% underwent a major urologic reconstruction. This was a well-followed patient population, with a median interval of 14 months between last visit with a pediatric urologist and established care with the adult clinic. They noted that the relatively high rate of reconstruction at the time of transfer could be related to differences in opinions between pediatric and adult-centered providers around reconstructive counseling. It could also be due to changes in patient preferences at a different stage in life.

BARRIERS TO TRANSITION

Alongside the importance of transition, recognition of the barriers to affecting transition of patients with SB began in the early 2000s. Several early reviews including those by Binks and colleagues[49] and Viner[50] described several considerations specific to all stakeholders in a young adult's transition process. Pediatric providers were described as harboring a distrust of adult providers and having a preference to maintain long-standing relationships with families. Concern was raised that patients and families may feel abandoned. Adult providers had a real and/or perceived lack of training and potentially, interest in patients with chronic pediatric illness. Balancing the care of

chronic illness and unrelated acute concerns is challenging. There may also be a lack of available resources for adult providers and clinics that are easier to obtain in a pediatric setting, ranging from dedicated care coordinators to equipment such as Hoyer lifts, and the struggle to run a dedicated multidisciplinary clinic in an adult facility.

Personnel

Most adult practices and insurance providers require patients to establish care separately with each subspecialty. This may be under the guidance of a PCP who may or may not have specific knowledge of these patients. Nutritionists and occupational therapists who may have been routine during pediatric care may decline to see these patients, in the absence of an acute concern. The disjointed nature of adult-oriented care results in patients being responsible for repeatedly recounting their medical history rather than having it curated by their multidisciplinary team. The need to initiate care outside the familiar pediatric multidisciplinary group is made more difficult by aging out of pediatric institutions, living outside their childhood home, potential educational or employment status, and changing insurance coverage.

The care of SB-specific concerns in adults is reliant on providers with a special interest in this population, for which there is a demonstrable paucity. A survey of urologists who were members of societies with an interest in SB reported varied practice patterns concerning timing and types of studies included in routine follow-up.[51] Guidelines have been offered for each subspecialty involved in SB care, including urologic guidelines.[52] The authors self-described these guidelines as "best practice" consensus statements in the absence of Level I evidence. Even so, we hope that these will help standardize care in the future. However, their implementation is reliant on savvy providers. There remains no clear guideline for the global care of adults with SB for the general practitioner, who is more likely to encounter these patients.

Success is also influenced by cognitive status and other social determinants of health including health literacy.[9] Health literacy has been shown to correlate with patient-reported readiness via TRAQ scores, including after adjusting for demographic and clinical factors, and to correlate with compliance with CIC regimens.[53,54] There is also increasing insight into the importance of fostering self-management skills and how these, together with compliance and problem-solving skills, interplay with family structure, parenting style, and other social structures.[55–58]

INSURANCE

Insurance status has been cited as a primary driver of transition failure.[59,60] This makes sense because a lack of continuous coverage alters expenses related to visits and dictates whether a patient can be seen at a given provider's office. The Affordable Care Act's Dependent Care Provision (DCP) introduced in 2010 offered an opportunity for eligible patients to achieve continuous coverage particularly around the time of transition. However, Loftus and colleagues[61] found that the DCP was not associated with improved insurance status of those young adults with SB requiring hospital admission and that, after implementation, there was a significant increase in the proportion of admissions for potentially preventable conditions.

Those with private insurance are more likely to have positive health outcomes related to SB[62] but are more likely to have an ED visit for a urologic condition.[38] However, having private insurance does not seem to significantly improve other metrics used to evaluate transition. Groskaufmanis and colleagues[63] reported that only 30% of privately insured patients with cerebral palsy or SB had an annual wellness visit, and rates of physical therapy, occupational therapy (PT/OT) visits were no higher than 20%. This is in comparison with 26% to 58% of young adults aged 18 to 25 years who had an annual visit in the general population.[64] Additionally, some patients and their families prefer public insurance even in childhood. Semistructured interviews of patients and parents/caregivers found that those participants on Medicaid were generally happy with their coverage, whereas those with private insurance had more varied experiences.[65]

Patient Preferences

Patient preferences also play a major role in deferred transition. Hettel and colleagues[66] surveyed adult patients with SB who had not been seen in more than 18 months at 2 tertiary centers, with established adult multidisciplinary clinics. Half of all barriers were patient related, with patient preference being the most prevalent. These included being tired of seeing doctors, feeling fine, and feeling that they must see too many doctors. One-quarter of respondents identified no specific barriers but still did no transition in a timely manner. Acuity of any condition likely affects preference to seek care and where to present.[47,51] Geographic distance from care may affect the ability and willingness to participate in long days of coordinated visits versus more frequent but shorter visits.[46]

These preferences may be driven by financial toxicity associated with SB. It is known that financial toxicity leads to delayed treatment and decreased treatment adherence, and other negative outcomes.[67] Aksenov and colleagues[65] performed semistructured interviews of patients and parents or caregivers, with an average patient age of 18 years. In addition to insurance-related costs as mentioned earlier, they provide lived examples of the substantial costs. These not only include direct costs, for example, travel expenses and care supplies such as catheters, but also include indirect costs, including missed time at work, loss of career opportunity, and mental challenges related to these financial stressors. Roughly, three-fourths of patients reported significant cognitive and time burden related to appointment and resource navigation, and roughly three-fourths of patients reported negative effect on affect and mood. Notably, these surveys included pediatric patients and could feasibly be even worse for independent adult patients.

A VISION FOR THE FUTURE

The last 2 decades have seen a tremendous amount of support for providers, patients, and families in their transition. The benefit of a multidisciplinary team is well established, in both the pediatric space and the transitional space. There seems to be a consensus that the transition process must be highly individualized and should be introduced well in advance, before a transfer. The importance of patient education and helping bridge the jump between pediatric-centered and adult-centered care is relatively well established. Despite significant advances in the field, the continued low success in transition rates—as defined by presentation to an adult specialist—together with the barriers described earlier suggest continued innovation is required. New initiatives may require deepening existing connections and enhancing collaboration outside of subspecialists.

There is an opportunity for continued collaboration between pediatric and adult providers. This should continue to involve trusted referral patterns and attentive patient handoffs—with a clear plan of care. This collaboration could be broadened to include collaborative long-term plans for given patients. Pediatric providers should seek continual education on the long-term outcomes of their patients and interventions, whereas adult providers might benefit from insight into the lived experiences of their patients. Both types of providers should work to ensure that patients are aware of their health conditions (and prior treatments) and understand how signs and symptoms of complications might manifest, at different points in their life.

We might also consider starting conversations around transition sooner than early adolescence. Although these may be difficult to have with parents overwhelmed with a new diagnosis and new skills, parents must be armed with the tools necessary to ensure successful transfer of skills, self-responsibility, and engagement of children as children grow with their condition. They may require coaching in how to discuss their child's condition. They must continue to be offered tools to adequately support patients—financially, socially, and emotionally. For those with diminished motivation or other psychosocial barriers to self-management, the study from Bradstreet and colleagues[10] offers several examples of an individualized approach, encouraging patients to engage with self-management tasks.

Among all subspecialists, urologists have the most forward role in the care of an individual with SB across their lifetime. Although medical homes have been demonstrated to be an effective means of care delivery for complex patients, it is not a model accessible to all.[22,68] Therefore, despite a clear need for patients, we must also realize that even with maximal education and excellent intentions, we are not primarily responsible for patient adherence to routine care. We must partner with other specialists, PCPs, and urgent care and emergency room physicians who may encounter our patients at a higher rate than ourselves. Tools must be developed to assist urologists without special training care for these patients, as well as nonurologists who might encounter these patients for other reasons.

It is important to embrace the individual needs of patients. Although the TRAQ-SB is well utilized in some programs, such as by Hopson and colleagues,[69] it may not provide sufficient granularity for health care providers to understand the needs of individuals for targeted intervention. Other metrics such as the Rotterdam Transition Profile have been proposed for use in young adults with cerebral palsy who have normal intelligence.[70] This offers several more domains, including finances, housing, intimate relationships, services aids, leisure, and social activities. It is also worth considering that self-assessment questionnaires may not correlate well with a readiness assessment performed by parents, nurses, or case workers. Indeed, adolescents with cerebral palsy consistently scored their global functioning higher when compared to their parents.[71] Holmbeck and colleagues[72] proposed a model in which nurses identified vulnerability factors during comprehensive assessments, rather than utilizing patient self-assessment, to allow for an individualized approach.

Our success in designing transition care programs will remain difficult to measure without determining metrics for success. Even when measured simply as establishment of care with an adult-centered provider, it is apparent that patient education and intersubspecialist communication is an insufficient approach. The ultimate goals of transition should further include timely access to care, improved patient outcomes by limiting preventable complications, while maximizing the patient's quality of life and independence. We must lean into a patient-directed approach grounded in active patient involvement. **Fig. 1** describes an expected transition trajectory summarizing the above, and the critical components for each stage's success. This will require continued resources, interest, and innovation, as well as partnership with our patients, general practitioners, and other

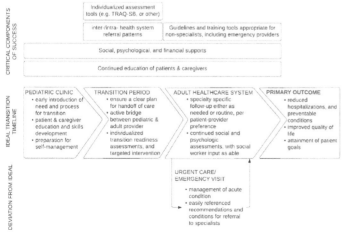

Fig. 1. A summary of the transition process, factors for success and deviations from the ideal pathway.

subspecialists, with a shared goal of maximizing patient outcomes.

CLINICS CARE POINTS

- These patients need lifelong urological and multidisciplinary care
- Ensuring preparation for transition will help to keep patients engaged with the healthcare they need
- When making treatment decision it is important to discuss and set realistic expectations
- It is important to discuss all aspects of a patients life with them including urinary function, fecal continence and sexual health/function

DISCLOSURE

None.

REFERENCES

1. Canfield MA, Mai CT, Wang Y, et al. The Association Between Race/Ethnicity and Major Birth Defects in the United States, 1999–2007. Am J Public Health 2014;104(9):e14–23.
2. Fremion EJ, Dosa NP. Spina bifida transition to adult healthcare guidelines. J Pediatr Rehabil Med 2019; 12(4):423–9.
3. American Academy of Pediatrics, American Academy of Family Physicians, American College of Physicians-American Society of Internal Medicine. A consensus statement on health care transitions for young adults with special health care needs. Pediatrics 2002;110(6 Pt 2):1304–6.
4. Woodhouse CR. The fate of the abnormal bladder in adolescence. J Urol 2001;166(6):2396–400.
5. Koch VH, Lopes MT, Furusawa E, et al. Multidisciplinary management of people with spina bifida across the lifespan. Pediatr Nephrol 2023;39(3): 681–97.
6. Wiener JS, Suson KD, Castillo J, et al. Bladder Management and Continence Outcomes in Adults with Spina Bifida: Results from the National Spina Bifida Patient Registry, 2009 to 2015. J Urol 2018;200(1): 187–94.
7. Szymanski KM, Cain MP, Whittam B, et al. All Incontinence is Not Created Equal: Impact of Urinary and Fecal Incontinence on Quality of Life in Adults with Spina Bifida. J Urol 2017;197(3 Part 2):885–91.
8. Lemelle JL, Guillemin F, Aubert D, et al. A Multicenter Evaluation of Urinary Incontinence Management and Outcome in Spina Bifida. J Urol 2006;175(1):208–12.
9. Lindquist B, Jacobsson H, Strinnholm M, et al. A scoping review of cognition in spina bifida and its consequences for activity and participation throughout life. Acta Paediatr 2022;111(9):1682–94.
10. Bradstreet LE, Ludwig N, Koterba C, et al. Supporting the Transition to Adulthood for Youth With Spina Bifida: A Call for Neuropsychology-Informed Interventions. Top Spinal Cord Inj Rehabil 2022;28(3):59–62.
11. Wasserman RM, Holmbeck GN. Profiles of Neuropsychological Functioning in Children and Adolescents with Spina Bifida: Associations with Biopsychosocial Predictors and Functional Outcomes. J Int Neuropsychol Soc 2016;22(8):804–15.
12. Bong GW, Rovner ES. Sexual health in adult men with spina bifida. Sci World J. 2007;7:1466-1469.
13. Choi EK, Ji Y, Han SW. Sexual Function and Quality of Life in Young Men With Spina Bifida: Could It Be Neglected Aspects in Clinical Practice? Urology 2017;108:225–32.
14. Palmer JS, Kaplan WE, Firlit CF. Erectile dysfunction in patients with spina bifida is a treatable condition. J Urol 2000;164(3 Pt 2):958–61.
15. Streur CS, Corona L, Smith JE, et al. Sexual Function of Men and Women With Spina Bifida: A Scoping Literature Review. Sex Med Rev 2021; 9(2):244–66.
16. Akre C, Light A, Sherman L, et al. What young with people with SB want to know about sex, and aren't being told. Child Care Health Dev 2015;41(6):963–9.
17. Alexander SC, Fortenberry JD, Pollak KI, et al. Sexuality talk during adolescent health maintenance visits. JAMA Pediatr 2014;168(2):163–9.
18. Auger N, Arbour L, Schnitzer ME, et al. Pregnancy outcomes of women with spina bifida. Disabil Rehabil 2019;41(12):1403–9.
19. Venna A, Valovska MT, Estrada CR, et al. False-positive urine pregnancy screening tests are uncommon in the hospital setting among patients with bowel-containing urinary tract reconstruction. J Pediatr Urol 2023;19(3):312.e1–4.
20. Visconti D, Noia G, Triarico S, et al. Sexuality, preconception counseling and urological management of pregnancy for young women with spina bifida. Eur J Obstet Gynecol Reprod Biol 2012;163(2):129–33.
21. McPherson AC, Chen L, O'Neil J, et al. Nutrition, metabolic syndrome, and obesity: Guidelines for the care of people with spina bifida. J Pediatr Rehabil Med 2020;13(4):637–53.
22. Shepard CL, Doerge EJ, Eickmeyer AB, et al. Ambulatory Care Use among Patients with Spina Bifida: Change in Care from Childhood to Adulthood. J Urol 2018;199(4):1050–5.
23. Alabi NB, Thibadeau J, Wiener JS, et al. Surgeries and Health Outcomes Among Patients With Spina Bifida. Pediatrics 2018;142(3).

24. Liu T, Ouyang L, Walker WO, et al. Education and employment as young adults living with spina bifida transition to adulthood in the USA: A study of the National Spina Bifida Patient Registry. Dev Med Child Neurol 2023;65(6):821–30.

25. Woodhouse CRJ, Neild GH, Yu RN, et al. Adult Care of Children From Pediatric Urology. J Urol 2012;187(4):1164–71.

26. Barf HA, Post MWM, Verhoef M, et al. Is cognitive functioning associated with subjective quality of life in young adults with spina bifida and hydrocephalus? J Rehabil Med 2010;42(1):56–9.

27. Hopson B, Rocque BG, Joseph DB, et al. The development of a lifetime care model in comprehensive spina bifida care. J Pediatr Rehabil Med 2018;11(4):323–34.

28. Davis MC, Hopson BD, Blount JP, et al. Predictors of permanent disability among adults with spinal dysraphism. J Neurosurg Spine 2017;27(2):169–77.

29. Wang HHS, Wiener JS, Ross SS, et al. Emergent care patterns in patients with spina bifida: a case-control study. J Urol 2015;193(1):268–73.

30. Mahmood D, Dicianno B, Bellin M. Self-management, preventable conditions and assessment of care among young adults with myelomeningocele. Child Care Health Dev 2011;37(6):861–5.

31. Stein R, Fisch M, Ermert A, et al. Urinary diversion and orthotopic bladder substitution in children and young adults with neurogenic bladder: a safe option for treatment? J Urol 2000;163(2):568–73.

32. Beierwaltes P, Church P, Gordon T, et al. Bowel function and care: Guidelines for the care of people with spina bifida. J Pediatr Rehabil Med 2020;13(4):491–8.

33. Mann JR, Royer JA, Turk MA, et al. Inpatient and emergency room visits for adolescents and young adults with spina bifida living in South Carolina. Pharm Manag PM R 2015;7(5):499–511.

34. Domino JS, Lundy P, Glynn EF, et al. Estimating the prevalence of neurosurgical interventions in adults with spina bifida using the Health Facts data set: implications for transition planning and the development of adult clinics. J Neurosurg Pediatr 2022;29(4):371–8.

35. Matta R, Wallis CJD, Etches J, et al. Healthcare utilization during transition to adult care in patients with spina bifida: A population-based longitudinal study in Ontario, Canada. Canadian Urological Association Journal 2023;17(6).

36. Dicianno BE, Wilson R. Hospitalizations of Adults With Spina Bifida and Congenital Spinal Cord Anomalies. Arch Phys Med Rehabil 2010;91(4):529–35.

37. Kinsman SL, Doehring MC. The cost of preventable conditions in adults with spina bifida. Eur J Pediatr Surg 1996;6(Suppl 1):17–20.

38. Lai LY, Lopez AD, Copp HL, et al. Access and Utilization of Health Care by Adults with Spina Bifida. Urology 2023;181:174–81.

39. White PH, Cooley WC; Transitions Clinical Report Authoring Group; American Academy of Pediatrics; American Academy of Family Physicians; American College of Physicians. Supporting the Health Care Transition From Adolescence to Adulthood in the Medical Home. Pediatrics. 2018;142(5):e20182587. Pediatrics 2019;143(2):e20183610.

40. Wood DL, Sawicki GS, Miller MD, et al. The Transition Readiness Assessment Questionnaire (TRAQ): its factor structure, reliability, and validity. Acad Pediatr 2014;14(4):415–22.

41. Wood D, Rocque B, Hopson B, et al. Transition Readiness Assessment Questionnaire Spina Bifida (TRAQ-SB) specific module and its association with clinical outcomes among youth and young adults with spina bifida. J Pediatr Rehabil Med 2019;12(4):405–13.

42. Kelly MS, Thibadeau J, Struwe S, et al. Evaluation of spina bifida transitional care practices in the United States. J Pediatr Rehabil Med 2017;10(3–4):275–81.

43. Choi EK, Bae E, Jang M. Transition programs for adolescents and young adults with spina bifida: A mixed-methods systematic review. J Adv Nurs 2021;77(2):608–21.

44. Campbell F, Biggs K, Aldiss SK, et al. Transition of care for adolescents from paediatric services to adult health services. Cochrane Database Syst Rev 2016;2016(4).

45. Manohar S, Staggers KA, Huang X, et al. The impact of a health care transition clinic on spina bifida condition management and transition planning. Disabil Health J 2023;16(4):101508.

46. Lindsay S, Fellin M, Cruickshank H, et al. Youth and parents' experiences of a new inter-agency transition model for spina bifida compared to youth who did not take part in the model. Disabil Health J 2016;9(4):705–12.

47. Summers SJ, Elliott S, McAdams S, et al. Urologic problems in spina bifida patients transitioning to adult care. Urology 2014;84(2):440–4.

48. McManus MA, Pollack LR, Cooley WC, et al. Current status of transition preparation among youth with special needs in the United States. Pediatrics 2013;131(6):1090–7.

49. Binks JA, Barden WS, Burke TA, et al. What do we really know about the transition to adult-centered health care? A focus on cerebral palsy and spina bifida. Arch Phys Med Rehabil 2007;88(8):1064–73.

50. Viner R. Barriers and good practice in transition from paediatric to adult care. J R Soc Med 2001;94(Suppl 40):2–4.

51. Agrawal S, Slocombe K, Wilson T, et al. Urologic provider experiences in transitioning spina bifida patients from pediatric to adult care. World J Urol 2019;37(4):607–11.

52. Joseph DB, Baum MA, Tanaka ST, et al. Urologic guidelines for the care and management of people

with spina bifida. J Pediatr Rehabil Med 2020;13(4): 479–89.

53. Rague JT, Kim S, Hirsch JA, et al. Assessment of Health Literacy and Self-reported Readiness for Transition to Adult Care among Adolescents and Young Adults with Spina Bifida. JAMA Netw Open 2021;4(9).

54. Cooper J, Chisolm D, McLeod DJ. Sociodemographic Characteristics, Health Literacy, and Care Compliance in Families With Spina Bifida. Glob Pediatr Health 2017;4. 2333794X17745765.

55. Psihogios AM, Kolbuck V, Holmbeck GN. Condition self-management in pediatric spina bifida: A longitudinal investigation of medical adherence, responsibility-sharing, and independence skills. J Pediatr Psychol 2015;40(8):790–803.

56. Psihogios AM, Murray C, Zebracki K, et al. Testing the Utility of a Bio-Neuropsychosocial Model for Predicting Medical Adherence and Responsibility during Early Adolescence in Youth with Spina Bifida. J Pediatr Psychol 2017;42(9):910–21.

57. Logan LR, Sawin KJ, Bellin MH, et al. Self-management and independence guidelines for the care of people with spina bifida. J Pediatr Rehabil Med 2020;13(4):583–600.

58. Holbein CE, Lennon JM, Kolbuck VD, et al. Observed differences in social behaviors exhibited in peer interactions between youth with spina bifida and their peers: neuropsychological correlates. J Pediatr Psychol 2015;40(3):320–35.

59. Sawyer SM, Macnee S. Transition to adult health care for adolescents with spina bifida: research issues. Dev Disabil Res Rev 2010;16(1):60–5.

60. Gray WN, Schaefer MR, Resmini-Rawlinson A, et al. Barriers to Transition From Pediatric to Adult Care: A Systematic Review. J Pediatr Psychol 2018;43(5): 488–502.

61. Loftus CJ, Ahn J, Hagedorn JC, et al. The impact of the dependent care provision on individuals with spina bifida transitioning to adulthood. J Pediatr Urol 2021;17(3):289.e1–9.

62. Schechter MS, Liu T, Soe M, et al. Sociodemographic attributes and spina bifida outcomes. Pediatrics 2015;135(4):e957–64.

63. Groskaufmanis L, Lin P, Kamdar N, et al. Racial and Ethnic Inequities in Use of Preventive Services Among Privately Insured Adults With a Pediatric-Onset Disability. Ann Fam Med 2022;20(5):430–7.

64. Adams SH, Park MJ, Irwin CE. Adolescent and Young Adult Preventive Care: Comparing National Survey Rates. Am J Prev Med 2015;49(2):238–47.

65. Aksenov LI, Fairchild RJ, Hobbs KT, et al. Financial toxicity among individuals with spina bifida and their families: A qualitative study and conceptual model. J Pediatr Urol 2022;18(3):290.e1–8.

66. Hettel D, Tran C, Szymanski K, et al. Lost in transition: Patient-identified barriers to adult urological spina bifida care. J Pediatr Urol 2018;14(6):535. e1–4.

67. de Souza JA, Conti RM. Mitigating Financial Toxicity Among US Patients With Cancer. JAMA Oncol 2017; 3(6):765–6.

68. Murphy NA, Carbone PS. Council on Children With Disabilities, American Academy of Pediatrics. Parent-provider-community partnerships: optimizing outcomes for children with disabilities. Pediatrics 2011;128(4):795–802.

69. Hopson B, Alford EN, Zimmerman K, et al. Development of an evidence-based individualized transition plan for spina bifida. Neurosurg Focus 2019;47(4): 4–9.

70. Donkervoort M, Wiegerink DJHG, van Meeteren J, et al, Transition Research Group South West Netherlands. Transition to adulthood: validation of the Rotterdam Transition Profile for young adults with cerebral palsy and normal intelligence. Dev Med Child Neurol 2009;51(1):53–62.

71. Büğüşan S, Kahraman A, Elbasan B, et al. Do adolescents with cerebral palsy agree with their caregivers on their participation and quality of life? Disabil Health J 2018;11(2):287–92.

72. Holmbeck GN, Kritikos TK, Stern A, et al. The Transition to Adult Health Care in Youth With Spina Bifida: Theory, Measurement, and Interventions. J Nurs Scholarsh 2021;53(2):198–207.

Sleep and Overactive Bladder in Parkinson's Disease

Yu Zheng, MD[a],*, Anne P. Cameron, MD[a]

KEYWORDS

- Nocturia • Parkinson's disease • Overactive bladder • LUTS • Sleep disturbances

KEY POINTS

- Nocturia and overactive bladder (OAB) are prevalent in patients with Parkinson's disease (PD) due to the bladder physiology changes and sleep disturbances associated with PD.
- The complex interplay of poor sleep quality, nocturia, and OAB lead to increased fall risk in patients with PD and severely impact not only their quality of life (QoL) but also QoL of their bed partners.
- Nocturia in patients with PD is multifactorial and often related to sleep disturbances from PD.
- Management of these patients requires a careful assessment of their PD status, available support structure, and tailoring of therapy that is feasible and effective.
- A multidisciplinary approach including neurologist, urologist, and sleep specialist should be considered to maximize treatment strategies for nocturia and OAB.

INTRODUCTION

Parkinson's disease (PD) is a progressive neurodegenerative disorder characterized by the loss of dopaminergic neurons in the substantia nigra leading to classic motor symptoms such as resting tremors, bradykinesia, rigidity, and postural instability. While significant progress has been made in addressing these motor dysfunctions, nonmotor symptoms are increasingly recognized as critical to the quality of life (QoL) in patients with PD[1] (Fig. 1). These include olfactory dysfunction, neuropsychiatric symptoms (depression, anxiety, and so forth), autonomic dysfunction (orthostatic hypotension [OH], constipation, and erectile dysfunction), sleep disorders, and lower urinary tract symptoms (LUTS).[2]

Studies show that LUTS are prevalent in 27% to 61% of patients with PD, and these symptoms are more prevalent in patients with PD when compared to an age-matched healthy cohort.[3] These symptoms, which worsen as PD progresses, include storage symptoms (urinary urgency, frequency, and nocturia) and/or voiding symptoms (urinary hesitancy, weak stream, and urinary retention). Notably, nocturia defined as the need to wake up at night more than once to void appears to be one of the most prevalent urinary symptoms with an overall prevalence of 59% in patients with PD.[2,4,5]

Nocturia has an obvious impact on total sleep time, quality of sleep, and sleep efficiency.[6] Unfortunately, patients with PD experience a broad spectrum of sleep disorders such as insomnia, rapid eye movement (REM) sleep behavior disorder, and circadian rhythm disturbances, which may occur in 60% to 90% of these patients.[7,8] Although it has been well established that the prevalence of nocturia and sleep disorders is high in the PD population, it is poorly understood whether the nocturia drives sleep disorders or whether the sleep disorders allow opportunistic nocturia. We therefore aim to describe the intersectionality of sleep disorders and OAB/nocturia in patients with PD to maximize treatment strategies for OAB/nocturia in this particular population.

[a] Department of Urology, University of Michigan, 1500 E Medical Center Drive, Ann Arbor, MI 48109, USA
* Corresponding author.
E-mail address: codapqat@med.umich.edu

Urol Clin N Am 51 (2024) 197–207
https://doi.org/10.1016/j.ucl.2024.02.005
0094-0143/24/© 2024 Elsevier Inc. All rights reserved.

urologic.theclinics.com

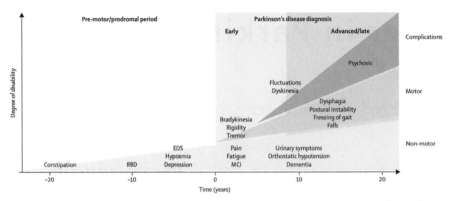

Fig. 1. Clinical symptoms and time course of PD progression. (*Reprinted* with permission from Elsevier. The Lancet, 2015 Aug 29;386(9996):896-912.)

PATHOPHYSIOLOGY OF OAB IN PD

Coordination of micturition requires an intricate interplay of the central and peripheral nervous system pathways with the bladder and urethra. Several of these pathways are disrupted in patients with PD. Normal voiding function involves the integration of sensory information, such as bladder fullness, which travels from the afferent fibers of the hypogastric, pelvic, and pudendal nerves up the spinal cord to the periaqueductal gray (PAG) in the midbrain. The PAG receives additional input like time, social situation, and emotions from the cortical regions such as the anterior cingulate gyrus and prefrontal cortex. Integration of bladder volume status with social context in the PAG will either promote urinary storage through inhibition of the pontine micturition complex or initiate the micturition reflex resulting in detrusor contraction with coordinated urethral sphincter relaxation. The micturition reflex is also affected by the nigrostriatal dopaminergic pathways. Stimulation of D1 receptors in the nigrostriatal dopaminergic pathway within the basal ganglia inhibits the micturition reflex while stimulation of D2 receptors does the opposite, but the overall dopinergic effect within the basal ganglia is to exert a tonic inhibitory effect on the micturition reflex.[1,9]

In PD, the degeneration of dopaminergic cells leads to the loss of dopamine-mediated inhibition on the micturition reflex. This often clinically manifests as OAB (urinary frequency, urgency, and urgency incontinence) and detrusor overactivity, which has been demonstrated in 67% of patients with PD on urodynamic testing.[10,11] Furthermore, patients with PD have been found to develop severe frontal cortex deficits over time.[1] Frontal cortex lesions in the anterior cingulate cortex and frontal gyri have been shown to produce detrusor overactivity.[12] Functional MRI studies have demonstrated

significant frontal cortex activity during bladder distension and micturition in healthy volunteers suggesting its significance in the regulation of micturition.[13] Therefore, lesions in these areas may disrupt sensory integration and alter bladder perception, leading to frequent, smaller volume voids and reduced bladder capacity. Furthermore, the frontal cortex has a bidirectional relationship with sleep. Lesions in the frontal cortex can impair REM sleep and disrupt sleep–wake cycles, potentially leading to conditions like narcolepsy and excessive daytime sleepiness, which in turn adversely affect frontal executive functions, including the processing of bladder sensory information and the planning of micturition.[14]

PD also affects the external urethral sphincter muscles, causing "sphincteric bradykinesia," which is the delayed or reduced ability to contract the sphincter in response to an urge to void.[15] This phenomenon coupled with detrusor overactivity often seen in PD compromises the individual's capacity to delay urination and prevent involuntary urine leakage. Conversely, some patients with PD may not relax their urethral sphincter rapidly or sufficiently when voiding, which can be perceived as urinary hesitancy or incomplete emptying.[15] This is a distinct and separate phenomenon to detrusor external sphincter dyssynergia, which is commonly found in spinal cord injury patients but rarely found in patients with PD.

PATHOPHYSIOLOGY OF NOCTURIA IN PD

The bladder physiology changes of detrusor overactivity, decreased functional bladder capacity, and bladder hypersensitivity offer an explanation for the increased prevalence of nocturia in patients with PD, but the exact cause of nocturia in patients with PD is likely multifactorial. Other contributors to nocturia include nocturnal polyuria, cardiovascular dysautonomia, disruption of the circadian rhythm, and sleep disorders. Nocturnal polyuria, defined by the International Continence Society (ICS) as greater than 33% of the entire daily (24 hours) voided volume occurring at night for the elderly, contributes to nocturia due to excessive production of urine and is highly prevalent in patients with PD.[5]

In patients with PD, the diminishment of postganglionic efferent sympathetic neurons in baroreceptors and the myocardium leads to an impairment in norepinephrine release and defective vasoconstriction during the transition from lying flat to standing upright, resulting in a neurogenic form of OH as well as supine hypertension.[16] OH, a sequelae of autonomic dysregulation, is present in 30% to 50% of patients with PD, and prevalence increases with disease duration and age.[17] Its association with nocturia lies in the body's compensatory mechanisms. When blood pressure drops due to OH, the body attempts to restore homeostasis through the release of antidiuretic hormone (ADH) and activating the renin-angiotensin-aldosterone system leading to sodium and water retention during the day. Once the individual lies down, increased renal blood flow due to the volume expansion leads to osmotic diuresis and consequently increased urine production.

Disruption of the circadian rhythm in PD also leads to excessive urine production. The circadian rhythm operates as the body's internal clock and dictates when individuals feel awake or sleepy based on external light cues. It is regulated by melatonin and arginine vasopressin (AVP) levels in response to day/night cycles. Under physiologic circumstances at night, melatonin levels rise to promote sleep while AVP levels rise to promote water reabsorption in the kidneys and thus reducing urine volume. In PD, neurodegenerative changes disturb the circadian rhythm, evident from prevalent sleep disorders and reduced melatonin levels in patients with PD.[18] This disturbance likely diminishes the nocturnal AVP surge, contributing to increased nighttime urine production and nocturia.

SLEEP DISTURBANCES AND NOCTURIA

Nocturia significantly impacts sleep quality in patients with PD, who often suffer from sleep disorders. A meta-analysis of polysomnographic findings of patients with PD compared to an age-matched cohort revealed that patients with PD consistently experience reduced total sleep time, sleep efficiency, sleep latency (time it takes to fall asleep), and total REM sleep compared.[19] Additionally, patients with PD with more than 2 episodes of nocturia are shown to worse sleep

metrics than those with fewer episodes.[6] Insomnia is a prevalent issue in PD, affecting 27% to 80% of patients, manifesting as difficulties in either falling or staying asleep.[20] Additionally, patients with PD frequently experience REM sleep behavior disorder (RBD), where the usual muscle relaxation during REM sleep is absent, leading to patients physically acting out their dreams, which can range from simple limb twitches to more violent movements, potentially harming themselves or bed partners.[21] This disorder, present in 33% to 46% of patients with PD, can precede PD's motor symptoms.[22,23] Restless legs syndrome (RLS), affecting about 15% of patients with PD, causes uncomfortable leg sensations, particularly in the evening, disrupting sleep onset. RLS prevalence tends to increase with PD progression and treatment duration.[22] Other notable sleep disturbances include parasomnias, excessive daytime sleepiness and obstructive sleep apnea, which is not thought to be associated with PD.[20] Nocturia is generally assumed to be bothersome because the urge to urinate is the primary reason for patients to wake up. However, given nocturia and sleep disorders often coexist in patients with PD, that assumption is not always correct. Patients who are awake due to sleep disturbances may not necessarily urinate because of an urge, but "convenience void" since they are already awake. This distinction suggests that improving sleep disorders could be more effective than focusing solely on nocturia management. For patients with PD, nocturia could stem from 2 distinct causes: fluid overload due to orthostatic hypotension and sleep disturbances; however, currently, no studies have definitively determined whether nocturia is due to nocturnal polyuria or sleep disturbances, though such distinctions could be explored in future research with voiding diaries.

WHY IT MATTERS?

The complex interplay of OAB, nocturia, and sleep disturbances in patients with PD drastically impairs sleep resulting in a reduction on QoL.[20,24] A Finnish population-based study found that nocturnal voiding twice or more per night correlates with poorer health-related QoL.[25] Additionally, nocturia and sleep impairment in patients with PD have been correlated with anxiety and depression.[26,27] The frequent need for nighttime bathroom visits also raises fall risks, which is particularly concerning due to PD-related motor instability. Compared to healthy counterparts, patients with PD have a higher fall incidence (54% vs 18%) and those experiencing nocturia have an increased risk of hip fractures, independent of age.[28,29] These sleep disruptions not only affect patients with PD but also extend to their bed partners, causing secondary sleep disorders.[30] Although underresearched, these secondary effects add to the emotional, physical, and financial burdens faced by caregivers of patients with PD.

WORKUP OF OAB AND NOCTURIA IN PD
History and Physical Examination

Often, PD is first diagnosed by a neurologist or internist, but some patients with undiagnosed PD may present to Urology clinic for assessment of their LUTS as the earliest sign of PD. A careful inventory of LUTS should be performed which can be categorized as storage symptoms or voiding symptoms. Patients with nocturia should be assessed as to whether they are woken up due to urinary urgency or are "convenience voiding." Other potential causes of LUTS should be assessed such as benign prostatic hyperplasia (BPH), obstructive sleep apnea (OSA), diabetes, and strokes. Functional impairment from the motor symptoms of PD, such as tremors, bradykinesia, or postural instability, and social situation and support should be carefully assessed. Patients with PD with severe mobility issues can have functional incontinence because it takes significantly longer to reach the toilet and undress. PD caregivers report a significant care burden so integrating their needs is critical to formulating a management plan that is acceptable and achievable to both parties.[30] Caregivers also provide valuable information about the patient's fluid intake and sleep patterns that may be unrecognized by patients. A detailed review of both PD-specific and other medications is essential, as these can affect bladder function. Evening fluid intake and consumption of caffeine or alcohol should be monitored as these can exacerbate symptoms.

A physical examination can aid in identifying the causes and severity of LUTS. Blood pressure measurements can reveal orthostatic hypotension. Skin excoriation of the urogenital area provides insight on severity of incontinence as well as degree of social support. During a digital rectal examination, not only can the prostate size be assessed but also a crude assessment of sphincteric bradykinesia can be performed by asking the patient to contract their anal sphincter with delays in anal sphincteric contraction being suggestive of bradykinesia. Overall mobility, hand dexterity, and cognition should be accessed as functional status often dictates symptom management strategies.

Diagnostic Tools

Voiding diaries allow objective quantification of OAB symptoms, fluid intake quantity and quality, and can be useful in initiating targeted behavioral modifications. They are crucial in the diagnosis of nocturia and nocturnal polyuria. A 3-day voiding diary has been found to provide reliable information without overburdening patients with excessive data collection.[31] Questionnaires such as the American Urological Association Symptom Index (AUA-SI) and Overactive Bladder Symptom Score have been used to objectively measure LUTS in patients with PD and can track symptom changes with each intervention. Urine analysis should be performed when evaluating OAB symptoms to rule out urinary tract infections. Low postvoid residuals (PVRs) can rule out overflow incontinence while elevated PVR can suggest detrusor underactivity or bladder outlet obstruction. Routine urodynamics are not necessary in patients with PD as there is minimal risk of upper tract deterioration.[32] Urodynamics can be helpful in evaluating concomitant BPH and OAB symptoms in male patients with PD or distinguishing stress urinary incontinence and OAB symptoms in female patients given full bladder cough stress test on pelvic examinations may be difficult to perform due to mobility issues. Urodynamic findings can be used to counsel patients with PD who seek more invasive therapy for OAB. A retrospective study of 390 patients with PD found detrusor overactivity with impaired contractility on urodynamics in 42% of patients, which may increase the risk of urinary retention in these patients who undergo bladder botulinum toxin (BTX) injections for OAB.[33]

MANAGEMENT OF OAB, NOCTURIA, AND CONSEQUENTLY SLEEP DISTURBANCES IN PD

The management of OAB and nocturia in patients with PD is challenging given these symptoms often do not exist in isolation, and there is a significant heterogeneity in PD severity and symptom presentation among patients. Therefore, addressing nocturia and OAB in patients with PD demands a diverse approach. Conservative measures such as behavioral modifications should always be considered first before progressing to medical or procedural interventions. Therapies targeted at maximizing sleep and PD-targeted therapies should also be considered. Collaboration with neurologists, physiotherapists, and sleep specialists is often necessary to optimize other aspects of PD such as sleep disturbances and motor symptoms, which have a cascading effect on LUTS. Such a comprehensive, team-based approach is paramount in navigating the complexities of LUTS in PD and optimizing patient outcomes (**Fig. 2**).

Behavioral Management

Behavioral modifications play a pivotal role in managing nocturia and OAB in patients with PD. These include minimizing fluid intake, especially 4 hours before sleeping, limiting caffeine and alcohol, and encouraging plain water for hydration. In a prospective study, a 25% reduction in baseline fluid intake improved urinary frequency, urgency, and nocturia.[34] Implementing timed voiding schedules every 3 to 4 hours during the day and voiding immediately before bed can minimize urinary urgency and nocturia. Patients with PD may benefit from structured pelvic floor physical therapy (PFPT) as well. Two pilot studies demonstrated improvement in urgency incontinence, nocturia, and overall QoL in patients who underwent pelvic floor exercises with electromyography (EMG) biofeedback for at least 8 weeks.[35] PFPT has almost no adverse events but can be burdensome for caretakers who must accompany patients with PD to the sessions. For patients with dependent edema, compression stockings, and elevating legs in the afternoon can facilitate fluid redistribution and reduce nocturnal diuresis. Most diuretics take effect in 6 to 8 hours, so their intake in the late afternoon or evening should be avoided to prevent excessive nighttime urination.[24] External collection catheters (condom catheter, Purewick, Becton-Dickinson (BD)- Franklin Lakes, NJ) and bedside commodes can provide as alternatives for those who struggle to reach the bathroom in time and are a much safer alternative than a foley catheter.[36] Installing night-lights in pathways to the bathroom and removing floor

obstacles such as rugs can reduce the risk of falls. Behavioral changes, such as minimizing daytime recumbency, sleeping with the head elevated at a 10° to 20° angle, and taking alpha-1 adrenoceptor agonists like midodrine, can effectively improve orthostatic hypotension, yet none of these interventions have been evaluated for their effectiveness in improving nocturia or OAB symptoms in patients with PD.[37] A study of 29 healthy volunteers noted a 146 mL decrease in nighttime voided volumes after 6 days of head up tilt sleeping.[38] Collectively, these behavioral and environmental modifications form an integrative strategy to manage nocturia and OAB while promoting both safety and sleep quality for patients with PD. Additionally, patients and their caregivers can greatly benefit from counseling on incontinence products and perineal skin care with barrier creams to help manage any incontinence.

Sleep-targeted Management

Improving the sleep quality in patients with PD can improve OAB and nocturia. General good sleep hygiene such as minimizing daytime naps (especially >20 minute naps), maintaining a consistent sleep schedule, reducing noise and light disturbances in the bedroom, and compliance with continuous positive airway pressure devices in those with OSA should be encouraged. With guidance from sleep specialists and neurologists, optimization of dopaminergic medication and sleep aids such as melatonin and antidepressants can improve sleep quality. Dopamine agonists have been shown to improve sleep parameters in multiple studies and appear especially effective for patients with PD with RLS.[23,39–41] Weaning off dopaminergic medication at night is theorized to

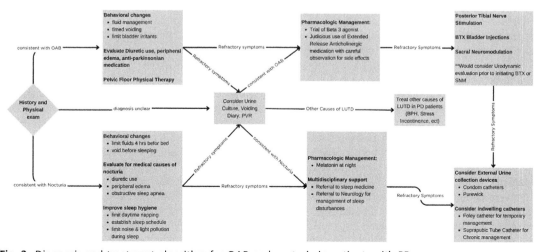

Fig. 2. Diagnosis and treatment algorithm for OAB and nocturia in patients with PD.

exacerbate insomnia as patients begin to notice the return of resting tremors and inability to get into comfortable positions in bed due to rigidity.[42] A study comparing extended-release levodopa versus placebo of 40 patients with PD demonstrated improvement in nocturnal akinesia and a trend toward increased total sleep time.[43] Extended-release levodopa at bedtime has also been reported to improve nocturia.[44] Varying doses of melatonin (1–12 mg) have been shown to be effective in improving nocturia with minimal side effects. A phase 2 study using 2 mg of sustained release melatonin in adults with PD demonstrated improvement in nighttime frequency of void from 3 to 1.67 after a 6 week period without any adverse events.[45] Other hypnotic medications such as trazodone, zolpidem, and clonazepam are effective at treating insomnia, RBD, and RLS, but the side-effect profile of these agents (dizziness, drowsiness, and cognitive impairments) suggests judicious use of these agents in patients with PD.[23] Given that melatonin is an over-the-counter supplement, the urologic provider can easily recommend this therapy.

Parkinson's Disease-targeted Therapy

Antiparkinsonian medication
The main classes of drugs used to treat the motor symptoms of PD include levodopa, dopamine agonist, and monamine oxidase type B (MAO-B) inhibitors. Treating the motor symptoms of PD has not been shown to improve OAB or nocturia, but these medications can impact LUTS. Therefore, it is important to be cognizant of the effects especially in patients who have recently started these medications. Urodynamics performed on 26 levodopa-naïve patients with PD 1 hour after the administration of levodopa demonstrated worsening detrusor overactivity and decrease bladder capacity (22% decrease).[46] However, after 2 months of levodopa therapy, repeat urodynamics on these patients demonstrated a delay in bladder sensation during filling, improvement in detrusor overactivity (93% improvement), and bladder capacity (33% improvement).[46] No randomized controlled trial (RCT) has evaluated the effects of dopamine agonist on LUTS, but one study suggested improvement in nocturia when patients with PD were switched from bromocriptine to pergolide and bladder capacity has been shown to increase in patients taking apomorphine.[47,48] Rasagiline, a second-generation MAO-B inhibitor, demonstrated an increase in bladder capacity by 16%, first desire to void by 34%, and decreased PVR by 53% when compared to placebo in patients with mild PD.[49] The effects of levodopa, dopamine

agonist, and MAO-B inhibitors on LUTS are mixed and undefined due to dopamine's varied affinity for the D1 and D2 receptors as well as downregulation of dopamine receptors over time.

Deep Brain Stimulation
Deep brain stimulation (DBS) of the substantia nigra has been shown to significantly improve motor symptoms in patients with PD, but its efficacy in treating LUTS is mixed.[50] A study comparing DBS to oral PD medications or apomorphine pump showed DBS patients experienced less nocturia, but their overall LUTS were the same.[51] A study involving urodynamics performed on 16 patients with PD before and after their DBS was turned on demonstrated a delay in the initial desire to void (199 vs 135 mL) and increase in bladder capacity (302 vs 174 mL) with the DBS turned on.[52] A study compared DBS of the globus pallidus pars interna versus subthalamic nucleus (STN) showed urinary incontinence and frequency trended toward improvement in either DBS location but was only statistically significant in the STN group.[53] However, nocturia did not improve for either group.[53] A recent study on 416 patients with PD concluded similar results of improved urinary urgency, frequency, and incontinence without any changes in nocturia.[54]

Bladder-targeted Therapy

Anticholinergic medication
Anticholinergic medications have been the basis of treatment of OAB and neurogenic detrusor overactivity. However, their side-effect profile (dry eyes, dry mouth, constipation, and cognitive dysfunction) can compound PD symptoms, which limits their use and adherence to the medication. The cognitive dysfunction of anticholinergic OAB medication is of particular concern given it adds to the anticholinergic burden for patients with PD who are taking anticholinergic medication for antiparkinsonian therapy. Additionally, patients with PD are inherently at risk for early cognitive decline and dementia.

Few anticholinergic medications have been studied specifically in patients with PD. Oxybutynin was evaluated in 7 patients with PD who were noted to have decreased frequency, nocturia, and incontinence with unchanged PVR after 12 weeks of therapy.[55] Tolterodine has been shown to increase bladder capacity, decrease number of voids, and urgency episodes without increasing PVR.[56,57] However, 20% of patients with PD discontinued the medication due to constipation, dizziness/headache, and lack of improvement in symptoms. An RCT comparing solifenacin (5–10 mg) to placebo in 23 patients with PD showed no significant improvement in mean number of voids per 24 hour period, but there was a significant decrease in urinary incontinence episodes from 1.3 to 0.5 episodes and nocturia (2.6–1.6 episodes over a 24 hour period) during the open label phase.[58] Side effects included constipation, xerostomia, and urinary retention, which resolved with the withdrawal of solifenacin. A recent RCT of fesoterodine (4 mg) versus placebo in 63 patients with PD demonstrated marginal decrease in voiding episodes in 24 hours (8.6 vs 7 episodes), nocturia (2.7 vs 2.3), and urgency incontinence episodes (1.8 vs 1.6).[59] Fesoterodine appears well tolerated as adverse events included xerostomia and constipation in 1 patient. There were no changes in baseline cognitive function or PVR after starting fesoterodine.[59] Although there is limited evidence to support the use of one anticholinergic over another in patients with PD, anticholinergics that do not cross the blood–brain barrier are generally recommended to minimize the potential cognitive side effects in patients at risk for cognitive impairment.[60] Given the marginal improvement of OAB/nocturia with anticholinergics in patients with PD and considering the substantial potential of these medications to worsen confusion and sleep–wake cycles in this group, we recommend the use of anticholinergics only if no other oral medication options are available and advise to use extended-release forms starting at the lowest possible dose.

Beta-3 agonist medication

Mirabegron and Vibegron are beta-3 agonists that have proven to be effective in managing idiopathic OAB. They offer an advantage over anticholinergic medications given their minimal side-effect profile, but their use can be limited by cost and lack of data on efficacy in PD. No RCT has been conducted on the efficacy and safety of beta-3 agonists in patients with PD. A retrospective study of 50 patients with PD started on 50 mg of mirabegron noted that 60% of the patients reported improvement or resolution of their OAB symptoms.[61] There was a statistically significant reduction of nocturia episodes. Only 2 adverse events were reported, which were dizziness and diaphoresis, which resolved after the medication was discontinued. However, compliance with mirabegron was reportedly low as only 46% of patients continued the medication after a median follow-up of 19 months. A prospective study of mirabegron 50 mg started in 30 patients with PD with OAB symptoms that have been refractory to anticholinergics demonstrated 80% of the patients reported improved incontinence

QoL scores without any adverse events.[62] Overall, beta-3 agonists offer a much better safety profile compared to anticholinergic medication for OAB/nocturia in patients with PD while the efficacy is likely comparable.

Vasopressin

Desmopressin is a synthetic analog of ADH and has been proven to be effective for nocturnal polyuria. However, extreme caution should be taken with its use in patients with PD due to severe risk of hyponatremia, confusion, and orthostatic hypotension. A study using intranasal desmopressin for nocturia in 8 patients with PD showed a significant decrease in nocturia in 5 out of the 8 patients.[63] Adverse events include 1 patient who stopped the medication due to severe hyponatremia and confusion, which resolved after the withdrawal of desmopressin.

Botulinum toxin

For patients with PD who either are unable to tolerate the side effects or are poorly compliant with pharmacotherapy for OAB/nocturia, BTX injections into the bladder can be considered. Literatures supporting the use BTX injections into the bladder are based on 2 formulations of BTX, which are onabotulinumtoxinA (Botox) and abobotulinumtoxinA (Dysport).[24] The most recent and largest study of BTX injections in patients with PD included 24 patients (17 men and 7 women) who underwent 100 U of Botox for urinary incontinence.[64] Twenty-nine percent of patients reported complete resolution of the urgency urinary incontinence, while 79% of the patients reported improvement in their OAB symptoms 1 month after their first injection. Adverse events included 25% of patients who had a urinary tract infection and 12.5% of the patients did have to start clean intermittent catheterization for incomplete bladder emptying. Smaller studies using 100 U of Botox or 500 U of Dysport for OAB in patients with PD concluded similar improvement in bladder capacity, urinary frequency, and urgency incontinence, but also noted the risk of increase in PVR.[65,66] Interestingly, a prospective study of 10 patients with PD (4 female and 6 male) who underwent 200 U of Botox for OAB symptoms refractory to pharmacotherapy shared similar improvements with OAB symptoms without a statistically significant increase in PVR after a follow-up of 4 months.[67] No conclusive evidence exists regarding BTX efficacy in improving nocturia in patients with PD, due to underpowered studies and a lack of specific focus on nocturia as an outcome. However, studies in other populations with OAB suggest that BTX does not significantly reduce nocturia. Therefore, we would advise against BTX for pure nocturia. When considering BTX bladder injections for patients with PD, it is crucial to assess baseline bladder contractility, PVR, and the potential for bladder outlet obstruction, particularly in males, due to the risk of urinary retention and challenges with self-catheterization if needed from limited hand dexterity. Additionally, Botox and Dysport are not interchangeable, and currently, there are no studies that directly compare their dose or efficacy in patients with PD. We would recommend any patient with PD undergo urodynamics prior to BTX injection to assess for risk of urinary retention and confirmation of diagnosis.

Neuromodulation

Several small studies have evaluated posterior tibial nerve stimulation (PTNS) and sacral neuromodulation (SNM) for patients with PD. A study of 47 patients with PD who underwent 12 weeks of PTNS demonstrated encouraging results with a mean decrease of daytime frequency episodes by 5.6 times and nocturia episodes by 2.7 times.[68] Other studies have supported these findings as well in addition to improvement in bladder capacity without any reported adverse events.[69] PTNS may improve OAB/nocturia symptoms acutely with almost no side effects, but the durability of the treatment remains unknown. Additionally, PTNS can be burdensome to patients due to the frequent clinic visits for the treatment, and implantable PTNS have not been studied in patients with PD. Very few studies have directly evaluated the use of SNM in patients with PD. A retrospective review of 34 patients with PD at a single institution who were evaluated for SNM with either peripheral nerve evaluation (7 patients) or stage 1 evaluation (27 patients) found that 82% of the patients proceeded to a permanent implant.[70] Of note, the indication for SNM in the majority of these patients was for refractory OAB symptoms (88%) while 12% of the patients were evaluated for nonobstructive urinary retention. Furthermore, 68% of the patients were able to discontinue their OAB medications after lead implantation. We do not routinely perform urodynamics in patients with PD who chose PTNS, but given the invasiveness of SNM, urodynamics is often performed before proceeding to ensure diagnostic accuracy.

Indwelling catheters

While several pharmacologic and procedural interventions exist to improve OAB and nocturia in patients with PD, these options may lose their efficacy over time given that PD is a progressive disease. Patients with severe OAB and nocturia that have been refractory to conservative measures or medications and/or unable to tolerate Botox, or neuromodulation, can consider indwelling catheters for severe incontinence management. It should be considered particularly when skin breakdown or hygiene becomes an issue or if their family can no longer manage the burden of the incontinence. Urethral Foley catheters can be considered acutely, but due to the risk of urethral erosion, long-term management is best with a suprapubic tubes (SPTs). The procedure has inherent risks, which include bowel injury, vascular injury at the time of placement, but special considerations for patients with PD include the risk of inadvertent tube dislodgment given the cognitive impairment, motor symptoms, and dementia associated with PD. Many patients and caregivers report high satisfaction with an SPT as the tube's location away from the urethra offers more freedom of movement and comfort during daily activities and sleep.[71]

SUMMARY

OAB and nocturia are highly prevalent in patients with PD due to bladder physiology alterations and sleep cycle disturbances that occur as the neurologic degenerative disease progresses. These symptoms severely affect the QoL both patients with PD and their bed partners. Management of these patients requires a careful assessment of their PD status, available support structure, and tailoring of therapy that is feasible and effective. Often, multiple interventions are required for success. Lastly, optimal management of these symptoms involves a coordinated effort from a multispecialty approach involving urologist, neurologist, sleep specialist, and pelvic floor specialist.

CLINICS CARE POINTS

- The pathophysiology of OAB and Nocturia in patients with PD is multifaceted.

- Managing sleep disturbances and OAB in patients with Parkinson's disease improves nocturia, overall QoL of the patient and their bed partners, and minmizes risk of falls.

- Melatonin is a low risk sleep aid that urologist can safely prescribe patients with PD with bothersome nocturia and sleep disturbances; however complex management of sleep disturbances in patients with PD should involve a sleep specialist.

DISCLOSURE

None.

REFERENCES

1. Kalia LV, Lang AE. Parkinson's disease. Lancet Lond Engl 2015;386(9996):896–912.
2. Martinez-Martin P, Schapira AHV, Stocchi F, et al. Prevalence of nonmotor symptoms in Parkinson's disease in an international setting; study using non-motor symptoms questionnaire in 545 patients. Mov Disord Off J Mov Disord Soc 2007;22(11):1623–9.
3. Campos-Sousa RN, Quagliato E, da Silva BB, et al. Urinary symptoms in Parkinson's disease: prevalence and associated factors. Arq Neuropsiquiatr 2003;61(2B):359–63.
4. Li FF, Cui YS, Yan R, et al. Prevalence of lower urinary tract symptoms, urinary incontinence and retention in Parkinson's disease: A systematic review and meta-analysis. Front Aging Neurosci 2022;14.
5. Hashim H, Blanker MH, Drake MJ, et al. International Continence Society (ICS) report on the terminology for nocturia and nocturnal lower urinary tract function. Neurourol Urodyn 2019;38(2):499–508.
6. Vaughan CP, Juncos JL, Trotti LM, et al. Nocturia and overnight polysomnography in Parkinson disease. Neurourol Urodyn 2013;32(8):1080–5.
7. Diaconu Ş, Irincu L, Ungureanu L, et al. Nocturia and Sleep in Parkinson's Disease. J Personalized Med 2023;13(7):1053.
8. Schütz L, Sixel-Döring F, Hermann W. Management of Sleep Disturbances in Parkinson's Disease. J Park Dis 2022;12(7):2029–58.
9. Brucker BM, Kalra S. Parkinson's Disease and Its Effect on the Lower Urinary Tract: Evaluation of Complications and Treatment Strategies. Urol Clin North Am 2017;44(3):415–28.
10. Uchiyama T, Sakakibara R, Yamamoto T, et al. Urinary dysfunction in early and untreated Parkinson's disease. J Neurol Neurosurg Psychiatry 2011;82(12):1382–6.
11. Araki I, Kitahara M, Oida T, et al. Voiding dysfunction and Parkinson's disease: urodynamic abnormalities and urinary symptoms. J Urol 2000;164(5):1640–3.
12. Yamamoto T, Sakakibara R, Nakazawa K, et al. Neuronal activities of forebrain structures with respect to bladder contraction in cats. Neurosci Lett 2010;473:42–7.
13. Herzog J, Weiss PH, Assmus A, et al. Subthalamic stimulation modulates cortical control of urinary bladder in Parkinson's disease. Brain J Neurol 2006;129(Pt 12):3366–75.
14. Hong J, Lozano DE, Beier KT, et al. Prefrontal cortical regulation of REM sleep. Nat Neurosci 2023;26(10):1820–32.
15. Xing T, Ma J, Ou T. Evaluation of neurogenic bladder outlet obstruction mimicking sphincter bradykinesia in male patients with Parkinson's disease. BMC Neurol 2021;21(1):125.
16. Park JW, Okamoto LE, Biaggioni I. Advances in the Pathophysiology and Management of Supine Hypertension in Patients with Neurogenic Orthostatic Hypotension. Curr Hypertens Rep 2022;24(3):45–54.
17. Palma JA, Kaufmann H. Orthostatic Hypotension in Parkinson Disease. Clin Geriatr Med 2020;36(1):53–67.
18. Breen DP, Vuono R, Nawarathna U, et al. Sleep and circadian rhythm regulation in early Parkinson disease. JAMA Neurol 2014;71(5):589–95.
19. Zhang Y, Ren R, Sanford LD, et al. Sleep in Parkinson's disease: A systematic review and meta-analysis of polysomnographic findings. Sleep Med Rev 2020;51:101281.
20. Loddo G, Calandra-Buonaura G, Sambati L, et al. The Treatment of Sleep Disorders in Parkinson's Disease: From Research to Clinical Practice. Front Neurol 2017;8:42.
21. Jozwiak N, Postuma RB, Montplaisir J, et al. REM Sleep Behavior Disorder and Cognitive Impairment in Parkinson's Disease. Sleep 2017;40(8):zsx101.
22. Gagnon JF, Bédard MA, Fantini ML, et al. REM sleep behavior disorder and REM sleep without atonia in Parkinson's disease. Neurology 2002;59(4):585–9.
23. Maggi G, Vitale C, Cerciello F, et al. Sleep and wakefulness disturbances in Parkinson's disease: A meta-analysis on prevalence and clinical aspects of REM sleep behavior disorder, excessive daytime sleepiness and insomnia. Sleep Med Rev 2023;68:101759.
24. Batla A, Phé V, De Min L, et al. Nocturia in Parkinson's Disease: Why Does It Occur and How to Manage? Mov Disord Clin Pract 2016;3(5):443–51.
25. Tikkinen KAO, Johnson TM, Tammela TLJ, et al. Nocturia frequency, bother, and quality of life: how often is too often? A population-based study in Finland. Eur Urol 2010;57(3):488–96.
26. Rana AQ, Paul DA, Qureshi AM, et al. Association between nocturia and anxiety in Parkinson's disease. Neurol Res 2015;37(7):563–7.
27. Breyer BN, Shindel AW, Erickson BA, et al. The association of depression, anxiety and nocturia: a systematic review. J Urol 2013;190(3):953–7.
28. Rudzińska M, Bukowczan S, Stożek J, et al. Causes and consequences of falls in Parkinson disease patients in a prospective study. Neurol Neurochir Pol 2013;47(5):423–30.
29. Temml C, Ponholzer A, Gutjahr G, et al. Nocturia is an age-independent risk factor for hip-fractures in men. Neurourol Urodyn 2009;28(8):949–52.
30. Macchi ZA, Koljack CE, Miyasaki JM, et al. Patient and caregiver characteristics associated with caregiver burden in Parkinson's disease: a palliative care approach. Ann Palliat Med 2020;9(Suppl 1):S24–33.
31. Cameron AP, Wiseman JB, Smith AR, et al. Are three-day voiding diaries feasible and reliable? Results from the Symptoms of Lower Urinary Tract Dysfunction Research Network (LURN) cohort. Neurourol Urodyn 2019;38(8):2185–93.

32. Ginsberg DA, Boone TB, Cameron AP, et al. The AUA/SUFU Guideline on Adult Neurogenic Lower Urinary Tract Dysfunction: Diagnosis and Evaluation. J Urol 2021;206(5):1097–105.

33. Kim M, Jung JH, Park J, et al. Impaired detrusor contractility is the pathognomonic urodynamic finding of multiple system atrophy compared to idiopathic Parkinson's disease. Parkinsonism Relat Disorders 2015;21(3):205–10.

34. Hashim H, Abrams P. How should patients with an overactive bladder manipulate their fluid intake? BJU Int 2008;102(1):62–6.

35. Vaughan CP, Burgio KL, Goode PS, et al. Behavioral therapy for urinary symptoms in Parkinson's disease: A randomized clinical trial. Neurourol Urodyn 2019; 38(6):1737–44.

36. Khosla L, Sani JM, Chughtai B. Patient and caretaker satisfaction with the PureWick system. Can J Urol 2022;29(4):11216–23.

37. Fanciulli A, Leys F, Falup-Pecurariu C, et al. Management of Orthostatic Hypotension in Parkinson's Disease. J Park Dis 2020;10(s1):S57–64.

38. Fan CW, O'Sullivan E, Healy M, et al. Physiological effects of sleeping with the head of the bed elevated 18 in. in young healthy volunteers. Ir J Med Sci 2008; 177(4):371–7.

39. Ray Chaudhuri K, Martinez-Martin P, Rolfe KA, et al. Improvements in nocturnal symptoms with ropinirole prolonged release in patients with advanced Parkinson's disease. Eur J Neurol 2012;19(1): 105–13.

40. Poewe WH, Rascol O, Quinn N, et al. Efficacy of pramipexole and transdermal rotigotine in advanced Parkinson's disease: a double-blind, double-dummy, randomised controlled trial. Lancet Neurol 2007; 6(6):513–20.

41. Calandra-Buonaura G, Guaraldi P, Doria A, et al. Rotigotine Objectively Improves Sleep in Parkinson's Disease: An Open-Label Pilot Study with Actigraphic Recording. Park Dis 2016;2016:3724148.

42. Chahine LM, Amara AW, Videnovic A. A systematic review of the literature on disorders of sleep and wakefulness in Parkinson's disease from 2005 to 2015. Sleep Med Rev 2017;35:33–50.

43. Wailke S, Herzog J, Witt K, et al. Effect of controlled-release levodopa on the microstructure of sleep in Parkinson's disease. Eur J Neurol 2011;18(4):590–6.

44. Brusa L, Ponzo V, Stefani A, et al. Extended release levodopa at bedtime as a treatment for nocturiain Parkinson's disease: An open label study. J Neurol Sci 2020;410:116625.

45. Batla A, Simeoni S, Uchiyama T, et al. Exploratory pilot study of exogenous sustained-release melatonin on nocturia in Parkinson's disease. Eur J Neurol 2021;28(6):1884–92.

46. Brusa L, Petta F, Pisani A, et al. Acute vs chronic effects of l-dopa on bladder function in patients with mild Parkinson disease. Neurology 2007;68(18): 1455–9.

47. Kuno S, Mizuta E, Yamasaki S, et al. Effects of pergolide on nocturia in Parkinson's disease: three female cases selected from over 400 patients. Parkinsonism Relat Disorders 2004;10(3):181–7.

48. Aranda B, Cramer P. Effects of apomorphine and L-dopa on the parkinsonian bladder. Neurourol Urodyn 1993;12(3):203–9.

49. Brusa L, Musco S, Bernardi G, et al. Rasagiline effect on bladder disturbances in early mild Parkinson's disease patients. Parkinsonism Relat Disorders 2014; 20(8):931–2.

50. Tabakin AL, Tunuguntla HSGR. Does deep brain stimulation improve Parkinson's disease-related lower urinary tract symptoms and voiding dysfunction? Bladder San Franc Calif 2021;8(2):e46.

51. Winge K, Nielsen KK. Bladder dysfunction in advanced Parkinson's disease. Neurourol Urodyn 2012;31(8):1279–83.

52. Seif C, Herzog J, van der Horst C, et al. Effect of subthalamic deep brain stimulation on the function of the urinary bladder. Ann Neurol 2004;55(1): 118–20.

53. Witte LP, Odekerken VJJ, Boel JA, et al. Does deep brain stimulation improve lower urinary tract symptoms in Parkinson's disease? Neurourol Urodyn 2018;37(1):354–9.

54. Zong H, Meng F, Zhang Y, et al. Clinical study of the effects of deep brain stimulation on urinary dysfunctions in patients with Parkinson's disease. Clin Interv Aging 2019;14:1159–66.

55. Bennett N, O'Leary M, Patel AS, et al. Can higher doses of oxybutynin improve efficacy in neurogenic bladder? J Urol 2004;171(2 Pt 1):749–51.

56. Watanabe M, Yamanishi T, Honda M, et al. Efficacy of extended-release tolterodine for the treatment of neurogenic detrusor overactivity and/or low-compliance bladder. Int J Urol Off J Jpn Urol Assoc 2010;17(11):931–6.

57. Palleschi G, Pastore AL, Stocchi F, et al. Correlation between the Overactive Bladder questionnaire (OAB-q) and urodynamic data of Parkinson disease patients affected by neurogenic detrusor overactivity during antimuscarinic treatment. Clin Neuropharmacol 2006;29(4):220–9.

58. Zesiewicz TA, Evatt M, Vaughan CP, et al. Randomized, controlled pilot trial of solifenacin succinate for overactive bladder in Parkinson's disease. Parkinsonism Relat Disorders 2015;21(5):514–20.

59. Yonguc T, Sefik E, Inci I, et al. Randomized, controlled trial of fesoterodine fumarate for overactive bladder in Parkinson's disease. World J Urol 2020;38(8):2013–9.

60. Nambiar AK, Arlandis S, Bø K, et al. European Association of Urology Guidelines on the Diagnosis and Management of Female Non-neurogenic Lower

Urinary Tract Symptoms. Part 1: Diagnostics, Overactive Bladder, Stress Urinary Incontinence, and Mixed Urinary Incontinence. Eur Urol 2022;82(1): 49–59.

61. Peyronnet B, Vurture G, Palma JA, et al. Mirabegron in patients with Parkinson disease and overactive bladder symptoms: A retrospective cohort. Parkinsonism Relat Disorders 2018;57:22–6.

62. Gubbiotti M, Conte A, Di Stasi SM, et al. Feasibility of mirabegron in the treatment of overactive bladder in patients affected by Parkinson's disease: A pilot study. Ther Adv Neurol Disord 2019;12. 1756286419843458.

63. Suchowersky O, Furtado S, Rohs G. Beneficial effect of intranasal desmopressin for nocturnal polyuria in Parkinson's disease. Mov Disord Off J Mov Disord Soc 1995;10(3):337–40.

64. Vurture G, Peyronnet B, Feigin A, et al. Outcomes of intradetrusor onabotulinum toxin A injection in patients with Parkinson's disease. Neurourol Urodyn 2018;37(8):2669–77.

65. Giannantoni A, Rossi A, Mearini E, et al. Botulinum toxin A for overactive bladder and detrusor muscle overactivity in patients with Parkinson's disease and multiple system atrophy. J Urol 2009;182(4): 1453–7.

66. Kulaksizoglu H, Parman Y. Use of botulinim toxin-A for the treatment of overactive bladder symptoms in patients with Parkinsons's disease. Parkinsonism Relat Disorders 2010;16(8):531–4.

67. Knüpfer SC, Schneider SA, Averhoff MM, et al. Preserved micturition after intradetrusor onabotulinumtoxinA injection for treatment of neurogenic bladder dysfunction in Parkinson's disease. BMC Urol 2016;16(1):55.

68. Kabay S, Canbaz Kabay S, Cetiner M, et al. The Clinical and Urodynamic Results of Percutaneous Posterior Tibial Nerve Stimulation on Neurogenic Detrusor Overactivity in Patients With Parkinson's Disease. Urology 2016;87:76–81.

69. Kabay SC, Kabay S, Yucel M, et al. Acute urodynamic effects of percutaneous posterior tibial nerve stimulation on neurogenic detrusor overactivity in patients with Parkinson's disease. Neurourol Urodyn 2009;28(1):62–7.

70. Martin S, Zillioux J, Goldman HB. Is sacral neuromodulation effective in patients with Parkinson's disease? A retrospective review. Neurourol Urodyn 2022;41(4):955–61.

71. Sheriff MK, Foley S, McFarlane J, et al. Long-term suprapubic catheterisation: clinical outcome and satisfaction survey. Spinal Cord 1998;36(3):171–6.

Bladder Compliance
How We Define It and Why It Is Important

Glenn T. Werneburg, MD, PhD[a],*, John T. Stoffel, MD[b]

KEYWORDS

- Compliance • Urodynamics • Neurogenic lower urinary tract dysfunction • Neurogenic bladder
- Voiding dysfunction • Detrusor pressure • Hydronephrosis

KEY POINTS

- Bladder compliance is the relationship between the change in bladder volume and the change in detrusor pressure.
- Several figures for the cutoff between normal and low compliance have been suggested but the guidance from several societies recommends a cutoff of 20 mL/cm H_2O, below which compliance is considered low.
- Low bladder compliance is associated with vesicoureteral reflux, upper urinary tract deterioration, and reduced renal function.
- Medical (anticholinergics and beta-3 agonists) and surgical (bladder augmentation) therapies have been shown to improve compliance and associated upper tract risk.
- Compliance is likely only one factor involved in upper tract deterioration, and we put forth a model wherein the proportion of time, during the micturition cycle at which detrusor pressure is greater than the ureteral pressure, is likely an excellent indicator of upper tract risk.

INTRODUCTION

Compliance is the ability of an organ to distend with increasing transmural pressure. The term has been used to describe lung, vessel, heart, and urinary bladder physiology. It is a measure of the elastic resistance of a system, or the system's ability to resist recoil to its initial dimensions. Compliance is the change in volume per the change in pressure of a system, $\Delta V/\Delta P$. In the urinary bladder, compliance is the change in detrusor pressure per unit volume. It can be thought of as resting detrusor tone causing intraluminal storage pressure changes in the bladder. Compliance of the bladder can be determined from a pressure–volume curve using cystometry (**Fig. 1**). The normal urinary bladder is highly compliant (see **Fig. 1**A), and low bladder compliance (see **Fig. 1**B and C) has been deemed an important risk factor in the prediction of renal function deterioration.

In this review, we discuss the definitions of compliance because it relates to the urinary tract. Further, we review the literature regarding the relationship between compliance and urologic pathophysiology. We discuss the relationship between urologic therapeutic modalities and compliance, with compliance being either an indication for treatment or outcome measure. We then discuss controversies and gaps in understanding, and opportunities for further research.

Funding: No external funding was associated with this study.
Clinical trial registration: This study is not a clinical trial and thus does not warrant registration as such.
Ethics of approval and patient consent: n/a.
[a] Department of Urology, Glickman Urological and Kidney Institute, Cleveland Clinic Foundation, 9500 Euclid Avenue, Cleveland, OH 44195, USA; [b] Department of Urology, Neurourology and Pelvic Reconstruction Division, University of Michigan, 3875 Taubman Center, 1500 East Medical Center Drive, Ann Arbor, MI 48109, USA
* Corresponding author.
E-mail address: wernebg@ccf.org

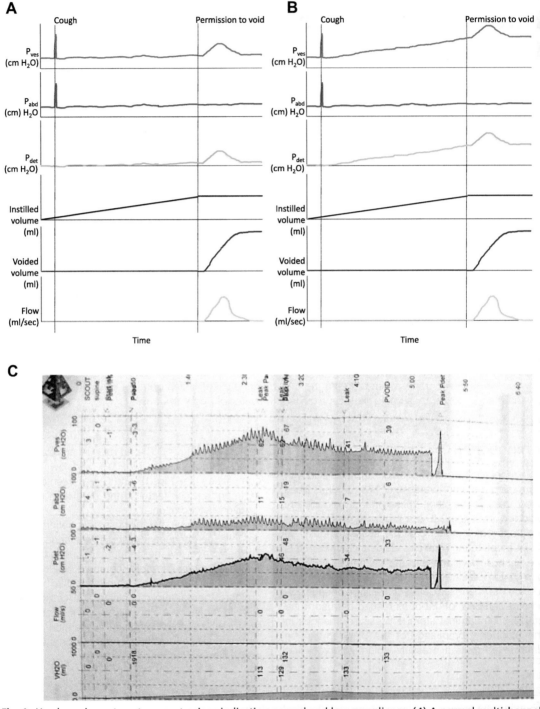

Fig. 1. Urodynamics cystometrogram tracings indicating normal and low compliance. (*A*) A normal multichannel cystometrogram. The P_{det} does not increase appreciably with increasing filling volume. (*B*) A multichannel cystometrogram schematic indicating low compliance. Here, the P_{det} increases markedly during the filling phase of voiding. (*C*) A multichannel cystometrogram tracing from an individual with low bladder compliance. Similar to the schematic in panel B, the P_{det} increases significantly with increased filling volume. P_{det} is the difference between P_{ves} and P_{abd}. Thus, when the subject coughs (*hashed line*), both the P_{ves} and P_{abd} increase but the P_{det} remains near zero. cm H_2O, centimeters water; mL, milliliters; P_{abd}, abdominal pressure; P_{det}, detrusor pressure; P_{ves}, vesical pressure.

HOW IS COMPLIANCE DEFINED?
Compliance Measurement and Terminology

According to the 2002 report from the International Continence Society, bladder compliance is "the relationship between change in bladder volume and change in detrusor pressure."[1] According to the report, compliance should be calculated by dividing the volume change (ΔV) by the detrusor pressure change (ΔP_{det}), during that change in volume. It states that is should be expressed in units of milliliters per centimeter H_2O. The report provides 2 recommended points from which compliance may be calculated: (1) the detrusor pressure at the initiation of bladder filling and the associated bladder volume (which is usually zero) and (2) the detrusor pressure and associated bladder volume at the maximum cystometric capacity, or just before the start of a detrusor contraction causing leakage (because this would disrupt the volume measurement, and therefore the calculation of compliance). The report states that both points should be measured excluding any detrusor contraction, and that the investigator may wish to define additional points from which to perform the calculation. In 2010, the International Urogynecological Association together with the International Continence Society published a joint report on terminology of pelvic floor dysfunction in the female population,[2] and in 2019, the International Continence Society provided a terminology report in the male population.[3] The reports reaffirmed the definition of compliance, which did not significantly change from the 2002 report, and also provided a series of factors that may affect compliance measurement: bladder filling, contractile and relaxant bladder detrusor properties (that be be affected by radiation, for example), and start and endpoints for compliance calculation. Variables and their considerations in compliance measurement are discussed in later discussion and indicated in **Table 1**.

Filling Medium and Filling Rate

The filling medium may affect the measurement of compliance.[4] Although early studies, such as those by McGuire and colleagues, had used gas cystometry, it is generally no longer used due to its compressibility, nonphysiologic state, and lack of utility in voiding studies. Liquid cystometry allows for accurate leak and leak point pressure determination, and therefore, accurate point determination from which compliance may be calculated. Specifically, liquid cystometry allows for adherence to the International Continence Society report's recommendation to perform the final compliance measurement before any detrusor

Variable	Recommendation
Points on urodynamics tracing	At the initiation and completion of filling, before leak
Physiologic diuresis	Catheterization at the initiation and conclusion of study will allow for accurate determination of the initial and final volumes for compliance calculation
Final volume	Assess compliance over the physiologic filling volume (based on voiding diaries and/or catheterization logs)
Medium	Liquid; generally water, saline, or contrast
Temperature	Physiologic temperature ideal but rarely practical. Room temperature (20°C–22°C/ 68°F –72°F) acceptable
Filling rate	Physiologic rate ideal but rarely practical. 20 mL/min if low compliance is suspected, 50 mL/min otherwise; adjust accordingly

Table 1
Variables for consideration and associated recommendation for the accurate measurement of compliance

contraction causing leakage.[1] Liquid medium choice is also important. For example, acidity may enhance detrusor overactivity, whereas alkalinity may reduce it.[5,6] Filling low compliance bladders with an alkaline solution has been shown to increase capacity by about 28%.[6] It has been suggested that the ideal medium is similar to urine at physiologic temperature[4] but differences between room and physiologic temperature filling media may not be clinically relevant in most patients.[7] In practice, room temperature (20°C–22°C/68°F–72°F) filling medium is often used.

In theory, filling should be performed by physiologic diuresis, but this is not practical in most centers. In practice in the adult population, filling rates generally range from 10 mL/min to 100 mL/min, the most common being 30 to 50 mL/min. It has been suggested that, in patients in whom low compliance is suspected, a filling rate of 20 mL/min should be used, otherwise a filling rate of 50 mL/min is acceptable.[4] Then, if low bladder compliance is seen, filling should be stopped and restarted at a lower fill rate (20 mL/min if the initial rate was 50 mL/min, or 10 mL/min if the initial rate was 20 mL/min) after 1 minute of observation for a fall in detrusor pressure. The International Continence Society also states that a faster rate may be more provocative, and that artifacts produced may settle when the filling is stopped.[2,3] Per the Good Urodynamic Practices guidance from the International Continence Society, a good urodynamics study should be performed interactively with the patient, which implies a dynamic reassessment of filling rate with a goal of reproducing the physiologic phenomena and symptoms of a given patient.[8]

Measurement Points and Calculation

To measure compliance, both the detrusor pressure and the bladder volume require accurate measurement. To measure the detrusor pressure (P_{det}), a catheter with a pressure sensor is placed in the bladder, and an additional sensor is placed in the rectum or vagina (or stoma, if present). Thus, the pressure in the bladder (vesical pressure, P_{ves}) is subtracted from the abdominal pressure (P_{abd}), to obtain the P_{det}. The P_{det} is thus measured at 2 points during filling—generally the beginning and the end (in the absence of a detrusor contraction, and before any associated leakage). For volume measurement, the cystometry is started in the empty state, at which the initial volume will typically be zero. The final volume will be similar to the total volume infused by the end of the filling phase, or maximum cystometric capacity. However, the volume of diuresis during the study is often not considered, and thus volume and compliance may be underestimated. Postvoid residual volume as determined by catheterization at the conclusion of the study would allow for the accurate determination of the true change in volume for compliance measurement. This may also be performed at study initiation to ensure an empty bladder at the study's initiation. Dray and Cameron note the importance of the assessment of compliance over the entirety of the volume range generally experienced by the bladder.[9] This range can be determined by either voiding diaries or a catheterization log (if patient performs intermittent catheterization). If a patient regularly harbors bladder volumes of 800 cc, compliance should be assessed over this range. Assessment of other measures of compliance, such as the area under the P_{det} curve (as indicated by the shading in **Fig. 1**C), is being evaluated.[10] Although such measures may hold value given its ability to consider the P_{det} over the entire filling phase, rather than only the start and end point, its association with upper tract deterioration and other outcomes requires further study.

Compliance is generally reported in the units of milliliters per centimeter H_2O, as recommended by the International Continence Society.[1] The compliance "cost," or the P_{det} required to hold 100 cm H_2O, has also been described. The compliance cost assesses the pressure per volume (the inverse of compliance), and thus a greater compliance cost is associated with lower compliance. Ghoniem and colleagues demonstrated that compliance cost was greater in myelomeningocele patients than that of controls and that those with vesicoureteral reflux and upper tract deterioration had greater compliance cost than those who did not have these findings.[11] Compliance cost is now not commonly used to describe the relationship between stored volume and P_{det} of the bladder, and compliance (in the units of milliliters per centimeter H_2O) is generally accepted.

There is no consensus on the optimal way to report compliance in cases wherein no significant increase in P_{det} was measured during filling.[4] For example, Harris and colleagues arbitrarily assigned the value of 1000 mL/cm H_2O in cases wherein there was no change in P_{det} (making the denominator of $\Delta V/\Delta P$ infinite).[12] Others have defined the compliance in these cases as the maximum cystometric capacity (assuming a ΔP 1 cm H_2O), or defined the ΔP as the smallest value that could be measured by their instrument.[13,14]

Another potential confounder in the calculation of compliance is potential "pop-off" mechanisms. As discussed, it is recommended to calculate compliance from points on the pressure/volume curve before any urinary leakage (an effective antegrade pop-off mechanism). However, the retrograde pop-off mechanism of ureteral reflux should also be considered. For example, a marked reduction in compliance in a subset of patients was seen when ureteral orifices were occluded during measurement.[15] An example is shown in **Fig. 2**, wherein a patient had a normal cystometrogram tracing but her fluoroscopy demonstrated that the majority of her urine was being stored in her upper tracts. Bladder diverticulae are another potential pop-off mechanism but their contribution to compliance measures is unclear, and correction for them is not straightforward.

Values for Normal and Abnormal Compliance

Bladder compliance is highly variable in the healthy population, with a mean in men of 56 mL/cm H_2O and a mean in women ranging from 71 to 241 mL/cm H_2O.[4,16] Given the wide ranges (and differences in quantitation approaches when there is no discernible increase in

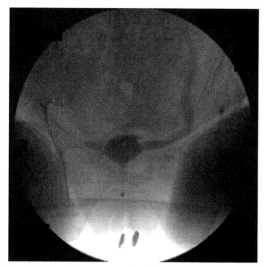

Fig. 2. Video fluoroscopy obtained at the time of urodynamics demonstrating a low capacity bladder and bilateral hydroureteronephrosis. The cystometrogram tracing in this individual was normal, as vesicoureteral reflux allowed for storage of the majority of her urine in the upper tracts.

P_{det}) of compliance in the healthy population, there is no widely accepted value for "normal" compliance. Similarly, cutoff values for low compliance are also variable but generally range from 10 to 40 mL/cm H_2O (**Table 2**). For example, Kaufman and colleagues used the value of 40 cm H_2O at maximum cystometric capacity as their cutoff for low compliance[17] but this figure relates to a cohort of children with myelomeningocele,[18] and its generalizability to other populations is not clear. Wahl and colleagues described the normal increase in P_{det} associated with filling to capacity as no more than 6 cm H_2O, independent of age and size of patients.[19] Weld and colleagues have described a compliance cutoff of 12.5 mL/cm H_2O, below which is considered low compliance.[20] Hackler and colleagues used the value of 20 mL/cm H_2O, below which was considered low, in their cohort of patients with spinal cord

Table 2
Values for normal compliance based on selected literature

Normal Compliance Value (mL/cm H_2O)	Reference
>10	Cho et al,[22] 2009
>12.5	Weld et al,[20] 2000
>20	Hackler et al,[21,] 1989; Stöhrer et al,[23] 1999; Pannek et al,[24] 2018
≥40	Kaufman et al,[17] 1996

injury.[21] Cho and colleagues used a cutoff of 10 mL/cm H_2O, below which was considered low compliance in their cohort.[22] The International Continence Society, the American Spinal Injury Association board, and the International Spinal Cord Society recommend a cutoff of 20 mL/cm H_2O).[23,24]

WHY IS COMPLIANCE IMPORTANT?
Compliance and Its Relationship with Vesicoureteral Reflux and Upper Tract Deterioration

Urinary bladder compliance was first described in 1981 by McGuire and colleagues. The group followed a cohort of patients with myelodysplasia.[18] Thirty of 42 patients in the cohort were found to have a "progressive increase in pressure with increasing volume" during urodynamics. The group noted that in this subgroup, if the pressure response to filling cannot be controlled (eg, using anticholinergic medication or intermittent catheterization), an addition to urethral closing pressure such as an artificial urinary sphincter, may lead to vesicoureteral reflux and renal deterioration, and ultimately recurrent incontinence.

Historically, compliance was categorized as normal or low, and a quantitative cutoff was not commonly used. Motivated by this, in a subsequent investigation by Ghoniem and colleagues in 1989, the group sought to analyze compliance in a group of children with myelomeningocele and compare the findings in a group of age-matched controls with enuresis.[11] The investigators described 2 components of compliance: a passive component, related to the intrinsic viscoelastic properties of the bladder, and an active component due to the contractility of smooth muscle, that is normally modulated in physiologic circumstances by reflex neural mechanisms. In an effort to study the 2 components, the group broke down compliance into 2 calculations: *initial compliance*, during the beginning of the filling phase when there was no appreciable change in intravesical pressure, and *terminal compliance*, at the end of the filling phase when there was a steep increase in pressure in response to small filling volume increments. The group measured the compliance using carbon dioxide cystometrograms with a filling rate of 50 mL per minute, during which there was gentle traction of the catheter on the bladder neck to occlude the urethra.

The investigators found a significant difference in the initial compliance between the control group and the group with myelomeningocele. Specifically, the mean initial compliance of the enuresis control group was 17 mL/cm H_2O, as compared with 32 mL/cm H_2O in the control group ($P < .005$). Terminal compliance also differed significantly between the groups ($P < .01$), with a mean of 11 mL/cm H_2O in the control group and 3 mL/cm H_2O in the myelomeningocele group. The investigators then stratified the myelomeningocele group into 2 groups: one with initial compliance values similar to controls (mean 30 mL/cm H_2O), and one with lower initial compliance than that of the control group (mean 7 cm H_2O). Vesicoureteral reflux was present in 7 patients (22% of their cohort), and 6 of these patients were in the low initial compliance subgroup. The mean terminal compliance of those with reflux was 2.1 mL/cm H_2O. Seven patients had upper tract deterioration, and the terminal compliance of this group was 2.1 mL/cm H_2O. The investigators stated that, were the ureteral orifices to be occluded during the urodynamics assessments, the compliance values may have been even lower. The investigators concluded that myelomeningocele patients with low compliance were prone to vesicoureteral reflux, upper tract deterioration, and poor renal function.

Also in 1989, Weston and colleagues reported on the outcomes of a cohort of 30 patients with neurologic pathology, the majority spina bifida, and known low compliance on urodynamic assessment.[25] Of this cohort, 20 patients had bilateral hydronephrosis, and 5 had severe impairment of renal function. After treatment (the majority with sphincterotomy or ileocystoplasty), all of the patients with normal renal function either stabilized or improved but those with impaired renal function all progressed to end-stage renal disease. The authors concluded, "poor compliance early in filling is an absolute indication for surgical intervention." They discuss that in their experience, the critical bladder pressure is about 20 cm H_2O, and that permanent pressures greater than this value may cause upper tract damage. They further note that the majority of their patients whose upper tracts deteriorated rapidly harbored pressures of at least 40 cm H_2O.

Hackler and colleagues sought to determine the incidence and effects of low bladder compliance on the upper urinary tract in individuals with spinal cord injury.[21] Their cohort included 254 patients who underwent urodynamic studies in a 3-year period, along with an excretory urogram and/or renal ultrasound. Seventeen percent of patients had low compliance, which they defined as 20 mL/cm H_2O. Hydronephrosis was present in 64% of the renal units in low compliance bladders as compared with only 21% of renal units in normal compliance bladders. Vesicoureteral reflux was present in 46% of renal units in low

compliance bladders, as compared with only 6% of renal units in normally compliant bladders. The authors concluded that after spinal cord injury, the development of low bladder compliance is not uncommon and is a risk factor for upper urinary tract deterioration. They note that attempts must be made to maintain low detrusor pressures, and that patients must undergo adequate and frequent surveillance.

As observed by Dray and Cameron,[9] the findings of the above studies supported a model for a mechanism by which elevated outlet pressures (eg, by a fixed sphincter or detrusor sphincteric dyssynergia) may contribute to progressive loss of compliance due to increased bladder pressure, and in turn impaired delivery of urine from the upper tracts to the bladder, and increased risk for vesicoureteral reflex, pyelonephritis, and upper tract deterioration.

Strategies to Improve Compliance and Thus Reduce Upper Tract Risk

Catheterization and urethral dilation

Weld and colleagues reported the outcomes of a cohort of 316 patients with spinal cord injury and neurogenic lower urinary tract dysfunction.[20] The investigators found that patients who managed their bladder drainage with clean intermittent catheterization, rather than indwelling catheter drainage, had a higher incidence of normal compliance. These findings were consistent across injury types. The study also found that low compliance was associated with vesicoureteral reflux, pyelonephritis, and upper tract stones. The authors concluded that clean intermittent catheterization protects bladder compliance over time and preventing the upper tract complications associated with low compliance.

Park and colleagues demonstrated that bladder compliance was improved through outlet pressure reduction using urethral dilation.[26] The group also showed that durable improvements in urodynamic parameters and upper tract function preservation were associated with urethral dilation but these were not seen in a subset in whom there was low compliance before the dilation. These findings were suggestive that in those with low compliance, there may be irreversible bladder changes due to outlet resistance, and that efforts should be taken to optimize compliance early to avoid such irreversible sequelae. However, reduction in outlet resistance through surgical therapy may also be associated with incontinence, and therefore such compliance management is limited to select patient groups, such as those who undergo sphincterotomy for detrusor sphincter dyssynergia and use a condom catheter.

Antimuscarinic agents

Safe compliance in those with NLUTD is commonly maintained by reducing bladder pressure medically or surgically.[27] Antimuscarinics and their role in improvement in bladder compliance and storage have been studied thoroughly. Along with compliance improvement, they have also been associated with the reduction in detrusor overactivity and incontinence. Although storage parameters are generally improved with antimuscarinic use, only a subset of studies has assessed compliance quantitatively and specifically. For example, when Guerra and colleagues performed a meta-analysis of the literature on antimuscarinic use in children with low bladder compliance and neurogenic lower urinary tract dysfunction, they found that only 2 of 8 studies reported compliance, both of which reported approximately 7.5 mL/cm H_2O increase[28–30] (**Table 3**). Madersbacher and colleagues showed that compliance was increased with the use of both trospium chloride and oxybutynin, and that there was no statistically significant difference in compliance between the 2 agents[31] (see **Table 3**). Antimuscarinic agents have also been demonstrated to be associated with increased compliance in those who use urinary catheters for bladder drainage assistance. Kim and colleagues reported on a cohort of 109 patients with a mean duration of catheter use of about 12 years.[32] The group found that of the 31 patients who had normal bladder compliance, 77% were using oxybutynin. This was a statistically significantly higher proportion than in those with low compliance.

Alpha-blocker agents

Alpha-blockers, commonly used in those with benign prostatic hyperplasia and lower urinary tract symptoms, have also been shown to improve bladder storage parameters including compliance. McGuire and Savastano observed that when the detrusor was decentralized (through dorsal rhizotomy) in cats and humans, there was a sympathetic-mediated change from a predominance of beta-adrenergic function (relaxation) to alpha-adrenergic function (contraction) during filling.[33] They thought that the reduced compliance associated with bladder decentralization may be mediated by alpha-receptors, and hypothesized that alpha blockade would improve compliance. In a primate model, the authors demonstrated that the alpha-blocker, phenoxybenzamine, improved bladder compliance in primates with dorsal rhizotomy, supporting their hypothesis.[33] Subsequently, Swierzewski and colleagues demonstrated that in a cohort of 12 patients with spinal cord injury who had low bladder compliance despite maximum

anticholinergic therapy and clean intermittent catheterization, the addition of the alpha-blocker terazosin was associated with improved bladder compliance in all patients.[34] There was a mean 73% improvement in compliance relative to baseline (see **Table 3**), and the effects were reversed on stopping the agent. The cohort also had improved continence, and the results together suggest that the compliance improvement may have been due to alpha blockade of receptors on the bladder wall or through central effects, rather than through reduced outlet resistance, again supporting the earlier hypothesis by McGuire and Savastano.[33] Although alpha-blocking agents are recommended in most major guidance documents for voiding in neurogenic lower urinary tract dysfunction,[35] they are not often considered for improvement in storage parameters.

Beta-3 agonists

Beta-3 agonists improve smooth muscle relaxation via sympathetic nervous system stimulation and are an effective therapy for patients with overactive bladder. There are early data for their efficacy in neurogenic lower urinary tract dysfunction. Groups have found improvements in compliance through the use of mirabegron, a beta-3 agonist[36] (see **Table 3**). For example, a study that randomized 78 patients with spinal cord injury or multiple sclerosis to either mirabegron or placebo found a statistically significant higher compliance in the mirabegron group (59 vs 30 mL/cm H_2O).[37] Another group found that, in a cohort of children with spina bifida with neurogenic lower urinary tract dysfunction, mirabegron was associated with improved compliance when substituted or added to an anticholinergic agent.[38]

Table 3		
Change in bladder compliance following therapies for neurogenic lower urinary tract dysfunction therapies from selected literature		
Therapy	**Mean Change in Compliance from Baseline**	**Reference**
Antimuscarinic therapy	7.5–23 mL/cm H_2O increase	28–31
Alpha-blocker agent	73% increase	34
Beta-3 agonist	12–24 mL/cm H_2O increase	37,41
Botulinum toxin	7–35 mL/cm H_2O increase	44,47,48
Augmentation cystoplasty	20 mL/cm H_2O increase	52

Wollner and colleagues also found that mirabegron was associated with elevated compliance in their review of a cohort with spinal cord injury.[39] Another beta-3 agonist, vibegron, may also be effective at improving compliance. For example, in a case report, compliance was improved in an individual with myelomeningocele who performed clean intermittent catheterization after switching from an anticholinergic agent to vibegron.[40] Subsequently, in a retrospective review of 31 patients with spinal cord injury and neurogenic lower urinary tract dysfunction, vibegron was associated with an increased compliance of about 12 mL/cm H_2O[41] (see **Table 3**). Bladder compliance improvement with vibegron was also demonstrated in a cohort of patients with spina bifida and antimuscarinic-resistant neurogenic lower urinary tract dysfunction.[42] In the 2 individuals with vesicoureteral reflux of the 15 patient cohort, reflux resolved with the initiation of vibegron.

Combination medical therapy
Combinations of medical therapy have also been investigated in those with NLUTD. For example, Cameron and colleagues showed that combination medical therapy was associated with multifold improvements in bladder compliance.[43] The group studied the effects of combinations of antimuscarinic agents, imipramine, and alpha-blockers. Specifically, they found a 5-fold increase in compliance in the group of patients who went from 0 to 2 agents, a 9.7-fold increase in compliance in the group that went from 0 to 3 agents, and a 3-fold increase in compliance in the group that went from an anticholinergic agent to triple drug therapy. Improvement in vesicoureteral reflux was also observed.

Botulinum toxin intravesical injection therapy
Intravesical injection of botulinum toxin has been shown to have good effect on compliance in those with NLUTD. For example, in a pediatric cohort of patients, average compliance increased from a baseline of 16 to 51 mL/cm H_2O. The treatment was associated with a reduction in maximum P_{det} and increase in bladder capacity.[44] Other studies in the pediatric population with neurogenic lower urinary tract dysfunction have also demonstrated improved compliance following botulinum toxin. For example, a systematic literature review by Gamé and colleagues found that in most studies, compliance improved greater than 20 mL/cm H_2O without adverse effects.[45] The findings have also been reflected in the adult population. Karsenty and colleagues performed a systematic review in adults with neurogenic lower urinary tract dysfunction, and identified several studies that demonstrated improved compliance following botulinum toxin as compared with baseline.[46] For example, in a cohort with detrusor overactivity, Kessler and colleagues reported an increase in compliance from a baseline of 20 to 55 mL/cm H_2O following botulinum toxin intravesical injection.[47] In those with spinal cord lesions who used intermittent catheterization for bladder drainage, Klaphajone and colleagues demonstrated significant improvements in compliance with botulinum toxin injection, even in a patient subset with very low compliance at baseline.[48]

Surgical management
Surgical management for low compliance bladders is generally reserved for those who are refractory to medical therapy and intravesical botulinum toxin. Management options include bladder augmentation and urinary diversion. Although there are many techniques and variations, bladder augmentation is a surgical approach wherein the urinary bladder is augmented with bowel or other organ. Augmentation is indicated for individuals who have refractory detrusor overactivity, loss of bladder compliance, and elevated detrusor leak point pressures, or in those with severely reduced bladder capacity that is causing prohibitively frequent intermittent catheterization or requires indwelling catheter drainage.[49] Bladder augmentation is associated with improved capacity, reduced detrusor pressures and compliance, and reduced incontinence.[50,51] In one study, augmentation cystoplasty was associated with a 20 mL/cm H_2O improvement in compliance.[52] (see **Table 3**). In a subset of patients, refractory symptoms and/or quality of life concerns may be best served with a urinary diversion. Indications for this intervention may include refractory urinary tract infections in the setting of low compliance, severe urethral and bladder neck erosion due to chronic catheterization, incontinence causing severe skin problems including decubitus ulcers, and/or an inability to manage bladder drainage assistance such as chronic or intermittent catheterization.[49]

Etiology of Reduced Compliance

In one investigation, mechanical properties of bladder strips from individuals with neurogenic pathology and low bladder compliance were studied and compared with strips of bladders from control patients, with presumed normal compliance. Based on assessment of strips from 11 patients in the neurogenic pathology group and 11 patients in the control group, the investigation found that there were only modest differences in some of the mechanical properties (peak tensions) and no differences in others (tension decay) between the

2 groups. The team concluded that these modest differences could not alone account for the marked differences in compliance between the groups, and that their results pointed to the importance of neurogenic rather than mechanical factors in the etiology of low compliance.[53] These findings were reflected in a guinea pig model of compliance, wherein the investigators found that the passive, rather than active, properties of the bladder wall.[54] Other studies suggests that bladder perfusion is important for the maintenance of compliance, and that ischemia may play a role in structural changes in the bladder role leading to low compliance.[55,56]

A series of other studies have led to a model in which bladder compliance is driven by several factors: intrinsic muscle properties, spinal parasympathetic reflex, vesical plexus intrinsic reflex activity, inhibition from the spinal cord.[4] Based on investigations from Edvarsen and from Marsh and colleagues,[57,58] Wyndaele and colleagues posit that at the onset of filling, the compliance is primarily driven by the properties of the bladder wall, and that later filling phases are registered neurologically and regulated by spinal reflexes.4

Compliance Limitations, a New Model, and Future Research

The importance of compliance lies in its association with upper urinary tract deterioration. However, there are low compliance bladders that are not subject to upper tract damage. For example, although Weld and colleagues demonstrated that low compliance was associated with upper tract risk, less than 30% of low compliance bladders had vesicoureteral reflux and less than 40% had any upper tract abnormality.[20] As discussed, other studies have also demonstrated the association of low compliance with upper tract risk but again a subset of low compliance bladders did not develop any upper tract abnormalities. For example, in the study by Hackler and colleagues, hydronephrosis was present in 64% of kidneys and reflux in 46% of kidneys in patients with low compliance bladders.[21] The remaining renal units did not harbor abnormalities, despite their association with low compliance bladders.

Motivated by these findings and others, we hypothesize that low compliance (and the elevated detrusor pressures and low volumes used for its calculation) plays an incomplete role in conferring risk to the upper urinary tract. *Rather, we think that the pressure differential between the lower urinary tract and upper urinary tract carries importance and that bladder compliance is a proxy for this pressure differential.*

The pressure differential between the upper and lower urinary tracts is a difficult entity to measure directly, and it will differ as a function of bladder filling volume. A more practical measurement would be the bladder volume at which the vesical pressure equals the upper tract pressure. This volume could then be normalized to the bladder's functional capacity based on voiding diaries of catheterization logs, or normalized to the maximum cystometric capacity. For example, the value, which we term V_{Peq}, and the percent of functional capacity (termed $V_{Peq\%}$) could be described and interpreted as follows:

V_{Peq} = 550, Functional capacity 700 cc, $V_{Peq\%}$ = 79%. In other words, at 79% of an individual's functional capacity, the lower and upper tract pressures are equal. Therefore, during the portion of the filling phase that this individual's bladder is above this critical volume, the pressure of the bladder could exceed the pressure of the upper urinary tract, and reflux/columnation could develop. Individuals with lower $V_{Peq\%}$ may be subject to more rapid upper tract deterioration because their upper tracts may remain at risk for a longer portion of their micturition cycle.

The above example is a hypothetical scenario, and research investigations must test these hypotheses directly. Specifically, the critical point may not be the point at which the pressures are equal but perhaps a point at which the vesical pressure is at some fraction of the upper tract pressure.

The role of detrusor leak point pressure also will likely play a role in this model. For example, physiologically, a leak point pressure lower than the pressure of the upper tract would prevent V_{Peq} from being reached, and protective of the upper tract. Those with low compliance but without upper tract deterioration may have a greater pressure differential between their lower and upper urinary tracts over their physiologic filling volumes. This differential may be due to their length and angle of their ureteral tunneling and/or other biomechanical factors. La Place's Law relates transmural pressure to both radius and wall thickness (**Fig. 3**). However, this assumes a spherical composition, whereas the bladder shape is commonly a flattened ellipse.[59] Whether bladder shape and differential wall thickness between the bladder trigone ureteral insertion points versus the bladder dome play a role in reflux and upper tract deterioration warrants investigation.

SUMMARY

Bladder compliance is the relationship between the change in bladder volume and the change in P_{det}. When calculating bladder compliance (ΔV/

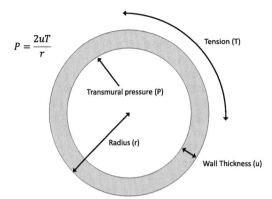

$$P = \frac{2uT}{r}$$

Tension (T)

Transmural pressure (P)

Radius (r)

Wall Thickness (u)

Fig. 3. Law of Laplace describes the relationship between the transmural pressure, radius, and wall thickness. The law assumes a spherical shape. Whether variability of bladder shape or wall thickness play a role in upper tract deterioration remains to be determined.

ΔP_{det}), the point at the initiation of filling and the point at the completion of filling should be used. Filling rate, filling medium, volume of diuresis, and the patient's functional bladder capacity should be considered when obtaining compliance measurements. Low bladder compliance has been demonstrated to be associated with adverse sequelae including vesicoureteral reflux, upper urinary tract deterioration, and reduced renal function. Different treatments have been shown to be effective for the improvement of bladder compliance and these sequelae. Such treatments include catheterization, medical therapy with anticholinergic agents or beta-3 agonists, botulinum toxin intravesical injection, and bladder augmentation. Compliance is likely only one part of the equation through which upper tract deterioration may be predicted, and we put forth a model wherein the proportion of time during the micturition cycle at which P_{det} is greater than the ureteral pressure is likely an excellent indicator of upper tract risk.

CLINICS CARE POINTS

- Bladder compliance is the ratio of change in filling volume to the change in detrusor pressure ($\Delta V/\Delta P_{det}$)
- The standard unit of bladder compliance is milliliters per centimeter H_2O
- A commonly used value for low compliance is a value less than 20 mL/cm H_2O
- Bladder compliance should be measured over the bladder's functional capacity, based on voiding diaries and/or catheterization logs

- Bladder compliance should be measured at the following 2 points from cystometry: (1) the detrusor pressure at the initiation of bladder filling and the associated bladder volume (which is usually 0) and (2) the detrusor pressure and associated bladder volume at the maximum cystometric capacity, or just before the start of a detrusor contraction causing leakage
- Catheterization at the beginning and/or end of cystometry may be used to accurately assess the change in volume for compliance calculation
- Low bladder compliance is associated with vesicoureteral reflux and upper urinary tract deterioration
- Low bladder compliance should prompt the initiation of therapeutic intervention with the goal of reducing the risk to the upper urinary tract

DISCLOSURE

G.T. Werneburg declares that he has no conflict of interest. J.T. Stoffel: Scientific Advisor Flume Catheter, Spine X; Site investigator Coloplast clinical trial.

REFERENCES

1. Abrams P, Cardozo L, Fall M, et al. The standardisation of terminology in lower urinary tract function: report from the standardisation sub-committee of the International Continence Society. Urology 2003; 61(1):37–49.
2. Haylen BT, De Ridder D, Freeman RM, et al. An International Urogynecological Association (IUGA)/International Continence Society (ICS) joint report on the terminology for female pelvic floor dysfunction. Neurourol Urodyn: Official Journal of the International Continence Society 2010;29(1):4–20.
3. D'Ancona C, Haylen B, Oelke M, et al. The International Continence Society (ICS) report on the terminology for adult male lower urinary tract and pelvic floor symptoms and dysfunction. Neurourol Urodyn 2019;38(2):433–77.
4. Wyndaele JJ, Gammie A, Bruschini H, et al. Bladder compliance what does it represent: can we measure it, and is it clinically relevant? Neurourol Urodyn 2011;30(5):714–22.
5. Peterson A, Webster G. Urodynamic and videourodynamic evaluation of voiding dysfunction. Campbell-Walsh Urol 2007;9:1986–2010.
6. Sethia K, Smith J. The effect of pH and lignocaine on detrusor instability. Br J Urol 1987;60(6):516–8.

7. Chin-Peuckert L, Rennick JE, Jednak R, et al. Should warm infusion solution be used for urodynamic studies in children? A prospective randomized study. J Urol 2004;172(4):1657–61.

8. Schäfer W, Abrams P, Liao L, et al. Good urodynamic practices: uroflowmetry, filling cystometry, and pressure-flow studies. Neurourol Urodyn: Official Journal of the International Continence Society 2002;21(3):261–74.

9. Dray EV, Cameron AP. Identifying patients with high-risk neurogenic bladder: beyond detrusor leak point pressure. Urologic Clinics 2017;44(3):441–52.

10. Tiryaki S, Tekin A, Avanoglu A, et al. A pilot study assessing average detrusor pressure garnered from area under a urodynamic curve: Evaluation of clinical outcomes. J Pediatr Urol 2022;18(3):325.e1–9.

11. Ghoniem GM, Bloom DA, McGuire EJ, et al. Bladder compliance in meningomyelocele children. J Urol 1989;141(6):1404–6.

12. Harris RL, Cundiff GW, Theofrastous JP, et al. Bladder compliance in neurologically intact women. Neurourol Urodyn: Official Journal of the International Continence Society 1996;15(5):483–8.

13. Gilmour RF, Churchill BM, Steckler RE, et al. A new technique for dynamic analysis of bladder compliance. J Urol 1993;150(4):1200–3.

14. Sandri S, Marino V, Castiglioni M, et al. The normal bladder compliance. Neurourol Urodyn 1990;9:207–8.

15. Garriboli M, Solomon E. On-table urodynamic with ureteric occlusion: A resource for measuring bladder capacity and compliance in the management of patients with gross vesico-ureteric reflux. Neurourol Urodyn 2022;41(1):448–55.

16. Pauwels E, De Wachter S, Wyndaele J. Normality of bladder filling studied in symptom-free middle-aged women. J Urol 2004;171(4):1567–70.

17. Kaufman AM, Ritchey ML, Roberts AC, et al. Decreased bladder compliance in patients with myelomeningocele treated with radiological observation. J Urol 1996;156(6):2031–3.

18. McGuire EJ, Woodside JR, Borden TA, et al. Prognostic value of urodynamic testing in myelodysplastic patients. J Urol 1981;126(2):205–9.

19. Wahl EF, Lerman SE, Lahdes-Vasama TT, et al. Measurement of bladder compliance can be standardized by a dimensionless number: theoretical perspective. BJU Int 2004;94(6):895–7.

20. WELD KJ, GRANEY MJ, DMOCHOWSKI RR. Differences in bladder compliance with time and associations of bladder management with compliance in spinal cord injured patients. J Urol 2000;163(4):1228–33.

21. Hackler RH, Hall MK, Zampieri TA. Bladder hypocompliance in the spinal cord injury population. J Urol 1989;141(6):1390–3.

22. Cho SY, Yi JS, Oh SJ. The clinical significance of poor bladder compliance. Neurourol Urodyn: Official Journal of the International Continence Society 2009;28(8):1010–4.

23. Stöhrer M, Goepel M, Kondo A, et al. The standardization of terminology in neurogenic lower urinary tract dysfunction with suggestions for diagnostic procedures. Neurourol Urodyn: Official Journal of the International Continence Society 1999;18(2):139–58.

24. Pannek J, Kennelly M, Kessler TM, et al. International spinal cord injury urodynamic basic data set (version 2.0). Spinal cord series and cases 2018;4(1):98.

25. Weston P, Robinson L, Williams S, et al. Poor compliance early in filling in the neuropathic bladder. Br J Urol 1989;63(1):28–31.

26. Park JM, Mcguire EJ, Koo HP, et al. External urethral sphincter dilation for the management of high risk myelomeningocele: 15-year experience. J Urol 2001;165(6 Part 2):2383–8.

27. Cameron AP. Medical management of neurogenic bladder with oral therapy. Transl Androl Urol 2016;5(1):51.

28. Guerra LA, Moher D, Sampson M, et al. Intravesical oxybutynin for children with poorly compliant neurogenic bladder: a systematic review. J Urol 2008;180(3):1091–7.

29. Ferrara P, d'Aleo C, Tarquini E, et al. Side-effects of oral or intravesical oxybutynin chloride in children with spina bifida. BJU Int 2001;87(7):674–8.

30. Guerra L, Raju G, Milks J, et al. Review of experience with intravesical oxybutynin at the Children's hospital of Eastern Ontario. Ottawa, Ontario, Canada: Department of Clinical Epidemiology and Community Health, University of Ottawa; 2007. master's thesis, chapt 2.

31. Madersbacher H, Stöhrer M, Richter R, et al. Trospium chloride versus oxybutynin: a randomized, double-blind, multicentre trial in the treatment of detrusor hyper-reflexia. Br J Urol 1995;75(4):452–6.

32. Kim YH, Bird ET, Priebe M, et al. The role of oxybutynin in spinal cord injured patients with indwelling catheters. J Urol 1997;158(6):2083–6.

33. McGuire EJ, Savastano JA. Effect of alpha-adrenergic blockade and anticholinergic agents on the decentralized primate bladder. Neurourol Urodyn 1985;4(2):139–42.

34. Swierzewski SJ III, Gormley EA, Belville WD, et al. The effect of terazosin on bladder function in the spinal cord injured patient. J Urol 1994;151(4):951–4.

35. Werneburg GT, Welk B, Averbeck MA, et al. Neuro-Urology: Call for Universal, Resource-Independent Guidance. Biomedicines 2023;11(2):397.

36. El Helou E, Labaki C, Chebel R, et al. The use of mirabegron in neurogenic bladder: a systematic review. World J Urol 2020;38:2435–42.

37. Krhut J, Borovička V, Bílková K, et al. Efficacy and safety of mirabegron for the treatment of neurogenic detrusor overactivity—Prospective, randomized, double-blind, placebo-controlled study. Neurourol Urodyn 2018;37(7):2226–33.

38. Park JS, Lee YS, Lee CN, et al. Efficacy and safety of mirabegron, a β3-adrenoceptor agonist, for treating neurogenic bladder in pediatric patients with spina bifida: a retrospective pilot study. World J Urol 2019;37:1665–70.

39. Wöllner J, Pannek J. Initial experience with the treatment of neurogenic detrusor overactivity with a new β-3 agonist (mirabegron) in patients with spinal cord injury. Spinal Cord 2016;54(1):78–82.

40. Kato T, Mizuno K, Nishio H, et al. Urodynamic effectiveness of a beta-3 adrenoreceptor agonist (vibegron) for a pediatric patient with anticholinergic-resistant neurogenic detrusor overactivity: a case report. J Med Case Rep 2021;15:1–7.

41. Matsuda K, Teruya K, Uemura O. Urodynamic effect of vibegron on neurogenic lower urinary tract dysfunction in individuals with spinal cord injury: A retrospective study. Spinal Cord 2022;60(8):716–21.

42. Aoki K, Momose H, Gotoh D, et al. Video-urodynamic effects of vibegron, a new selective β3-adrenoceptor agonist, on antimuscarinic-resistant neurogenic bladder dysfunction in patients with spina bifida. Int J Urol 2022;29(1):76–81.

43. Cameron AP, Clemens JQ, Latini JM, et al. Combination drug therapy improves compliance of the neurogenic bladder. J Urol 2009;182(3):1062–7.

44. Schulte-Baukloh H, Michael T, Stürzebecher B, et al. Botulinum-a toxin detrusor injection as a novel approach in the treatment of bladder spasticity in children with neurogenic bladder. Eur Urol 2003;44(1):139–43.

45. Gamé X, Mouracade P, Chartier-Kastler E, et al. Botulinum toxin-A (Botox®) intradetrusor injections in children with neurogenic detrusor overactivity/neurogenic overactive bladder: a systematic literature review. J Pediatr Urol 2009;5(3):156–64.

46. Karsenty G, Denys P, Amarenco G, et al. Botulinum toxin A (Botox®) intradetrusor injections in adults with neurogenic detrusor overactivity/neurogenic overactive bladder: a systematic literature review. Eur Urol 2008;53(2):275–87.

47. Kessler TM, Danuser H, Schumacher M, et al. Botulinum A toxin injections into the detrusor: an effective treatment in idiopathic and neurogenic detrusor overactivity? Neurourol Urodyn: Official Journal of the International Continence Society 2005;24(3):231–6.

48. Klaphajone J, Kitisomprayoonkul W, Sriplakit S. Botulinum toxin type A injections for treating neurogenic detrusor overactivity combined with low-compliance bladder in patients with spinal cord lesions. Arch Phys Med Rehabil 2005;86(11):2114–8.

49. Gor RA, Elliott SP. Surgical management of neurogenic lower urinary tract dysfunction. Urologic Clinics 2017;44(3):475–90.

50. Gurung PM, Attar KH, Abdul-Rahman A, et al. Long-term outcomes of augmentation ileocystoplasty in patients with spinal cord injury: a minimum of 10 years of follow-up. BJU Int 2012;109(8):1236–42.

51. Kilic N, Celayir S, Elicevik M, et al. Bladder augmentation: Urodynamic findings and clinical outcome in different augmentation techniques. Eur J Pediatr Surg 1999;9(01):29–32.

52. Mast P, Hoebeke P, Wyndaele J, et al. Experience with augmentation cystoplasty. A review. Spinal Cord 1995;33(10):560–4.

53. German K, Bedwani J, Davies J, et al. An assessment of the contribution of visco-elastic factors in the aetiology of poor compliance in the human neurophathic bladder. Br J Urol 1994;74(6):744–8.

54. Macneil H, Brading A, Williams J. Cause of low compliance in a guinea-pig model of instability and low compliance. Neurourol Urodyn 1992;11(1):47–52.

55. Kershen RT, Azadzoi KM, Siroky MB. Blood flow, pressure and compliance in the male human bladder. J Urol 2002;168(1):121–5.

56. Vince R, Tracey A, Deebel NA, et al. Effects of vesical and perfusion pressure on perfusate flow, and flow on vesical pressure, in the isolated perfused working pig bladder reveal a potential mechanism for the regulation of detrusor compliance. Neurourol Urodyn 2018;37(2):642–9.

57. Edvardsen P. Nervous control of urinary bladder in cats: I. The collecting phase. Acta Physiol Scand 1968;72(1-2):157–71.

58. Marsh DJ, Suzuki G, Meyers FH. Role of afferent activity from the bladder in regulating its activity. American Journal of Physiology-Legacy Content 1959;196(2):351–3.

59. Rule AD, Sauver JLS, Jacobson DJ, et al. Three-dimensional ultrasound bladder characteristics and their association with prostate size and lower urinary tract dysfunction among men in the community. Urology 2009;74(4):908–13.

Detrusor Sphincter Dyssynergia

Marc A. Furrer, MD, FEBU[a,b,c,d],*, Thomas M. Kessler, MD, FEBU[e],
Jalesh N. Panicker, MD, DM, FRCP[f]

KEYWORDS

- Pontine micturition center • Spinobulbospinal pathway • Pelvic floor electromyography
- Videocystometrography • Catheterization • Pharmacotherapy • Botulinum toxin
- Sacral neuromodulation

KEY POINTS

- High voiding pressures can lead to significant complications if DSD is not treated and followed-up regularly.
- Combined diagnostic modalities can improve detection of DSD * Non-invasive and invasive treatment options are centered around symptomatic management rather that addressing the underlying causative mechanisms.
- Regular followed-up is required in the long-term from both, a urological and neurological perspective.
- Surveillance alone is possible in some patients but treatment must be considered in patients at risk for upper tract damage.

INTRODUCTION

Neurologic disorders commonly cause lower urinary tract (LUT) dysfunction affecting both the voiding and storage phase and, subsequently, cause various degree of LUT symptoms. The site and nature of the neurologic lesion affects the pattern of dysfunction such as detrusor overactivity, detrusor underactivity, and/or detrusor sphincter dyssynergia (DSD), which have a pronounced effect on quality of life.[1]

Definition of Detrusor Sphincter Dyssynergia

The International Continence Society (ICS) has defined DSD, also called detrusor external-sphincter dyssynergia or detrusor striated-sphincter dyssynergia, as "a detrusor contraction concurrent with an involuntary contraction of the urethral and/or periurethral striated muscle and typically occurs in patients with a supra-sacral lesion, and is uncommon in lesions of the lower cord."

Although a straightforward and pragmatic definition, controversies remain when considering complex and challenging neurourological patients and the type of DSD is poorly categorized. Given that none of the proposed DSD-classifications (**Table 1**)[2–4] allow for an appropriate assessment of upper urinary tract risk following spinal cord injury, the ICS recommends that DSD is assessed as a binary yes-no variable, whether present or not, which is considered logical and practical to assess and treat patients in daily practice.

[a] Department of Uro-Neurology, National Hospital for Neurology and Neurosurgery and UCL Institute of Neurology, Queen Square, London, UK; [b] Department of Urology Inselspital, University of Bern, Bern 3010, Switzerland; [c] Department of Urology, Solothurner Spitäler AG, Kantonsspital Olten, Olten 4600, Switzerland; [d] Department of Urology, Solothurner Spitäler AG, Bürgerspital Solothurn, Solothurn 4500, Switzerland; [e] Department of Neuro-Urology, Balgrist University Hospital, University of Zürich, Zürich 8008, Switzerland; [f] Faculty of Brain Sciences, UCL Queen Square Institute of Neurology, University College London, London, WC1N 3BG, UK
* Corresponding author. Department of Urology, Kantonsspital Olten, Baslerstrasse 150, 4600 Olten, Switzerland
E-mail address: marc.furrer@nhs.net

Urol Clin N Am 51 (2024) 221–232
https://doi.org/10.1016/j.ucl.2024.01.001

Table 1
Proposed detrusor sphincter dyssynergia classification systems

Classification	Description	Grades/Types
Yalla et al,[2] 1977	Grading (Grade 1–3) to determine degree of DSD and its influence on voiding function	*Grade 1:* high intravesical voiding pressures resulting from the resistance offered by the semicompliant striated sphincter *Grade 2:* either inappropriate or clonic striated sphincter contractions resulting in interrupted voiding *Grade 3:* nonvoiding secondary to sustained spasticity of the external sphincter with complete closure of the outlet
Blaivas & Fisher,[36] 1981	Adapted classification (Type 1–3) focusing on electromyographic profile	*Type 1:* crescendo increase in EMG activity that suddenly relaxes at peak of detrusor contraction *Type 2:* clonic sphincter contractions interspersed throughout detrusor contraction *Type 3:* sustained sphincter contraction that persists throughout bladder contraction
Weld et al,[4] 2000	Intermittent (Type 1) vs continuous (Type 2) sphincter contractions (no significant relationship of the DSD-type with symptom severity found)	*Type 1:* intermittent sphincter contraction interspersed throughout detrusor contraction *Type 2:* continuous sphincter contraction that persists throughout bladder contraction

Although DSD is commonly found in patients with spinal cord lesions (eg, multiple sclerosis), there is no clear relationship between the severity of the condition and the type of DSD.[5] Although it has been argued that a spinal cord lesion resulting in incomplete sensory and motor findings is more often associated with Blaivas type 1 DSD as compared with complete spinal cord injuries,[6] this has not been a consistent finding and studies have found no relationship between the type of DSD and degree of mobility.[7] Of note, classifications described in **Table 1** cannot compete with the ICS-definition. Gross and colleagues[8] described that, first, none of the systems can differentiate between patients with and without an underlying neurologic disorder. Second, these classifications cannot distinguish patients with a maximum storage detrusor pressure at urethral leakage of either 40 cm H_2O or lesser or greater than 40 cm H_2O (or only maximum storage detrusor pressure in case of no urethral leakage), which is a risk factor for upper urinary tract damage and for a poor neurourological course. Urodynamic testing should be performed to allow for an adequate characterization of DSD and the clinical relevance of these classification systems in the clinical assessment and treatment of patients is debatable at present.

Cause and Prevalence of Detrusor Sphincter Dyssynergia

Although the exact prevalence of DSD is unknown, this can occur in any significant neurologic disease affecting the suprasacral spinal cord and most commonly occurs in patients with spinal cord injury, spinal dysraphism (spina bifida), multiple sclerosis, multiple system atrophy (MSA), and myelopathy postspinal surgery. DSD prevalence in spinal cord injury is influenced by the level and severity of injury. Following suprasacral spinal cord injury, the prevalence can range between 70% and 100% after the spinal shock phase.[9] In multiple sclerosis, 20% to 25% of patients will eventually develop DSD, whereas DSD is reported in up to 50% of infants with spina bifida. The reported prevalence of DSD is lower in patients with progressive neurologic disorders,[10] such as human T-lymphotropic virus-1 (HTLV-1)-related myelopathy, and following transverse myelitis.[11–13]

MSA is a rare, progressive neurodegenerative disorder affecting multiple regions of the central nervous system (CNS), including the autonomic nervous system and spinal cord. Bloch and colleagues reported DSD rates in both men and women to be 49% and 46%, respectively.[14] In Parkinson disease, DSD rates are much lower (0%–21%). Moreover, DSD seems significantly earlier in MSA (<2 years) compared with PD (>5 years).[14–16] One study reported a prevalence of DSD of 8% in hereditary spinocerebellar ataxia. In general, DSD is an uncommon condition following cerebral diseases. However, it has been reported following stroke with spasticity of the external urethral sphincter being a possible pathophysiologic mechanism.[17]

PHYSIOLOGY AND PATHOPHYSIOLOGY
Physiology of Bladder Storage and Micturition Phase

Reviewing the physiologic control of LUT functions provides a framework to understand the mechanisms responsible for DSD following neurologic disease. The neural networks regulating bladder filling and voiding function act as an on–off switching circuit, establishing a reciprocal relationship between the urinary bladder and the urethral outlet. During bladder filling, storage reflexes, primarily located in the spinal cord, are engaged, whereas voiding is governed by reflex mechanisms organized in the brain.

Storage phase
Throughout the phase of urine storage, bladder distension triggers an increase in vesical afferent firing and sensory nerves convey information about bladder wall pressure. A-fibers are activated by low-intensity stimuli via stretch-sensitive mechanoreceptors during passive distension during filling, and active contraction, and C-fibers, which remain dormant in physiologic conditions and primarily respond to high-intensity stimuli such as a maximum stretch of the bladder, become active following neurologic conditions. Signals travel through the pelvic/hypogastric/pudendal nerves to the lumbosacral spinal cord and through a spinobulbospinal reflex pathways involving brain stem nuclei such as the pontine micturition center (PMC) and midbrain periaqueductal gray region, which maintain the storage phase. Feedback from the limbic system and prefrontal cortex to the midbrain facilitates ongoing bladder storage.

The maintenance of continence during urine storage involves an interplay between the internal and external urethral sphincter. Although the internal sphincter (smooth muscle) contracts, and the bladder neck closes through sympathetic (hypogastric) innervation during the filling phase, the external urethral sphincter (striated muscle) remains contracted by stimulation through the pudendal nerve (signals originating from the Onuf's nucleus located in the anterior horn of the S2–S4 segment). This coordinated activity is orchestrated by urethral reflexes collectively referred to as the "guarding reflex," which is initiated through afferent signals to the sacral spinal cord, where pudendal motoneuron efferents (and therefore and both the smooth and striated components of the urethral sphincter) are activated by interneuronal circuitry in the spinal cord.

Expressed more specifically at a muscular level, the guarding reflex maintains urinary continence with synergic activation of internal (extension of the trigone/detrusor encircling the bladder neck) and external urethral sphincter (striated muscle group positioned distal to the internal sphincter) to achieve a pressure in the proximal urethra that is higher than within the bladder.[18]

Additionally, sympathetic firing has an inhibitory effect (relaxation) on the detrusor and influences signal transmission in bladder ganglia. Notably, a specific region in the rostral pons, referred to as the pontine storage center or "L" region, amplifies activity in the external urethral sphincter and may play a role in sphincter reflexes or involuntary sphincter control. In animals, reflex activation of the lumbar sympathetic pathway inhibits bladder smooth muscle, contracts the bladder outlet, and inhibits parasympathetic activity at the autonomic ganglia level. However, the significance of sympathetic control during filling and storage, and the ganglionic inhibition in humans is less clear (compared with animal models where this has been worked out), as sympatholytic drugs or sympathetic chain resection have minimal effects on bladder storage.

Micturition phase
To initiate the voiding process "the guarding reflex" has to be inhibited. Excitation of the PMC activates descending pathways leading to stimulation of sacral parasympathetic (S2–S4) outflow with subsequent relaxation of the internal urethral sphincter (resulting in lower proximal urethral pressures) and, after a brief delay, synergic detrusor contraction. Concurrently, sympathetic and pudendal outflow to the urethral region (external urethral sphincter) is inhibited. This sequence results in bladder contraction, increased intravesical pressure, and urine flow. Secondary reflexes, prompted by urine flow through the urethra, further aid in bladder emptying.

Of note, the periaqueductal gray (PAG) is active in both storage and voiding phases of the micturition cycle but the extent of its activity differs between these 2 phases. During the storage phase, the PAG is activated but the PMC is inactive, and during the voiding, the PMC maintains activation, and the activation of the PAG enhances.

Pathophysiology of Detrusor Sphincter Dyssynergia

DSD occurs following a disruption of the spinobulbospinal reflex between the pontine and sacral micturition center. The PMC is no longer able to coordinate the functioning of the centers in the sacral spinal cord, resulting in simultaneous (dyssynergic) contraction of the external urethral sphincter and the detrusor when voiding.[5,19] The detrusor contracts against a closed bladder outlet due to involuntary contraction of the external urinary sphincter, and this lack of coordination between the detrusor and the external urethral sphincter leads to a neurologically induced bladder outlet obstruction. Simultaneous activation of the external urethral sphincter and detrusor with consequently elevated detrusor leak point pressure reflects an increased resistance in the proximal urethra, which does not allow the bladder pressures to decrease through voiding.

Could Detrusor Sphincter Dyssynergia Following Spinal Cord Injury Represent a Return of an Infantile Pattern of Voiding?

In healthy infants and young children aged younger than 3 to 5 years, bladder emptying is regulated by a reflex pathway that is organized in the spinal cord and mediated through C-fiber afferents.[20] Voiding occurs incompletely owing to discoordination between the detrusor and sphincter[21] and urodynamic studies in healthy infants demonstrate fluctuating voiding pressures often with a polyphasic contraction, which is associated with increased pelvic floor activity.[22,23] As the child becomes older, the C-fiber mediated voiding reflex becomes suppressed and dormant, and in its place thinly myelinated A delta fiber, which has a lower threshold for mechanosensitive activation, begins to convey sensations from the bladder and become responsible for responding to passive distension and active contraction; voiding becomes mediated through the spinobulbospinal reflex under higher cortical control discussed earlier.

Following spinal cord injury, these dormant C-fibers become sensitized, and a segmental spinal reflex emerges that is mediated by C-fiber afferent nerves resulting in involuntary detrusor contractions at low bladder volumes that presents as neurogenic detrusor overactivity (NDO).[20,24] Spinal cord injury also results in voiding dysfunction due to dyscoordination between the detrusor and sphincter, similar to the infantile pattern of voiding. It could be postulated therefore that DSD could represent a return of the voiding pattern seen in infants that had been suppressed following CNS maturation. Further research is required to explore this possibility further.

CLINICAL CONSEQUENCES OF DETRUSOR SPHINCTER DYSSYNERGIA

High urethral closure pressures during the detrusor contraction lead to high intravesical voiding pressure and large postvoid residual, which can end up with serious complications in up to 50% of patients if DSD is not treated and followed-up regularly and appropriately.[4] High voiding pressures (in case of continued voiding with underlying DSD) can lead to structural alterations in the bladder wall such as increased thickness and trabeculations. Furthermore, a loss of bladder compliance may result with sustained detrusor pressures greater than 40 cm H_2O with or without urethral leakage of urine as shown in spina bifida.[25] Consequently, vesico-uretero-renal reflux with high upper tract pressures and hydronephrosis may develop. The combination of elevated postvoid residuals and pathologic upper tract changes lead to recurrent urinary tract infections with potential further complications such as urosepsis. Additionally, there is a risk for stone formation in the ureters, kidneys, and bladder.[1] Furthermore, patients with spinal cord lesion at or above T6 level are at risk for developing autonomic dysreflexia and its potential sequelae.[26] DSD is therefore associated with several complications and recognition and treatment of DSD is of utmost importance. The continuous DSD phenotype may be more associated with developing loss of bladder compliance and consequently renal compromise in patients with spinal cord injury.[27]

The risk for lower and upper urinary tract damage, with subsequent end-stage renal disease is highest in individuals with spinal dysraphism (ie, spina bifida) and spinal cord injury.[1] In patients with multiple sclerosis, the association of DSD and upper tract changes remains a matter of debate. Although some studies report low incidence of upper tract damage and low compliance bladder despite DSD being apparent,[28] others show an increasing risk of upper tract complications in symptomatic individuals as the disease progresses, with sequelae occurring after 6 to 8 years from diagnosis.[29]

DIAGNOSIS

Despite being of high relevance, no single gold standard technique exists to diagnose DSD. Of note, data on sensitivity and specificity remain sparse, and centers of excellence worldwide use varied techniques for diagnosis. Diagnosis can be made either through neurophysiological tests or through uroimaging. However, the former is considered more sensitive because it specifically assesses functional impairment and not only morphologic changes.[30,31] Combined diagnostic modalities can improve the detection of DSD[32] such as urodynamic studies with concomitant pelvic floor electromyography (EMG), voiding cystourethrogram (VCUG), that is, video-urodynamics (VCMG) to supplement quantitative measurement with imaging, with or without urethral pressure profile during detrusor contraction and pressure-flow studies. Importantly, results should be interpreted by health-care professionals experienced in urodynamic testing.

Electromyography

Pelvic floor EMG testing is one approach for assessing DSD. Concentric needle EMG recording with the electrodes inserted into the striated external urethral sphincter is regarded as the gold standard for EMG recordings. The advantage of this method is that it records specifically the muscle activity of the striated external urethral sphincter. However, electrode placement is invasive, can pose technical challenges, and can cause discomfort for patients.

Alternatively, perineal and perianal surface electrode placement is commonly performed and less invasive and offers easier application and increased comfort for the patient. However, the surface electromyographic signal records EMG activity from different pelvic floor muscles, not specifically the external urethral sphincter. Furthermore, the signal quality may be contaminated by artifacts due to body habitus from inadequate electrode adhesion to the skin and electrode displacement or the urinary stream in women tracking down the perineum that may hamper clear EMG reading. The presence of adipose tissue between the muscle and the electrode may dampen the EMG signal.[32]

DSD is diagnosed with increased visual or audible EMG activity from the external urethral sphincter at the time of voiding and detrusor contraction (based on a pathologically increased recruitment of motor units). More specifically, Blaivas and colleagues established a considerable part of current urodynamic technique with the application of concentric needle electrodes in the external urethral sphincter, and defined DSD as increased EMG-activity during an involuntary detrusor contraction.[3] Earlier, Yalla and colleagues described DSD as inappropriate contraction or failure of relaxation of either the internal (smooth muscle) or external (striated muscle) urethral sphincter or both coincident with detrusor contraction, recording simultaneously the activity of the external urethral sphincter by EMG. However, Mayo and colleagues defined DSD as increased EMG-activity from an anal unipolar needle electrode with instruction to void or following a Valsalva maneuver.[33] As discordance was demonstrated between the anal and urethral sphincter in 39% of patients with spinal cord injury, urethral sphincter EMG is recommended for a proper DSD diagnosis.[34]

Recognizing the potential complexities in detecting muscle activity through EMG, the ICS Guidelines on urodynamic equipment standardization advise that EMG recordings during urodynamics should adhere to specific criteria. These criteria include a high input impedance exceeding 100 MΩ, a common-mode rejection ratio greater than 80, and the incorporation of a filtering program. These specifications aim to optimize the consistency of EMG recordings during testing.[35] However, despite this effort of ICS in standardization, published statements regarding EMG technique and reporting vary considerably. One of the reasons of varying terms is that most of the work to establish techniques, which are nowadays used for DSD diagnosis, was performed long before a consensus existed for the definition of DSD. Furthermore, information on standard methodology and recommendations (eg, surface patch electrodes or wire electrodes [monopolar or bipolar] versus needle and type of needle [coaxial versus concentric] for the recording of external sphincter activity) is lacking. In this sense, the standardization of terminology on DSD has been established but as yet no acceptable consensus regarding diagnostic technique exists. Therefore, interpretation of the current literature has to be made cautiously.

Voiding Cystourethrography

Of late, other techniques such as VCUG and VCMG when combined with pressure recordings have been developed. The objective of VCUG is to illustrate both the anatomy and functionality of the urethra and the bladder. This dynamic procedure provides insights into the functioning and coordination of the lower urinary system. More specifically, fluoroscopy shows the effect of myogenic contraction in the external urethral sphincter area.

When using VCUG, DSD is diagnosed in the presence of a dilated bladder neck and posterior urethra proximal to the level of the external urethral sphincter during detrusor contraction on fluoroscopy. Blaivas and colleagues described DSD by VCUG as a dilated posterior urethra obstructed by the external sphincter,[3,36] and Yalla as narrowing of the external sphincter zone.[2]

Advantages of VCUG include the simplicity of the procedure and minimal invasiveness compared with EMG, with less patient discomfort. A disadvantage is that bladder neck dyssynergia (BND) or outlet obstruction from the prostate may preempt visualization of the external sphincter on VCUG, which could explain the higher prevalence of DSD in male patients. Moreover, when performing this investigation, drawbacks such as exposure to (harmful) radiation and increased time and costs of the investigation (eg, additional equipment) have to be considered. In addition, discordance between variables exists. For instance, a closed bladder neck on VCUG makes visualization of the external urethral sphincter impossible.

Urodynamic Investigation (Videocystometrography)

Urodynamic investigation alongside VCUG (so-called VCMG) fundamentally delivers sufficient information to accurately diagnose DSD. Common pathologic findings during filling cystometry include leak-point pressure greater than 40 cm H_2O and low bladder compliance (<20 mL/cm H_2O).

Urethral pressure profilometry
Measurement of the urethral pressure at the level of the external sphincter, and even more simplified, when using a multiple transducer catheter measuring urethral and intravesical pressure simultaneously can help in diagnosing DSD. However, it remains a matter of debate whether urethral (external urethral sphincter) pressure measurement and profilometry should be routinely used to diagnose DSD. Some groups have performed this at the internal and external sphincter level as a complementary measurement, or coupled with EMG recording from the periurethral striated muscles.[2,5,37] Pathognomonic findings on urethral pressure profile are intermittent pressure increases during voiding.[38] Other studies found an additional value of intraurethral pressure measurement to characterize DSD, with a urethral pressure increase greater than 20 cm H_2O (ie, relatively specific cutoff) being a single indicator of DSD in 86% of examined patients.[39,40] Others defined DSD as any urethral pressure increase, maintenance or decrease less than 10 cm H_2O of urethral pressure during voiding phase.[41] Conversely, Suzuki and colleagues concluded that urethral pressure measurement alone is inaccurate to assess DSD.[41]

Continuous urethral pressure profilometry Continuous recording of the urethral pressure profile simultaneously with intravesical pressure has been used to diagnose DSD. Pressures are recorded using 2 microtransducers enclosed in a thin catheter, which is moved at a constant speed through the urethra with the aid of a specially designed withdrawal instrument. As such, closure pressure can be measured simultaneously with the intravesical and intraurethral pressure. The functional as well as the absolute length of the urethra can be estimated with an accuracy of 0.5 mm.

Belluci and colleagues reported false-negative rate of 85% and low positive and negative predictive values for DSD diagnosis.[41] Nevertheless, urethral pressure measurement is commonly used to assess decrease in external urethral sphincter pressure after DSD treatment (eg, intrasphincteric botulinum toxin injection). In summary, the ICS considers it investigational.[42]

Sonography

Transrectal ultrasound as part of the routine examination may play a role in DSD diagnosis as well. Studies from the 1980s suggest superiority in diagnostic accuracy of sonography when compared with VCUG, with additional advantages such as absence of radiation exposure and imaging the periurethral and bladder soft tissue. However, information in the literature remain sparse.

Comparison of All Diagnostic Tools

Although some authors suggest that the burden of EMG might be replaced by urodynamic studies alone (including ice water tests during the filling cystometry),[43,44] the combination of EMG and VCMG is still considered the most acceptable and widely agreed diagnostic method to achieve accurate DSD diagnosis because the combined use of both modalities for diagnosis can identify more DSD cases than either modality alone.[36]

Mayo and colleagues noted 50% agreement between EMG and VCUG for DSD diagnosis. A more recent study demonstrated a 46% disagreement and 54% agreement between patch EMG and VCUG,[32] others report agreement up to 60%.[45]

Moreover, even though external urethral sphincter pressure measurement might theoretically provide sufficient information for DSD-diagnosis and could facilitate urodynamic investigation by replacing combined pelvic floor EMG and VCUG, it is not recommended in daily clinical practice.

In case of clinical suspicion for DSD and absence of EMG activity, VCUG findings should be affirmed with cystoscopic findings alongside with detrusor pressures during contraction and presence of potential autonomic dysreflexia during a contraction, and bladder compliance to confirm the condition of DSD.[45]

DIFFERENTIAL DIAGNOSIS

There are several conditions that can mimic DSD. Importantly, although some authors suggest that DSD can also be observed in patients without spinal cord damage but nonneurological pathologic conditions, and even healthy volunteers,[46] others state that DSD has to be differentiated from BND and from external sphincter dyscoordination (ie, detrusor sphincter dyscoordination, dysfunctional voiding, and nonrelaxing urethral sphincter obstruction) in patients without neurologic disease.[47] BND implicates incomplete opening of the bladder neck during voiding, also named as detrusor-internal sphincter dyssynergia, or proximal sphincter dyssynergia when occurring secondary to a neurologic lesion, and is a failure of the smooth muscle of the bladder neck and proximal urethra to relax during detrusor contraction in the voiding phase,[48] which leads to functional subvesical obstruction.

However, if a clinical DSD picture (particularly with simultaneous detrusor overactivity) is observed in patients without diagnosed neurologic disease, further careful neurologic assessment should be performed to rule out any potential underlying neurologic condition.

Gross and colleagues, however, argue that application of different terms for the same urodynamic observation may not be appropriate, given that patients are not treated according to a definition but based on their genitourinary symptoms, and that the urodynamic phenomenon of a detrusor contraction is only considered by the DSD definition but not by the other terms.[8]

Of note, BND and DSD simultaneously occur in almost all patients with complete spinal cord injury (>T12), whereas paraplegics with incomplete lesions had DSD without BND.[37]

CLINICAL APPROACH

History taking and clinical examination provide valuable information for diagnosis of DSD; however, specialized tests are required to confirm the diagnosis.

History Taking

Patients with DSD may experience urinary retention, urinary urgency, incontinence, and incomplete voiding, among other symptoms. These symptoms can significantly affect quality of life and have to be assessed with a comprehensive evaluation. Medication use, availability of support and circumstances at work and at home should also factored into the assessment.

Of note, assessment of LUT symptoms in neurologic patients (especially with spinal dysraphism or after spinal cord injury) with DSD may be characteristically difficult given their reduced awareness of the LUT.[49] Moreover, normal clinical findings do not exclude underlying pathologic conditions of the CNS.

Clinical Examination

Voluntary pelvic floor (and anal sphincter) contraction and tone, sacral reflexes (eg, bulbocavernosus reflex), perineal examination and sensations of the sacral dermatomes, and the prostate size in men should be examined. Furthermore, patient's ability to perform intermittent self-catheterization should be assessed, for example, by the pencil and paper test.[50] Importantly, the underlying neurologic findings should be reviewed.[51]

Noninvasive Investigations

Noninvasive investigation such as uroflowmetry (intermittent or low flow), postvoid residual (documenting bladder emptying), and bladder diary (eg, documenting voiding volumes and incontinence episodes) provide information about the LUT dysfunction and are interpreted together with more invasive investigations.

Screening urine cultures in the asymptomatic patient are not recommended because it is associated with a risk of overtreating bacterial colonization.

TREATMENT

DSD treatment options are centered around symptomatic management rather that addressing the underlying causative mechanisms. Surveillance alone is however possible in some patients with DSD; however, treatment must be considered in patients with high intravesical storage pressures, postvoid residual, or when urinary symptoms are associated with impaired quality of life. As such, the management plan must be patient centered. Yet, more clinical studies are warranted to improve identification of optimal candidates and to reduce procedural morbidity. Stoffel and colleagues suggest that treating physicians should first identify management goals (eg, quality of life and patient's safety) before initiating any therapy.[5]

Noninvasive Treatment Options

Catheterization

Bladder drainage, preferably with intermittent self-catheterization in combination with antimuscarinics or onabotulinumtoxinA injections into the detrusor (to minimize detrusor pressure) or into the external urethral sphincter (to minimize infravesical resistance) is the most widely adopted approach to treating symptomatic DSD.[52,53] This is specifically indicated in patients with low compliance bladder or significant postvoid residuals to prevent chronic urinary tract infections and progressing hydronephrosis. Frequency of catheterization should be adjusted according to postvoid residual volumes. As mentioned above, it has to be considered whether patients can safely perform intermittent catheterization beforehand to prevent false tracts from occurring. In particular, the catheter should not be advanced beyond the sphincter level, until any spasm is relieved.

If patients are unable to perform intermittent catheterization, long-term urethral or suprapubic indwelling catheter drainage is an option with the latter being preferred given indwelling catheters may cause damage to the LUT if patients report reduced sensations.[54] Treatment options for urinary incontinence in DSD include using a condom catheter in men. However, no satisfactory external collection device exists for women. Long-term indwelling catheterization may be considered as well.

Pharmacotherapy

Oral drugs, in particular alpha-blockers but also antispasmodic medications, such as baclofen, benzodiazepines, or intravesical oxybutynin, have been used in the past; however, there are limited data, no randomized trials, and no information on long-term benefits. As such, the role of pharmacologic agents in DSD treatment is limited.[27,55]

Invasive Treatment Options

Inability to catheterize or the occurrence of complications secondary to DSD is a strong indication to proceed with invasive interventions.

OnabotulinumtoxinA injections into the external urethral sphincter

Injections of onabotulinumtoxinA into the external urethral sphincter induce muscle relaxation and paralysis by preventing the release of acetylcholine from presynaptic vesicles at the neuromuscular junction and causing reduction of the outflow resistance. In general, the duration of its effects is 3 to 4 months. The detrusor can be injected concomitantly into the detrusor to address NDO.[56]

Cystoscopic or ultrasound-guided transperineal injection involves injecting at 2 to 4 places across the dorsal aspect (9–3 o'clock) of the external urethral sphincter and within the detrusor. Administered doses vary from 80 to 250 units onabotulinumtoxinA among different centers.[57,58] Importantly, the effectiveness of repeat injections was found to be similar to that of the initial injection. Therefore, in case of poor response to the first injection patients are less likely to respond to subsequent injections.[59]

A systematic review has analyzed outcomes and efficacy of onabotulinumtoxinA injection as the primary intervention strategy in patients (84% men) suffering from DSD. One month after injection, improvement of urodynamic parameters (ie, reduction in mean urethral pressure, detrusor leak point pressure, and postvoid residual) was reported in 60% to 78% of patients. Reinjection was required in the majority of patients after 4 to 9 months.[52] In a recent study, one-third of patients were also able to resume spontaneous voiding without indwelling catheters.

OnabotulinumtoxinA injections are considered safe without any significant adverse events. Its usage may also improve quality of life. As such, it is a valuable option for patients that wish to avoid, or those who cannot perform, intermittent self-catherization but it is still an off-label treatment in most countries. Injection into the external urethral sphincter may however increase incontinence severity, frequency, and also lead to de novo urinary urgency.[60]

Further research, ideally prospective randomized studies of different doses and type of injection modality with long-term follow-up of repeated sphincter and detrusor injections are needed, especially given that long-term use of detrusor injections may impede detrusor contractility, thereby influencing future treatment options.

Sacral neuromodulation

Minardi and colleagues reported improved refractory urgency urinary incontinence and urinary retention in patients with DSD following SNM. They demonstrated significant decrease in residual volume and incontinence episodes and increased voided volume and number of voiding per day.[61] A systematic review has revealed evidence that sacral neuromodulation (SNM) may be effective and safe for the treatment of patients with neurogenic LUTD, indicating success rates of 77%, 92%, and 100% in patients with spinal cord injury, multiple sclerosis, and Parkinson disease, respectively. Symptom-specific success rates were 73% (chronic urinary retention), 74% (urgency incontinence), 86% (urgency-frequency syndrome), and 84% (combination of chronic urinary retention and urgency-frequency syndrome or urgency incontinence).[62] Several studies report favorable outcomes in patients with neurogenic LUT dysfunction, especially for storage symptom control.[63] However, the effect of SNM on voiding dysfunction is less clear and small open-label studies have demonstrated improvement in DSD[63] but not in patients with detrusor underactivity.[64]

According to the ICS, sacral neuromodulation in patients with spinal cord injury should be limited to ASIA D (incomplete injury with some preservation of motor function below the level) and E (normal sensory and motor function below the injury level) patients with preserved bladder filling sensation.[65] As such, the International Consultation on Incontinence has provided a Grade C recommendation for SNM,[65] whereas the European Association of Urology (EAU guidelines have provided no recommendation.[66] However, there will be relevant recommendation changes in the near future since Liechti and colleagues recently showed in a sham-controlled, double-blind, multicenter trial that SNM effectively corrected refractory neurogenic LUT dysfunction in the short term in well-selected neurologic patients.[67]

Nevertheless, standardized clinical or urodynamic criteria regarding ideal patient selection and success definition for SNM are lacking. Even though most of the evidence is based on DSD patients with multiple sclerosis and incomplete spinal cord injury, data on its use in Parkinson disease, cerebrovascular accident, or brain trauma exist as well.[62] Urodynamic evaluation after stage 1 implantation would help to affirm the disappearance of the DSD before confirming stage 2 implantation.[63]

Urethral stents
Insertion of a temporary or permanent rigid, noncompressible urethral stent across the external sphincter is a controversial option. Although urodynamic parameters may improve (eg, reduced post-void residuals and voiding pressures), the risk for complications (eg, stent removal due to migration, erosion, or autonomic dysreflexia) is considered high, and long-term efficacy seems to be limited.[68]

Endoscopic urethral sphincterotomy
Resection of the external urethral sphincter at the 12 o'clock position (cold knife or electrocautery) is another even more invasive treatment option. It is associated with significant hemorrhage and urinary extravasation at the resection site requiring

catheter drainage for several days. Moreover, the risk for developing other complications (eg, recurrent UTI) is considerable. When considering this procedure, treating physicians should consider that bladder neck obstruction may become more evident following treatment, and that patients may require external urinary collection devices (eg, condom catheter) if the treatment is successful. Although patients may need to undergo repeat procedures, long-term rates greater than 50% have been reported.[69]

Other invasive treatment options
If these therapies mentioned above fail, long-term indwelling urinary catheterization or even urinary diversion with an ileal conduit, or dorsal root rhizotomy with sacral anterior nerve root stimulation may need to be considered to prevent end-stage renal failure.[50]

FOLLOW-UP

Patients with neurogenic LUT dysfunction should be followed-up regularly and in the long-term from both urologic and neurologic perspectives. Given the association between DSD and upper urinary tract involvement, patients at high risk should undergo close monitoring including periodic urodynamic studies to determine whether interventions directed at improving or resolving the condition remain durable over time. It is crucial to prevent complications and to preserve renal function before irreversible damage to the lower and upper urinary tract occurs.[8,49,66,70]

CLINICS CARE POINTS

- High urethral closure pressures during the detrusor contraction can lead to significant complications if DSD is not treated and followed-up regularly.
- Urodynamics with concomitant EMG or fluoroscopy are the most commonly used diagnostic DSD tests.
- Combination of EMG and VCMG is the most acceptable diagnostic method to achieve accurate DSD diagnosis.
- DSD treatment options are centered around symptomatic management rather that addressing the underlying causative mechanisms.
- Bladder drainage in combination with antimuscarinics or onabotulinumtoxinA injections into the detrusor or into the external

urethral sphincter is the most widely adopted approach to treating symptomatic DSD.

- Alternative invasive treatment options include sacral neuromodulation, urethral stents, and endoscopic urethral sphincterotomy.

ACKNOWLEDGMENTS

J.N. Panicker is supported in part by funding from the United Kingdom's Department of Health and Social Care, United Kingdom NIHR University College London Hospitals Biomedical Research Centres funding scheme.

DISCLOSURE

Competing interests: the authors declare no competing interests.

REFERENCES

1. Panicker JN, Fowler CJ, Kessler TM. Lower urinary tract dysfunction in the neurological patient: clinical assessment and management. Lancet Neurol 2015; 14(7):720–32.
2. Yalla SV, Blunt, Fam, et al. Detrusor-urethral sphincter dyssynergia. J Urol 1977;118(6):1026–9.
3. Blaivas JG, Sinha, Zayed, et al. Detrusor-external sphincter dyssynergia: a detailed electromyographic study. J Urol 1981;125(4):545–8.
4. Weld KJ, Graney MJ, Dmochowski RR. Clinical significance of detrusor sphincter dyssynergia type in patients with post-traumatic spinal cord injury. Urology 2000;56(4):565–8.
5. Stoffel JT. Detrusor sphincter dyssynergia: a review of physiology, diagnosis, and treatment strategies. Transl Androl Urol 2016;5(1):127–35.
6. Schurch B, Schmid, Karsenty, et al. Can neurologic examination predict type of detrusor sphincter-dyssynergia in patients with spinal cord injury? Urology 2005;65(2):243–6.
7. Bellucci CH, Wöllner, Gregorini, et al. Acute spinal cord injury–do ambulatory patients need urodynamic investigations? J Urol 2013;189(4):1369–73.
8. Gross O, Leitner, Rasenack, et al. Detrusor sphincter dyssynergia: can a more specific definition distinguish between patients with and without an underlying neurological disorder? Spinal Cord 2021;59(9):1026–33.
9. Wang Z, Deng, Li, et al. The Video-Urodynamic and Electrophysiological Characteristics in Patients With Traumatic Spinal Cord Injury. Int Neurourol J 2021; 25(4):327–36.
10. Araki I, Matsui, Ozawa, et al. Relationship of bladder dysfunction to lesion site in multiple sclerosis. J Urol 2003;169(4):1384–7.
11. Gliga LA, Lavelle, Christie, et al. Urodynamics findings in transverse myelitis patients with lower urinary tract symptoms: Results from a tertiary referral urodynamic center. Neurourol Urodyn 2017;36(2):360–3.
12. Bauer SB, Hallett, Khoshbin, et al. Predictive value of urodynamic evaluation in newborns with myelodysplasia. JAMA 1984;252(5):650–2.
13. Castro NM, Freitas, Rodrigues, et al. Urodynamic features of the voiding dysfunction in HTLV-1 infected individuals. Int Braz J Urol 2007;33(2): 238–45 [discussion: 244–5].
14. Bloch F, Pichon, Bonnet, et al. Urodynamic analysis in multiple system atrophy: characterisation of detrusor-sphincter dyssynergia. J Neurol 2010;257(12): 1986–91.
15. Kitta T, Ouchi, Chiba, et al. Animal Model for Lower Urinary Tract Dysfunction in Parkinson's Disease. Int J Mol Sci 2020;21(18).
16. Yeo L, Singh, Gundeti, et al. Urinary tract dysfunction in Parkinson's disease: a review. Int Urol Nephrol 2012;44(2):415–24.
17. Meng NH, Lo, Chou, et al. Incomplete bladder emptying in patients with stroke: is detrusor external sphincter dyssynergia a potential cause? Arch Phys Med Rehabil 2010;91(7):1105–9.
18. Fowler CJ. Integrated control of lower urinary tract–clinical perspective. Br J Pharmacol 2006; 147(Suppl 2):S14–24.
19. Pullen AH, Tucker D, Martin JE. Morphological and morphometric characterisation of Onuf's nucleus in the spinal cord in man. J Anat 1997;191(Pt 2): 201–13.
20. Fowler CJ, Griffiths D, de Groat WC. The neural control of micturition. Nat Rev Neurosci 2008;9(6): 453–66.
21. Nevéus T, Sillén U. Lower urinary tract function in childhood; normal development and common functional disturbances. Acta Physiol 2013;207(1): 85–92.
22. Bachelard M, Sillén, Hansson, et al. Urodynamic pattern in asymptomatic infants: siblings of children with vesicoureteral reflux. J Urol 1999;162(5):1733–8 [discussion: 1737-8].
23. Yeung CK, Godley, Dhillon, et al. Urodynamic patterns in infants with normal lower urinary tracts or primary vesico-ureteric reflux. Br J Urol 1998;81(3): 461–7.
24. de Groat WC, Kawatani, Hisamitsu, et al. Mechanisms underlying the recovery of urinary bladder function following spinal cord injury. J Auton Nerv Syst 1990;30:S71–7.
25. McGuire EJ, Woodside, Borden, et al. Prognostic value of urodynamic testing in myelodysplastic patients. J Urol 1981;126(2):205–9.
26. Perkash I. Urodynamic patterns after traumatic spinal cord injury. J Spinal Cord Med 2015;38(2):134.

27. Bacsu CD, Chan L, Tse V. Diagnosing detrusor sphincter dyssynergia in the neurological patient. BJU Int 2012;109(Suppl 3):31–4.

28. Fletcher SG, Dillon, Gilchrist, et al. Renal deterioration in multiple sclerosis patients with neurovesical dysfunction. Mult Scler 2013;19(9):1169–74.

29.. de Sèze M, Ruffion A, Denys P, et al. The neurogenic bladder in multiple sclerosis: review of the literature and proposal of management guidelines. Mult Scler 2007;13(7):915–28.

30. Petersen JA, Spiess, Curt, et al. Spinal cord injury: one-year evolution of motor-evoked potentials and recovery of leg motor function in 255 patients. Neurorehabil Neural Repair 2012;26(8):939–48.

31. Zörner B, Blanckenhorn WU, Dietz V, et al. Clinical algorithm for improved prediction of ambulation and patient stratification after incomplete spinal cord injury. J Neurotrauma 2010;27(1):241–52.

32. Spettel S, Kalorin C, De E. Combined diagnostic modalities improve detection of detrusor external sphincter dyssynergia. ISRN Obstet Gynecol 2011; 2011:323421.

33. Mayo ME. The value of sphincter electromyography in urodynamics. J Urol 1979;122(3):357–60.

34. Koyanagi T, Arikado, Takamatsu, et al. Experience with electromyography of the external urethral sphincter in spinal cord injury patients. J Urol 1982;127(2):272–6.

35. Gammie A, Bosch, Djurhuus, et al. Do we need better methods of assessing urethral function: ICI-RS 2013? Neurourol Urodyn 2014;33(5):587–90.

36. Blaivas JG, Fisher DM. Combined radiographic and urodynamic monitoring: advances in technique. J Urol 1981;125(5):693–4.

37. Schurch B, Yasuda K, Rossier AB. Detrusor bladder neck dyssynergia revisited. J Urol 1994;152(6 Pt 1): 2066–70.

38. Yalla SV, Yap W, Fam BA. Detrusor urethral sphincter dyssynergia: micturitional vesicourethral pressure profile patterns. J Urol 1982;128(5):969–73.

39. Bary PR, Day, Lewis, et al. Dynamic urethral function in the assessment of spinal injury patients. Br J Urol 1982;54(1):39–44.

40. Corona LE, Cameron, Clemens, et al. Urethral Pressure Measurement as a Tool for the Urodynamic Diagnosis of Detrusor Sphincter Dyssynergia. Int Neurourol J 2018;22(4):268–74.

41. Suzuki Bellucci CH, Wöllner, Gregorini, et al. External urethral sphincter pressure measurement: an accurate method for the diagnosis of detrusor external sphincter dyssynergia? PLoS One 2012; 7(5):e37996.

42. Lose G, Griffiths, Hosker, et al. Standardisation of urethral pressure measurement: report from the Standardisation Sub-Committee of the International Continence Society. Neurourol Urodyn 2002;21(3): 258–60.

43. Geirsson G, Fall M. The ice-water test in the diagnosis of detrusor-external sphincter dyssynergia. Scand J Urol Nephrol 1995;29(4):457–61.

44.. Schäfer W, Abrams P, Liao L, et al. Good urodynamic practices: uroflowmetry, filling cystometry, and pressure-flow studies. Neurourol Urodyn 2002;21(3):261–74.

45. De EJ, Patel, Tharian, et al. Diagnostic discordance of electromyography (EMG) versus voiding cystourethrogram (VCUG) for detrusor-external sphincter dyssynergy (DESD). Neurourol Urodyn 2005;24(7): 616–21.

46. Leitner L, Walter, Sammer, et al. Urodynamic Investigation: A Valid Tool to Define Normal Lower Urinary Tract Function? PLoS One 2016;11(10):e0163847.

47.. Hoang-Böhm J, Lusch A, Sha W, Alken P. Biofeedback bei kindlichen Blasenfunktionsstörungen. Indikationen, praktische Durchführung und Therapieergebnisse [Biofeedback for urinary bladder dysfunctions in childhood. Indications, practice and the results of therapy]. Urologe A 2004;43(7):813–9.

48. Tosaka A, Murota-Kawano A, Ando M. Video urodynamics using transrectal ultrasonography for lower urinary tract symptoms in women. Neurourol Urodyn 2003;22(1):33–9.

49.. Schöps TF, Schneider MP, Steffen F, et al. Neurogenic lower urinary tract dysfunction (NLUTD) in patients with spinal cord injury: long-term urodynamic findings. BJU Int 2015;115(Suppl 6):33–8.

50. Mahfouz W, Corcos J. Management of detrusor external sphincter dyssynergia in neurogenic bladder. Eur J Phys Rehabil Med 2011;47(4):639–50.

51. Rosier P, Schaefer, Lose, et al. International Continence Society Good Urodynamic Practices and Terms 2016: Urodynamics, uroflowmetry, cystometry, and pressure-flow study. Neurourol Urodyn 2017;36(5):1243–60.

52. Goel S, Pierce, Pain, et al. Use of Botulinum Toxin A (BoNT-A) in Detrusor External Sphincter Dyssynergia (DESD): A Systematic Review and Meta-analysis. Urology 2020;140:7–13.

53. Schurch B, Hauri, Rodic, et al. Botulinum-A toxin as a treatment of detrusor-sphincter dyssynergia: a prospective study in 24 spinal cord injury patients. J Urol 1996;155(3):1023–9.

54. Stoffel JT, McGuire EJ. Outcome of urethral closure in patients with neurologic impairment and complete urethral destruction. Neurourol Urodyn 2006;25(1): 19–22.

55. Klausner AP, Steers WD. The neurogenic bladder: an update with management strategies for primary care physicians. Med Clin North Am 2011;95(1): 111–20.

56. Apostolidis A, Dasgupta, Denys, et al. Recommendations on the use of botulinum toxin in the treatment of lower urinary tract disorders and pelvic floor

dysfunctions: a European consensus report. Eur Urol 2009;55(1):100–19.

57. Utomo E, Groen J, Blok BF. Surgical management of functional bladder outlet obstruction in adults with neurogenic bladder dysfunction. Cochrane Database Syst Rev 2014;(5):Cd004927.

58. Schurch B, de Sèze, Denys, et al. Botulinum toxin type a is a safe and effective treatment for neurogenic urinary incontinence: results of a single treatment, randomized, placebo controlled 6-month study. J Urol 2005;174(1):196–200.

59. Soler JM, Previnaire JG, Hadiji N. Predictors of outcome for urethral injection of botulinum toxin to treat detrusor sphincter dyssynergia in men with spinal cord injury. Spinal Cord 2016;54(6):492–6.

60. Kuo HC. Satisfaction with urethral injection of botulinum toxin A for detrusor sphincter dyssynergia in patients with spinal cord lesion. Neurourol Urodyn 2008;27(8):793–6.

61. Minardi D, Muzzonigro G. Sacral neuromodulation in patients with multiple sclerosis. World J Urol 2012; 30(1):123–8.

62. Kessler TM, La Framboise, Trelle, et al. Sacral neuromodulation for neurogenic lower urinary tract dysfunction: systematic review and meta-analysis. Eur Urol 2010;58(6):865–74.

63. Chaabane W, Guillotreau, Castel-Lacanal, et al. Sacral neuromodulation for treating neurogenic bladder dysfunction: clinical and urodynamic study. Neurourol Urodyn 2011;30(4):547–50.

64. Lombardi G, Nelli, Mencarini, et al. Clinical concomitant benefits on pelvic floor dysfunctions after sacral neuromodulation in patients with incomplete spinal cord injury. Spinal Cord 2011;49(5):629–36.

65. Goldman HB, Lloyd, Noblett, et al. International Continence Society best practice statement for use of sacral neuromodulation. Neurourol Urodyn 2018; 37(5):1823–48.

66. EAU Guidelines on Neuro-Urology. edn presented at the EAU Annual Congress Milan. 2023. SBN 978-94-92671-19-6. March 10-13, 2023, The Allianz MiCo Conference Center; Milan, Italy.

67. Liechti MD, van der Lely S, Knüpfer SC, et al. Sacral Neuromodulation for Neurogenic Lower Urinary Tract Dysfunction. NEJM Evid 2022;1(11). EVIDoa2200071.

68. Mehta SS, Tophill PR. Memokath stents for the treatment of detrusor sphincter dyssynergia (DSD) in men with spinal cord injury: the Princess Royal Spinal Injuries Unit 10-year experience. Spinal Cord 2006;44(1):1–6.

69. Vainrib M, Reyblat P, Ginsberg DA. Long-term efficacy of repeat incisions of bladder neck/external sphincter in patients with spinal cord injury. Urology 2014;84(4):940–5.

70. van der Lely SL, Bachmann, Mehnert. Quantitative electrical pain threshold assessment in the lower urinary tract. Neurourol Urodyn 2020;39(1):420–31.

Questionnaires for Neurogenic Lower Urinary Tract Dysfunction

Blayne Welk, MD, MSc[a,b],*

KEYWORDS

- Neurogenic bladder • Patient-reported outcomes • Spinal cord injury • Multiple sclerosis
- Questionnaire

KEY POINTS

- Disease and symptom-specific quality of life (QOL) questionnaires are available for the neurogenic lower urinary tract dysfunction (NLUTD) population.
- Examples of urinary-specific questionnaires in this population include Qualiveen, Neurogenic Bladder Symptom Score, Actionable Bladder Symptom Screening Tool-Short Form, Incontinence Quality of Life Questionnaire, SCI-QOL bladder management difficulties/bladder complications, Incontinence severity index-pediatric, and the Urinary Symptom Questionnaire for individuals with neurogenic bladder.
- Although many NLUTD studies historically used unvalidated QOL questionnaires, the availability of established patient-reported outcome measures that are psychometrically validated allows researchers to use appropriate tools to assess urinary-related QOL and symptoms in the NLUTD population.
- Future research should further develop and integrate these QOL questionnaires into clinical practice to enhance the care and decision-making processes for individuals with NLUTD.

INTRODUCTION

In clinical research, our goal is often to measure an exposure or outcome accurately. In some cases, this is easy; for example, blood pressure and weight, are physical characteristics that are readily and accurately assessable. However, the measurement of something that is a concept rather than a physical characteristic, for example, quality of life (QOL), is more challenging. In this situation, we can use patient-reported outcome measures that seek to assess this abstract concept in a valid and reliable manner.

The field of neurogenic lower urinary tract dysfunction (NLUTD) research is one that is well suited to including a measure of QOL. There are of course objective parameters that drive management of NLUTD, for example, urodynamic parameters or measures of renal function or anatomy; however, there are also important QOL considerations that are included when contemplating a medical or surgical intervention. Patient-centered care and shared decision-making is an important model of care delivery that emphasizes that patients should consider their QOL when making decisions about NLUTD treatment.

The science of understanding QOL has evolved significantly during the last 70 years, and physicians and researchers should be aware of a few specific considerations when assessing QOL.

[a] Department of Surgery, Western University, 268 Grosvenor Street, London, Onatrio N6A 4V2, Canada;
[b] Department of Epidemiology and Biostatistics, Western University, 268 Grosvenor Street, London, Ontario N6A 4V2, Canada
* Corresponding author.
E-mail address: blayne.welk@sjhc.london.on.ca

Urol Clin N Am 51 (2024) 233–238
https://doi.org/10.1016/j.ucl.2024.01.004

First, is the concept of general QOL versus disease-specific QOL. In general QOL, the patient is asked about their overall physician and mental well-being; perhaps, one of the most commonly used questionnaires is the SF-12.[1] It has questions that address body pain, limitations in the person's physical/social/usual role because of physical/emotional problems, and vitality. This questionnaire asks the person to consider their overall ability to function in life due to the sum of all the health factors that may affect them. In disease-specific QOL, the patient is asked to focus on the impact of a specific disease process or body organ on their health (ie, "Is your life regulated by your bladder problems?"). Second is the perspective from which QOL is measured; this can be the viewpoint of the patient, those around the patient, or the health-care professional. In medicine, and NLUTD, most QOL questionnaires are designed to be completed by the patient and to measure their viewpoint because this is patient-focused and arguably the most important viewpoint.

Once the decisions about whether to measure general or disease-specific QOL, and which viewpoint to measure it from, have been made, then the specific characteristics of the possible QOL measures become relevant.[2] Some are designed to be cross-sectional (ie, differentiate QOL at a single time point or administration), predictive (ie, predict something such as the need for referral or further treatment), or responsive (ie, demonstrate a change after an intervention). The validity of the QOL measurement for the researcher's/clinician's purpose can be best assessed by reviewing the development of the QOL questionnaire. Understanding how the items were generated, and how they were tested is important. It is important to ensure that the proposed tool is valid (by assessing face validity, numerical tests such as Cronbach's alpha or interclass coefficient, and construct validity with tests of relationships to other questionnaires or variables) and reliable (meaning that it is consistent in its ability to measure QOL, and usually demonstrated by asking the patient to complete the questionnaire at 2 time points, and ensuring the answers are appropriately correlated). Additional factors, such as the feasibility (how easy will it be for people to complete the questionnaire based on factors such as readability, time requirement, and educational level), responsiveness (whether the score change in the expected direction after an intervention), and interpretability (how to relate a numerical score change to a real-world "anchor" such as need for treatment, or whether the change is apparent to the patient) may be relevant.

NATURE OF THE PROBLEM

A systematic review article examined the use of QOL questionnaires in NLUTD between 2000 and 2014.[3] It found that there were only 39 articles in this time period that used QOL questionnaires, and aside from the use of the Qualiveen questionnaire (in 6 out of 39 of the studies),[4] all the rest of the questionnaires were not specifically developed for NLUTD (although the Incontinence Quality of Life Questionnaire [I-QOL] was developed for women with stress/mixed urinary incontinence, it was used in 4 out of 39 studies and has been cross-validated in people with multiple sclerosis (MS) and spinal cord injury [SCI][5]). This review highlighted the limited research on QOL in NLUTD, and the lack of questionnaire development in this patient population. However, during the last decade, new questionnaires that measure QOL in NLUTD have been developed. The objective of this article is to review the questionnaires and QOL measures that are of specific relevance to NLUTD.

CURRENT EVIDENCE

The following questionnaires are of special relevance to the NLUTD population because they focus specifically on bladder-related QOL or symptoms. A brief overview of the questionnaires, their purpose, and the specific populations they have been studied in is shown in **Table 1**.

1. Qualiveen and Qualiveen-SF: This questionnaire was the first validated, bladder-specific QOL questionnaire specific to an NLUTD population (in this case SCI).[4] This questionnaire was originally developed in French, and the English language version was validated in 2006.[6] The full version has 30 questions, and a short form (SF) with 8 questions has also been published.[7] It has 4 QOL domains that it assesses: bother with limitations, fears, feeling, and frequency of limitations. It has since been validated in people with MS,[8] and the ability to transform the SF score from ordinal data to interval data has been proven with Rasch modeling.[9] When scores for each domain are converted to a summary score of 0 to 4, a change of 0.5 was found to be the minimally important difference, and a change of 0.7 was a moderate change in QOL.[10] As a result of its maturity, it has been used in several studies in the NLUTD population, and validated translations/cultural adaptations have been published (including Arabic, German, Turkish, Russian, Greek, Polish, Dutch, Spanish, Italian, Portuguese, and Persian).

Table 1
Basic characteristics, including the intended purpose and validated population of NLUTD-related questionnaires

Questionnaire	SF Available	Translations	Purpose	Validated NLUTD Populations
Qualiveen	Yes	Multiple	Assess NLUTD-related QOL	SCI and MS
NBSS	Yes	Multiple	Assess NLUTD-related symptoms/consequences, and QOL	SCI, MS, SB, and cerebral palsy
ABSST	Yes	Multiple	Predict need for referral to a urologist	MS
I-QOL	No	Multiple	Assess incontinence-related QOL	SCI and MS
SCI-QOL bladder management difficulties	Yes/Computer-adaptive	No	Assess bladder-related QOL	SCI
SCI-QOL bladder complications	No	No	Assess UTI-related QOL	SCI
ISI-P	No	No	Assess incontinence-related QOL	Adolescents with SB
USQNB (USQNB-IC, USQNB-IDC, and USQNB-V)	No	No	Assess symptoms potentially related to NLUTD UTI	SCI, MS, and SB

2. Neurogenic bladder symptom score (NBSS): This is a validated questionnaire that can be used to assess symptoms in the NLUTD population (specifically those with SCI, MS, and spina bifida).[11,12] It has 3 domains (incontinence, storage and voiding, and consequences) with a total of 24 questions. These questions assess symptoms rather than QOL, similar to how prostate-related urinary symptoms can be scored based on their frequency with the American Urological Association (AUA) symptom score. It has a single, separate QOL question which asks, "If you had to live the rest of your life with the way your bladder (or urinary reservoir) currently works, how would you feel," which is scored from "pleased" to "unhappy" with a total of 5 possible answers. Additional research has validated it a second population of people exclusively with SCI[13] and demonstrated that it is responsive to change.[14] It has also been shown to be valid in people with cerebral palsy, although the nonscored question around type of toileting may need refinement.[15] A short form has been developed,[16] and similar to the Qualiveen, validated translations/cultural adaptations have been developed (including French, Spanish, Russian, Portuguese, Persian, Arabic, Japanese, Polish, Greek, and Turkish).

3. The I-QOL: This questionnaire was originally developed for use in women with stress incontinence and overactive bladder.[17] It has 22 items in total that address 3 domains related to QOL (avoiding and limiting factors, psychosocial impact, and social embarrassment). It was subsequently validated in people with SCI and MS[5] in order for it to be used in several of the large regulatory trials of onabotulinum toxin. It has been well studied in the non-NLUTD population, and there are several translations available. One important strength of this questionnaire is that a mapping algorithm has been developed for the EuroQol five-dimensional questionnaire index scores, which allows you to estimate health utilities and conduct health economic evaluations such as quality-adjusted life years.[18] Limitations of this tool include the fact that it only assesses incontinence symptoms, and it was not originally developed for NLUTD or for men.

4. Actionable Bladder Symptom Screening Tool-Short Form (ABSST): This tool was developed to screen people with MS and identify those with more significant urinary symptoms that may need further assessment.[19,20] It evaluates bladder symptoms, coping strategies, and the impact of bladder symptoms. The original full version suggested a score of 8 or greater on the 17 different questions would have a positive predictive value (PPV) of 76% and a negative predictive value (NPV) of 95% for correctly

identifying patients with MS receiving a referral to a urologist. The SF version (with only 8 items) and a simplified scoring system may be quicker to use; however, the PPV and NPV are lower.[21] Translations have been published in Turkish, Persian, Spanish, and Dutch.

5. The spinal cord injury quality of life (SCI-QOL) bladder management difficulties, and SCI-QOL bladder complications: These are 2 of the large number of computer adaptive questionnaires that were developed to measure physical, emotional, and social aspects of QOL after SCI.[22] Relevant to the bladder, 2 item banks were created that were specific to bladder dysfunction.[23] The final set of items for the bladder management difficulties included 15 possible questions, while a second set of 5 items, specific to urinary tract infections, was used to create the bladder complications questionnaire. Advantages of these questionnaires are that they are computer adaptive and therefore able to omit questions based on the answers to the initial questions in order to minimize the number of questions for a respondent.

6. Incontinence severity index-pediatric (ISI-P): This was originally developed for adults with incontinence and modified to account for insensate incontinence. It has 11 questions, which are categorized into 2 domains: urinary incontinence symptom severity and urinary incontinence impairment. In a small study of 33 adolescents with SB, it was found to be valid and reliable.[24]

7. Urinary Symptom Questionnaire for individuals with neurogenic bladder (USQNB): This questionnaire was developed to measure patient relevant symptoms in people living with SCI or SB who use intermittent catheters (USQNB-IC)[25] or who use indwelling catheter (USQNB-IDC) or are able to void (USQNB-V), with the later 2 developed in people with SCI or MS.[26,27] The questions focus on symptoms potentially related to urinary tract infections (UTIs). The goal is to use the USQNB questionnaire to better treat UTIs in this patient population. This is an intriguing, patient-centered approach to UTI identification in the NLUTD population, and initial study on the interpretability of the score shows promise.[28]

There are also questionnaires that are disease-specific and include different levels of assessment of bladder dysfunction as part of their overall assessment. Examples for common NLUTD diseases include the Multiple Sclerosis Quality of Life 54 item[29] scale, which has a question on bladder function. The Quality of Life in Spina Bifida[30] scale has questions for both the parent and the child and includes a question about suitability of washroom facilities. A more contemporary questionnaire for adults with spina bifida (QUALAS-A: QUAlity of Life Assessment in Spina bifida for Adults)[31] has an entire domain that addresses bladder and bowel-related QOL. For people living with SCI, the Spinal Cord Injury Functional Index[32] is a comprehensive questionnaire with 90 items on self-care (including bladder and bowel).

DISCUSSION

The goal of this article was to present questionnaires that tackle specific aspects of NLUTD. For the most part, these questionnaires are still used primarily for research purposes; however, hopefully future studies will allow these tools to move into the realm of clinical care, similar to how the AUA symptom score, or the International Consultation on Incontinence Questionnaires have transitioned into day-to-day clinical care because of their clear interpretability and ability to directly impact patient-level decision-making. A survey of urologists who provide care to people with NLUTD identified a need for further questionnaire development to support shared decision-making.[33]

Authors have summarized the evidence regarding questionnaires in NLUTD in prior systematic reviews. Tsang and colleagues identified questionnaires for people with SCI and MS that addressed NLUTD.[34] They identified 18 questionnaires, the vast majority of which were disease-specific general QOL questionnaires for people with MS; only the Qualiveen and I-QOL were published at the time of their search. Most of these questionnaires addressed physical function, psychosocial impact, and/or social relationships directly or peripherally in the context of NLUTD. A subsequent systematic review published in 2017 identified 42 studies that assessed NLUTD in people with SCI.[35] Importantly, most of the studies used general SCI QOL questionnaires, and among those that did use bladder-specific tools, many were not validated or designed for people with NLUTD.

A large group of content experts was assembled to review clinical assessments/diagnostic tools, common data sets, and questionnaires relevant to people with SCI.[36] Their goal was to define measures that should be used in SCI clinical care and research. They highly recommended the use of the Qualiveen questionnaire as a QOL endpoint due to its use in several studies involving people with SCI, and the fact that there are multiple published validation studies. The NBSS, SCI-QOL bladder management difficulties, and SCI-QOL bladder complications were recommended as supplemental measures.

In conclusion, there are now several established and developing patient reported outcome measures that are available for use in NLUTD research. They are supported by standard psychometric validation and reliability testing, and should be considered as the preferred way to assess urinary-related QOL or symptoms in this patient population.

CLINICS CARE POINTS

- The Qualiveen, NBSS, and SCI-QOL bladder management difficulties and bladder complications should be considered for use in clinical research.
- Further research is needed to better understand how these questionnaires can help guide clinical management.

DISCLOSURE

Dr B. Welk has been a consultant for BD Company.

REFERENCES

1. Ware J, Kosinski M, Keller SD. A 12-item short-form health survey: construction of scales and preliminary tests of reliability and validity. Med Care 1996;34(3): 220–33.
2. Hundleby JD, Nunnally J. Psychometric theory. Am Educ Res J 1968;5(3):431.
3. Patel DP, Elliott SP, Stoffel JT, et al. Patient reported outcomes measures in neurogenic bladder and bowel: a systematic review of the current literature. Neurourol Urodyn 2016;35(1):8–14.
4. Costa P, Perrouin-Verbe B, Colvez A, et al. Quality of life in spinal cord injury patients with urinary difficulties. development and validation of qualiveen. Eur Urol 2001;39(1):107–13.
5. Schurch B, Denys P, Kozma CM, et al. Reliability and validity of the incontinence quality of life questionnaire in patients with neurogenic urinary incontinence. Arch Phys Med Rehabil 2007;88(5):646–52.
6. Bonniaud V, Parratte B. Adaptation culturelle d'un questionnaire de qualité de vie : Qualiveen en langue anglaise. Ann Readapt Med Phys 2006; 49(3):92–9.
7. Bonniaud V, Bryant D, Parratte B, et al. Development and validation of the short form of a urinary quality of life questionnaire: SF-qualiveen. J Urol 2008;180(6): 2592–8.

8. Bonniaud V, Bryant D, Parratte B, et al. Qualiveen: a urinary disorder-specific instrument for use in clinical trials in multiple sclerosis. Arch Phys Med Rehabil 2006;87(12):1661–3.
9. Milinis K, Tennant A, Young CA, et al. Rasch analysis of SF-qualiveen in multiple sclerosis. Neurourol Urodyn 2017;36(4):1161–6.
10. Bonniaud V, Bryant D, Parratte B, et al. Qualiveen, a urinary-disorder specific instrument: 0.5 corresponds to the minimal important difference. J Clin Epidemiol 2008;61(5):505–10.
11. Welk B, Morrow S, Madarasz W, et al. The validity and reliability of the neurogenic bladder symptom score. J Urol 2014;192(2):452–7.
12. Welk B, Morrow SA, Madarasz W, et al. The conceptualization and development of a patient-reported neurogenic bladder symptom score. Res Rep Urol 2013;5:129–37.
13. Welk B, Lenherr S, Elliott S, et al. The neurogenic bladder symptom score (NBSS): a secondary assessment of its validity, reliability among people with a spinal cord injury. Spinal Cord 2018;56(3): 259–64.
14. Welk B, Carlson K, Baverstock R. A pilot study of the responsiveness of the neurogenic bladder symptom score (NBSS). Canadian Urological Association journal = Journal de l'Association des urologues du Canada 2017;11(12):376–8.
15. Pariser JJ, Welk B, Kennelly M, et al. (NBRG.org) for the NBRG. reliability and validity of the neurogenic bladder symptom score in adults with cerebral palsy. Urology 2019;128:107–11.
16. Welk B, Lenherr S, Elliott S, et al. The creation and validation of a short form of the Neurogenic Bladder Symptom Score. Neurourol Urodyn 2020; 35(1):8.
17. Patrick DL, Martin ML, Bushnell DM, et al. Quality of life of women with urinary incontinence: further development of the incontinence quality of life instrument (I-QOL). Urology 1999;53(1):71–6.
18. Kay S, Tolley K, Colayco D, et al. Mapping EQ-5D utility scores from the incontinence quality of life questionnaire among patients with neurogenic and idiopathic overactive bladder. Value Health 2013; 16(2):394–402.
19. Bates D, Burks J, Globe D, et al. Development of a short form and scoring algorithm from the validated actionable bladder symptom screening tool. BMC Neurol 2013;13:78.
20. Burks J, Chancellor M, Bates D, et al. Development and validation of the actionable bladder symptom screening tool for multiple sclerosis patients. Int J MS Care 2013;15(4):182–92.
21. Jongen PJ, Blok BF, Heesakkers JP, et al. Simplified scoring of the Actionable 8-item screening questionnaire for neurogenic bladder overactivity in multiple sclerosis: a comparative analysis of test

performance at different cut-off points. BMC Urol 2015;15(1):106.

22. Tulsky DS, Kisala PA, Victorson D, et al. Developing a contemporary patient-reported outcomes measure for spinal cord injury. Arch Phys Med Rehabil 2011; 92(10 Suppl):S44–51.

23. Tulsky DS, Kisala PA, Tate DG, et al. Development and psychometric characteristics of the SCI-QOL Bladder Management difficulties and bowel management difficulties item banks and short forms and the SCI-QOL bladder complications scale. Journal of Spinal Cord Medicine 2015;38(3):288–302.

24. Hubert KC, Sideridis G, Sherlock R, et al. Urinary incontinence in spina bifida: Initial instrument validation. Res Dev Disabil 2015;40:42–50.

25. Tractenberg RE, Groah SL, Rounds AK, et al. Preliminary validation of a urinary symptom questionnaire for individuals with neuropathic bladder using intermittent catheterization (USQNB-IC): a patient-centered patient reported outcome. PLoS One 2018;13(7):e0197568.

26. Tractenberg RE, Frost JK, Yumoto F, et al. Reliability of the Urinary Symptom Questionnaires for people with neurogenic bladder (USQNB) who void or use indwelling catheters. Spinal Cord 2021;59(9):939–47.

27. Tractenberg RE, Frost JK, Yumoto F, et al. Validity of the Urinary Symptom Questionnaires for people with neurogenic bladder (USQNB) who void or use indwelling catheters. Spinal Cord 2021;59(9):948–58.

28. Tractenberg RE, Groah SL, Rounds AK, et al. Clinical profiles and symptom burden estimates to support decision-making using the urinary symptom questionnaire for people with neurogenic bladder (USQNB) using intermittent catheters. PMR 2021; 13(3):229–40.

29. Vickrey BG, Hays RD, Harooni R, et al. A health-related quality of life measure for multiple sclerosis. Qual Life Res 1995;4(3):187–206.

30. Parkin PC, Kirpalani HM, Rosenbaum PL, et al. Development of a health-related quality of life instrument for use in children with spina bifida. Qual Life Res : An International Journal of Quality of Life Aspects of Treatment, Care and Rehabilitation 1997; 6(2):123–32.

31. Szymanski KM, Misseri R, Whittam B, et al. QUAlity of Life Assessment in Spina bifida for Adults (QUALAS- A): development and international validation of a novel health- related quality of life instrument. Qual Life Res : An International Journal of Quality of Life Aspects of Treatment, Care and Rehabilitation 2015;1–10. https://doi.org/10.1007/s11136-015-0988-5.

32. Jette AM, Slavin MD, Ni P, et al. Development and initial evaluation of the SCI-FI/AT. Journal of Spinal Cord Medicine 2015;38(3):409–18.

33. Fendereski K, Hebert KJ, Matta R, et al. Variation in provider practice patterns and the perceived need for a shared decision-making tool for neurogenic lower urinary tract dysfunction. Urology 2023;174: 185–90.

34. Tsang B, Stothers L, Macnab A, et al. A systematic review and comparison of questionnaires in the management of spinal cord injury, multiple sclerosis and the neurogenic bladder. Neurourol Urodyn 2016;35(3):354–64.

35. Best KL, Ethans K, Craven BC, et al. Identifying and classifying quality of life tools for neurogenic bladder function after spinal cord injury: A systematic review. J Spinal Cord Med 2017;40(5):505–29.

36. Tate DG, Wheeler T, Lane GI, et al. Recommendations for evaluation of neurogenic bladder and bowel dysfunction after spinal cord injury and/or disease. J Spinal Cord Medicine 2020;43(2):141–64.

An Overview of the Effect of Aging on the Female Urethra

Andrew S. Afyouni, BS[a], Yi Xi Wu, PhD[a], Ulysses G.J. Balis, MD[b],
John DeLancey, MD[c], Zhina Sadeghi, MD[a],*

KEYWORDS

- Female urethral aging • Urinary incontinence • Urethral striated muscle • Urethral imaging

KEY POINTS

- Aging causes a reduction in closure pressure in the female urethra, contributing to urinary incontinence (UI).
- Aging leads to the loss of striated muscle and increased connective tissue proportion, thereby reducing urethral closure pressure and increasing the risk of stress UI.
- Age-related alterations affect smooth muscle, causing weakening of urethral tone and resistance to intra-abdominal pressure.
- Aging influences vascular and neurophysiological aspects of the urethra, impacting its ability to maintain continence.
- MRI and ultrasound can provide essential insights into aging-related urethral changes, advancing our understanding of UI and informing prevention and treatment strategies.

INTRODUCTION

Recent evidence shows that the female urethra is pivotal in maintaining urinary continence throughout a woman's life.[1] However, as women age, the dynamics of the urethra and its surrounding structures can undergo significant changes, leading to various degrees of urinary incontinence (UI). This section explores the role of female urethra aging in UI, shedding light on the intricate interplay of factors that contribute to this common and often distressing condition.

Defining Urinary Incontinence

UI is defined as the involuntary leakage of urine, and it encompasses several subtypes, such as stress incontinence, urge incontinence, and mixed incontinence. Classical thinking held that stress urinary incontinence (SUI) results from abnormal urethral support, which is provided by suburethral tissues and regulated by pelvic floor reflexes and voluntary control.[1] Urge urinary incontinence (UUI) has been considered to be a consequence of detrusor overactivity, which is similarly governed by a complex interplay between somatic and visceral innervations.[2,3] Finally, recent large case-control studies have demonstrated that urethral failure, defined as the inability to provide adequate closure pressure within the urethra, is the most contributory cause of SUI and an important contributing factor for UUI, which possibly explains why many women experience mixed urinary

a Division of Neurourology and Reconstructive Pelvic Surgery, Department of Urology, University of California Irvine, 3800 W. Chapman Avenue, Suite 7200, Orange, CA 92868, USA; b Division of Pathology Informatics, Department of Pathology, University of Michigan Medical School, 2800 Plymouth Road, NCRC Building 35, Ann Arbor, MI 48109, USA; c Department of Obstetrics and Gynecology, University of Michigan Medical School, L4208 UH South, 1500 East Medical Center Drive, Ann Arbor, MI 48109, USA
* Corresponding author.
E-mail address: ZhinaS@hs.uci.edu

Urol Clin N Am 51 (2024) 239–251
https://doi.org/10.1016/j.ucl.2024.02.001

urologic.theclinics.com

symptoms.[4,5] This observation led to the proposal of a "three-factor paradigm," as first outlined by DeLancey and colleagues[6] (**Fig. 1**). Each of the 3 components of this paradigm contributes to continence—an issue with even one of the factors can cause a woman to become incontinent. Because urethral function declines by 15% each decade,[7] even in the absence of childbirth, understanding the role of urethral failure in the aging population is important.

The Prevalence and Significance of Urinary Incontinence in Aging Women

Nearly 25% to 50% of women will experience UI at some point during their lifetimes.[8,9] Both the prevalence and severity of incontinence increase with age. Current epidemiologic data suggest that the overall prevalence of UI ranges from 20% in women aged over 20 years and increases to roughly 40% to 50% in women aged older than 60 years.[10] However, these percentages may be higher due to the private nature and social stigma associated with this condition, making collecting reliable data more difficult.[11] Despite this high prevalence, it is estimated that only 30% to 40% of symptomatic women with UI seek care.[9]

The significance of UI in aging women extends beyond its prevalence. It has profound physical, emotional, and social consequences. Physically, it can lead to skin problems, urinary tract infections, and falls,[12] which are particularly detrimental for older individuals. Emotionally, UI can result in feelings of embarrassment, depression, and social isolation, as affected individuals may withdraw from social activities due to fear of leakage.

Socially, it can limit a woman's ability to participate in daily life, negatively affecting her independence and overall well-being.[9,10,13–15] All these affective symptoms contribute to higher overall morbidity, mortality, and health care costs both to patients and health care as a whole.

In the United States alone, an average of $10 to 15 billion dollars is spent each year on treatments for female UI.[16] The condition leads to increased health care costs, including doctor visits, medications, and, in some cases, surgical interventions. Additionally, the cost of absorbent products, such as adult diapers, can be substantial over time and further increase the annual expenditure of this condition. Therefore, addressing UI is essential for improving the quality of life for aging women and managing health care expenditures.

Aging and the Complexity of Urinary Incontinence

Aging exacerbates the complexity of UI, as it is often intertwined with age-related changes in the lower urinary tract. Additionally, aging women may experience coexisting medical conditions, such as pelvic organ prolapse, diabetes, or neurologic disorders, which can further complicate the evaluation and management of UI. While multiple factors can contribute to the development of UI in aging women, the condition's relationship with urethral aging is particularly noteworthy.

To date, urodynamics evaluations, other urethral function tests, and clinical epidemiologic studies have largely comprised the depth of our knowledge and understanding of alterations in urethral function throughout a woman's lifetime. However,

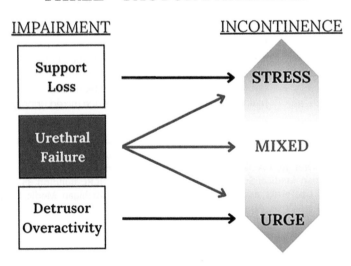

Fig. 1. The 3 factor paradigm. As De-Lancey and colleagues describe, urethral function is an important contributor to the pathogenesis of both stress and UI. (*From* Pipitone, F., Sadeghi, Z. & DeLancey, J. O. L. Urethral function and failure: A review of current knowledge of urethral closure mechanisms, how they vary, and how they are affected by life events. Neurourol Urodyn 40, 1869–1879 (2021)).

the relationship between structural and physio-logic changes in urethral tissue and aging remains a poorly studied area among existing literature.

The purpose of this review is to provide a broad exploration of the intricate relationship between aging and female urethra function, the implications of UI in aging women, and potential diagnostic modalities meant to advance our understanding of urethral failure. Our aim is to enhance the understanding of health care professionals, researchers, and the public by investigating the development of UI in the context of urethral aging. Understanding the multifaceted impact of aging on the female urethra and the resulting UI is essential for developing effective prevention and treatment strategies that will ultimately improve the quality of life for millions of aging women worldwide.

PHYSIOLOGIC CHANGES TO THE FEMALE URETHRAL WITH AGING
Striated Muscle Changes

Two groups of striated muscles contribute to UI. The striated muscles surrounding the female urethra (striated urogenital sphincter[17]) provide roughly one-third of urethral closure pressure.[18] The medial aspect of the levator ani muscles contributes support to the urethra and the bladder neck through their attachment to the vaginal wall and endopelvic fascia adjacent to the urethra.[1,19] The intrinsic urethral striated muscle partially circumscribes the urethra lumen in a horseshoe-like pattern almost along the entire length of the urethra.[18] On the other hand, the extrinsic periurethral striated muscles are separated from the intrinsic striated muscles by endopelvic connective tissue, which we will discuss in subsequent sections,[19,20] as shown in **Fig. 2**. As previously mentioned, aging can lead to the weakening and atrophy of these striated muscles, contributing to reduced urethral closure and urethral hypermobility, resulting in UI.

Additional anatomic and histochemical studies have also demonstrated differences in morphology and innervation patterns between the two types of striated muscles. Urethral striated muscle is densely innervated by small-diameter slow-twitch fibers that function to maintain tone over extended periods without fatigue.[21] Conversely, periurethral striated muscle is innervated by large-diameter fast-twitch and slow-twitch fibers that allow the pelvic floor muscles to contract with significant force quickly. This makes the pelvic floor striated musculature ideally suited to promptly halt micturition by increasing intraurethral resistance during sudden increases in intra-abdominal pressure elicited during coughing and sneezing.[19,20]

With age, the diameters of the muscle fibers in the urethra demonstrate greater degrees of variation while the quantity and density of the urethral striated fibers decline. It is estimated that an average of 2% to 4% of striated fibers are lost per year,[22] and muscle cell counts decrease by approximately 50% between the ages of 20 and 80 years,[23] possibly contributing to the higher incidence of lower urinary tract symptoms (LUTS) seen in the elderly population. As previously mentioned, striated muscle loss mirrors a decrease in innervation beginning in the upper urethra while sparing more distal regions and showing greater decreases in muscle thickness dorsally (adjacent to the vagina) rather than dorsally (adjacent to the pubic aspect)[24,25] (**Fig. 3A**).

Smooth Muscle Changes

Smooth muscle within the urethra contributes to its tone and closure mechanism, representing about one-third of the urethral closure function.[18] Smooth muscle surrounds the urethral mucosa and submucosa, forming a firm and dense tubular configuration. Numerous small smooth muscle bundles within this structure form a compact fibroelastic, collagenous tissue that makes up a more prominent longitudinal layer and a smaller outer circular layer that circles the urethra over its entire length.[23]

The impact of age on urethral smooth muscle is a quickly developing topic of research and remains a subject of debate. While some studies have reported no significant changes in urethral smooth muscle with age, recent studies have shown that the density of the circular smooth muscle layers decreases by 25% to 50% in women aged 70 to 89 years compared to women of reproductive age. Clobes and colleagues observed a reduction in the circular smooth muscle layer in older women.[23,26] Semmelink and colleagues noted hormonally induced age-independent atrophy in the smooth muscle layers of postmenopausal women, suggesting that age-related changes have a limited impact on decreased maximal urethral closure pressure (MUCP) associated with aging.[27]

Vascular Changes

The urethral mucosa (urothelium) and the greatly vascularized submucosa constitute a compressible and easily deformable layer spanning the entire length of the urethra that partially contributes to the intraluminal urethral pressure needed to keep the urethra closed at rest.[28] The lumen is surrounded by a prominent vascular plexus that is believed to contribute to continence by forming

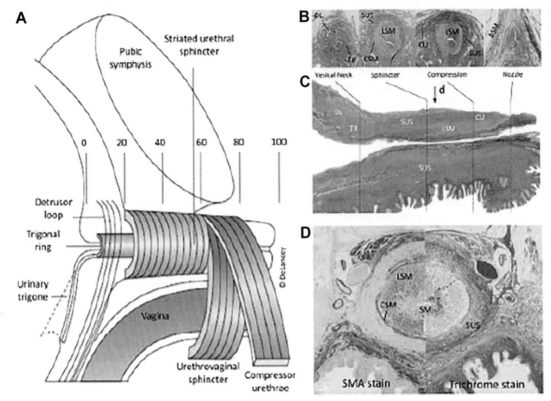

Fig. 2. Anatomy of the female urethra. (*A*) Graphical depiction of the urethra in mid-sagittal view and divided in fifths from 0 (internal urethral meatus) to 100 (external urethral meatus). (*B*) Examples of trichrome axial histologic sections of urethras. (*C*) Trichrome histologic sectioning of the mid-sagittal urethra. The arrow (d) indicates the cross-section level of panel D. (*D*) Mid-urethra axial section with SMA stain (*left*) and trichrome stain (*right*), where DL is Detrusor loop; TR is trigonal ring; SUS is striated urethral sphincter; LSM is longitudinal smooth muscle; CSM is circular smooth muscle; CU is compressor urethrae; BSM is bulbospongiosus muscle; SM is submucosa; SMA is smooth muscle actin and V is vagina. © DeLancey.

a watertight seal via coaptation of the mucosal surfaces.[29,30]

Following menopause, the number of arteriovenous anastomoses declines and is gradually replaced by a complex array of wide, thin-walled venous sinuses. Early studies by Berkow, Amboy, and Huisman[31] have also elucidated that, with age, the extent of blood supply and venous sinuses become excessive in relation to the baseline metabolic needs of urethral tissue seen in women of reproductive age[32] (**Fig. 3**B).

Neurophysiological Changes

The female urethra relies on complex neurovascular networks to maintain continence. The autonomic nervous system, consisting of both sympathetic and parasympathetic branches, and the somatic nervous system work in tandem to regulate urethral function.

As women age, there can be alterations to these neural pathways as age-related changes in neural innervation can result in diminished coordination

of the urethral sphincters and detrusor muscle, ultimately impacting continence. This compromised neural control may lead to an increase in urgency, frequency, and urgency incontinence.

It is currently believed that aging decreases the quantity and overall distribution of intramuscular nerves within the striated urethral sphincter, decreasing the number of striated muscle cells over time[33] (**Fig. 3**C). Notably, the patterns of nerve and striated muscle loss closely mirror one another, as smaller terminal nerve fibers present in peripheral areas furthest from the axon-rich compressor urethra and urethrovaginal sphincter are the first to become atrophied and denervated with aging.

Connective Tissue Changes

The connective tissues that surround the female urethra are crucial for providing structural support. As women age, these connective tissues may undergo alterations, including a decrease in elasticity and resilience. This can lead to the weakening of the urethral support structures, which are necessary for

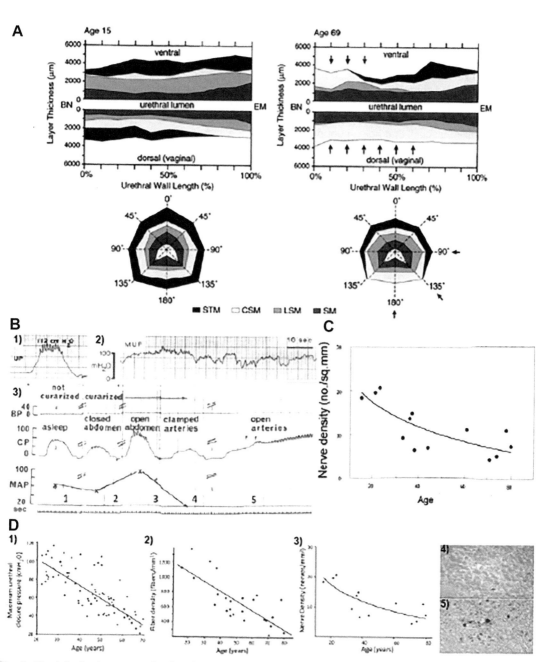

Fig. 3. Physiologic changes to the female urethra with aging. (*A*) Graphical representation of the aging-related muscle loss pattern in the urethral wall, as observed through histologic findings. The upper plots display changes in layer thickness in mid-sagittal sections, while the lower plots show corresponding mid-urethral cross-sections. Notably, there is a proximal reduction (indicated by *arrows*) in the thickness of striated muscle in both the dorsal wall and the mid-urethral cross-section with advancing age. BN, bladder neck; CSM, circular smooth muscle; EM, external meatus; LSM, longitudinal smooth muscle; SM, submucosa; STM, striated muscle. (*B*) Variations in urethral pressure are depicted. (1) Normal urethral pressure profile showing arterial pulsations in the high-pressure zone synchronized with the electrocardiogram (not shown). (2) Natural fluctuations in urethral pressure. (3) Urethral closure pressure profiles at various stages of the Rud experiment: (i) before curarization, (ii) after curarization, (iii) after opening the abdomen, (iv) after arterial clamping, and (v) upon reopening the arteries (continuous tracing). BP, bladder pressure; CP, closure pressure; MAP, mean arterial pressure; UP, urethral pressure. (*C*) Logarithmic regression analysis demonstrates the relationship between urethral nerve density and the age of cadavers. (*D*) The impact of age on the urethra is illustrated. Panel 1 shows the reduction in urethral closure pressure per decade, which corresponds to a decrease in striated muscle fiber density (panel 2) and nerve

maintaining proper anatomic positioning and continence. Consequently, the loss of support can result in urethral hypermobility and SUI.

The supportive connective tissue of the pelvic floor is composed of a complex network of smooth muscle, collagen, and elastin embedded in a non-fibrillar ground substance, commonly referred to as the "endopelvic fascia," that helps support the bladder base, urethra, and pelvic organs.[34,35] The endopelvic fascia spans from its fusion on the anterior vaginal wall to its connection on the lateral os pubis and arcus tendinous fascia pelvis, forming a hammock-like structure that compresses the urethra.[1,21,36]

In a recent study, our group applied Vectorized scale-Invariant Pattern Recognition (VIPR)[37,38] to quantitatively fractionate cell type composition of the urethra in old and young histologic specimens. Mid-sagittal, whole-urethra Masson trichrome histologic sections obtained from autopsies in young and older women were scanned at histologic resolution. Analysis was conducted on the muscular urethra below the bladder neck and above the distal fibrous "nozzle." VIPR was used to identify striated muscle, smooth muscle/fibroblast, and connective-tissue components of the urethral wall using an image computational pipeline that transforms each image location into a local kernel figure-of-merit heat-map for cell type, using K-Means clustering followed by boosting with early cuts. Striated muscle loss and a higher connective-tissue proportion are evident among the older female urethras compared to younger urethras. The substantial amount of unexplored connective tissue in older female urethra highlights a significant gap in our knowledge (**Fig. 4**).

Several studies have shown changes to the endopelvic fascia that present with aging. Research on the pathophysiology of genitourinary prolapse has elucidated a correlation with increased collagen turnover, causing a total reduction in collagen content and, thus, collagen solubility.[39] Other studies have postulated that abnormal extracellular matrix remodeling may be mitigated by a genetic component that is exacerbated by age-associated changes to hormones and mechanical stress.[40–43] However, the extent to which genetic factors and/or acquired defects contribute to age-related changes to connective tissue metabolism and fibroblast change remains debatable. Regardless, these changes play a significant role in decreasing connective tissue compliance and resilience over time and serve as catalysts for the pathogenesis of pelvic floor disorders.

URODYNAMIC FINDINGS OF FEMALE URETHRAL CHANGES WITH AGING

Urodynamic assessments play a critical role in understanding the impact of aging on the female urethra and urinary continence. This section delves into two key urodynamic parameters, MUCP and leak point pressure (LPP), to elucidate the changes that occur with aging and their clinical significance. Additionally, we explore the relationship between urodynamic studies and aging-related patterns of incontinence.

Maximal Urethral Pressure

MUCP is the urodynamic measurement that evaluates the maximal pressure within the urethra during various phases of the voiding cycle. MUCP is

---

density (panel 3). Panels d and e illustrate the decline in striated muscle cells from a young (d) to an elderly (e) stage. ([A] *From* Perucchini, D., DeLancey, J. O. L., Ashton-Miller, J. A., Peschers, U. & Kataria, T. Age effects on urethral striated muscle: I. Changes in number and diameter of striated muscle fibers in the ventral urethra. *Am J Obstet Gynecol* 186, 351–355 (2002); and Perucchini, D., DeLancey, J. O. L., Ashton-Miller, J. A., Galecki, A. & Schaer, G. N. Age effects on urethral striated muscle: II. Anatomic location of muscle loss. *Am J Obstet Gynecol* 186, 356–360 (2002); and [B1] Kulseng-Hanssen S. Prevalence and pattern of unstable urethral pressure in one hundred seventy-four gynecologic patients referred for urodynamic investigation. *Am J Obstet Gynecol*. 1983 Aug 15;146(8):895-900; and [B2, B3] Rud, T., Andersson, K. E., Asmussen, M., Hunting, A. & Ulmsten, U. Factors maintaining the intraurethral pressure in women. *Invest Urol* 17, 343–7 (1980); and Rud, T. Urethral pressure profile in continent women from childhood to old age. *Acta Obstet Gynecol* Scand 59, 331–335 (1980); and [C] PANDIT, M. et al. Quantification of intramuscular nerves within the female striated urogenital sphincter muscle. *Obstetrics and Gynecology* 95, 797–800 (2000); [D] Trowbridge, E. R., Wei, J. T., Fenner, D. E., Ashton-Miller, J. A. & DeLancey, J. O. L. Effects of aging on lower urinary tract and pelvic floor function in nulliparous women. *Obstetrics and gynecology* 109, 715–720 (2007); and Perucchini, D., DeLancey, J. O. L., Ashton-Miller, J. A., Peschers, U. & Kataria, T. Age effects on urethral striated muscle: I. Changes in number and diameter of striated muscle fibers in the ventral urethra. *Am J Obstet Gynecol* 186, 351–355 (2002); and Perucchini, D., DeLancey, J. O. L., Ashton-Miller, J. A., Galecki, A. & Schaer, G. N. Age effects on urethral striated muscle: II. Anatomic location of muscle loss. *Am J Obstet Gynecol* 186, 356–360 (2002); and PANDIT, M. et al. Quantification of intramuscular nerves within the female striated urogenital sphincter muscle. *Obstetrics and Gynecology* 95, 797–800 (2000). Sources:(d&e) Data obtained from samples collected for Perucchini 2002.)

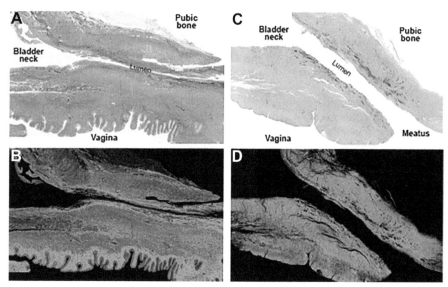

Fig. 4. Comparison of mid-sagittal whole female urethra histologic specimens in young (*left*) and older (*right*) women. (*A* and *C*) Masson trichrome, (*B* and *D*) VIPR was used to identify striated muscle (*red*), smooth muscle (*orange*), and collective-tissue (*blue*) components of the urethral wall using an image computational pipeline. Our early results demonstrate striated muscle loss and a higher connective-tissue proportion is evident among the older female urethras compared to younger female urethras.

determined through a catheter-based urodynamic study, where pressure sensors are positioned in the urethra to measure the highest recorded pressure.[44] It is the parameter whose decline is most clearly linked to advancing age. MUCP correlates well with LPP, urethral incompetence, and urethral hypermobility, which we previously discussed, making it a good predictor of incontinence severity.[45] Additionally, recent formative data have demonstrated that MUCP, rather than urethral support, is the factor most strongly associated with the diagnosis of SUI.[46] However, it is essential to note that individual factors, such as overall health, lifestyle, and genetic predisposition, can influence these variations.

Age-related decline in MUCP is observed in urodynamic studies of the female urethra.[47] While there is a lack of robust research in this area, findings suggest that MUP may decrease with age,[48] mirroring the changes in LPP.

Specifically, urine leakage with MUCP of 20 cm H_2O or lesser is prognostic of intrinsic sphincter deficiency UI and is associated with a higher risk of failure from stress incontinence surgery.[49–51] When compared to women aged 20 to 29 years, women aged 36 to 40 years and 61 to 65 years had 25% and 50% lower urethral closure pressure, respectively. Studies on nulliparous women have found that MUCP roughly 15 cm H_2O per decade and that age alone explained 57% of the variance in MUCP on linear regression modeling[7,52] (**Fig. 3**D).

Leak Point Pressure

LPP is a crucial urodynamic parameter that measures the pressure at which urinary leakage occurs. Specifically, it is defined as the intravesical pressure threshold before urine leakage occurs due to increased intra-abdominal pressure (which is why it is often also abbreviated as abdominal leak point pressure [ALPP]) in the absence of detrusor contraction.[53] In other words, it identifies the point at which this pressure exceeds the urethral closure pressure, leading to involuntary urine leakage. It is an overall assessment of how the several anatomic units work together to maintain continence.

Originally, LPP was developed to measure passive urethral resistance in children with spina bifida.[54–56] Later, it was modified to measure Valsalva or stress LPP and serve as a valuable diagnostic tool that aids in diagnosing and differentiating types of incontinence. Broadly, higher LPP values are typically indicative of better urethral closure, making it less likely for stress incontinence to occur. Conversely, lower LPP values suggest weaker urethral closure, increasing the likelihood of stress incontinence.[57]

With the natural process of aging, changes in the female urethra become evident in urodynamic assessments. Research has shown that LPP tends to decrease with age.[44,45,53,58] Elicited increases in LPP less than 60 cm H_2O have been shown to be suggestive of intrinsic sphincter deficiency and are related to the severity SUI, further correlating with a higher risk of failure following SUI surgery.[49,50] Furthermore, 80% of patients with LPPs between 60 cm H_2O and 90 cm H_2O continue to experience UI due to urethral hypermobility.[49]

This decline in LPP is attributed to the anatomic and physiologic changes in the urethra and its surrounding structures. The age-related weakening of the pelvic floor muscles and the connective tissue alterations can contribute to reduced urethral closure pressure, which we will discuss in the next section.

As LPP decreases with age, it makes aging women more susceptible to SUI, which is often triggered by everyday activities.[46,59,60] Therefore, age-related changes in LPP are of considerable clinical relevance. Clinicians should consider these changes when diagnosing and managing UI in older women.

IMAGING DATA ON CHANGES IN THE FEMALE URETHRA WITH AGING

Imaging technologies have played a pivotal role in advancing our understanding of the female urethra and how it changes with the aging process. In this section, we will delve into two crucial imaging methods, MRI and ultrasonography, and further examine their roles in assessing age-related alterations in the female urethra.

MRI Changes

There is variation in the growth and development of all organs in the body, and the urethra is no exception. Some women are born with a smaller and less robust urethra, while others are larger and more competent. Because urethral function deteriorates with age, knowing something about urethral morphology can add to our understanding of incontinence. MRI has emerged as a valuable tool for assessing the female urethra. Its noninvasive nature and high-resolution imaging capabilities make it ideal for visualizing the structural and functional aspects of the urethra. When employed in urethral assessment, MRI offers in-depth insights into the anatomy and dynamics of the urethra. It allows for the examination of the pelvic floor musculature, urethral sphincter integrity, and potential anatomic anomalies, making it an essential tool for researchers and clinicians alike.[61] Diffusion tensor imaging with fiber tractography performed on a recent MRI unit is a robust method for the three-dimensional visualization of the details and connections of the urethral female sphincters. Quantitative variations with age need to be considered.

MRI, due to its superior soft tissue contrast resolution, has demonstrated various findings related to urethral aging; even though the available data are diverse, it provides valuable insights into age-related alterations in the female urethra. Notable observations include the thinning of the urethral wall, a decrease in urethral length, and increased urethral mobility.[62] Findings of MRI that are predictive of urethral hypermobility include abnormal descent of the bladder neck, disruption of periurethral ligaments and vaginal attachments, and defects within the levator ani muscle.[63] Urethral internal sphincter deficiency may be represented in MRI as foreshortening or thinning of the sphincter muscle and bladder neck insufficiency manifested by funneling. These structural changes often correlate with UI, particularly stress incontinence.[64]

A preliminary study by Masteling and colleagues demonstrated[65] that aging is associated with changes to the MRI signal contrast noise ratio of the striated urethral sphincter independent of effects on muscle thickness. Their preliminary results suggest that MRI signal intensity decreases with aging, although the thickness of the region occupied by striated muscle does not. These MRI-visible changes were consistent with histologic findings of fiber dropout seen with aging and represent a way to measure this phenomenon in living women, as shown in **Fig. 5**.

Ultrasound Changes

1. Role of ultrasound in urethral imaging

Ultrasound imaging, specifically transperineal or transvaginal ultrasound, offers a cost-effective and widely available method for assessing the female urethra. It provides real-time and dynamic imaging, allowing for the comprehensive evaluation of the urethra's behavior during various activities, such as rest, stress, or the Valsalva maneuver.

The role of ultrasound in urethral imaging is significant, especially in the context of aging. It excels at capturing changes in urethral mobility and support, which are essential in understanding SUI. By measuring the angle and mobility of the urethra and bladder neck, ultrasound aids in the diagnosis and characterization of incontinence patterns, thereby guiding treatment decisions.[66]

2. Aging-related ultrasound observations of the female urethra

Ultrasound observations of the female urethra in aging women reveal several noteworthy findings.

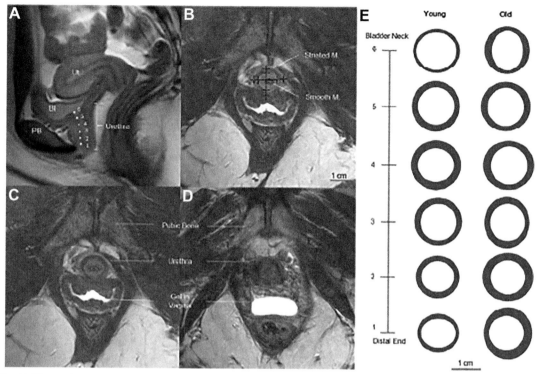

Fig. 5. Tissue characterization using MRI contrast-to-noise ratio. (*A*) Sagittal representation of 6 equally spaced cross-sections of the urethra; Notable structures: PB, pubic bone; B, bladder; Ut, uterus. (*B*) Anteroposterior and transverse measurements of the striated muscle in the external urethral sphincter (indicated by *short black lines*). (*C, D*) Axial MRI comparing tissue characteristics and signals in young (*C*) and older (*D*) nulliparous females. (*E*) A comparison of the average diameters and thickness of the striated sphincter at 6 equally spaced locations along the urethra.

Most prominently, age-related changes in urethral mobility and support are frequently observed. The increased mobility of the urethra and bladder neck with age is a key factor contributing to reduced urethral closure pressure and the development of stress incontinence.[67]

Recent ultrasound research has explored the vascular aspects of the continence mechanism, but our understanding of this area is in its infancy. For example, multiparous women demonstrate a significant decrease in Doppler ultrasound parameters related to vascular factors in the mid-urethra compared to newly parous controls. Similar findings were observed when comparing incontinence with continent and postmenopausal with perimenopausal women.[68,69]

Furthermore, ultrasound provides valuable insights into the condition of the pelvic floor muscles. Similar to MRI, ultrasound often shows signs of muscle atrophy and alterations in muscle tone in aging women.[70] These observations highlight the weakening of urethral support structures, offering a clear link to the increased susceptibility to SUI in older individuals.

GAPS IN KNOWLEDGE ABOUT FEMALE URETHRA CHANGES WITH AGING

Understanding how the female urethra changes with aging remains an evolving field, and several significant gaps in knowledge persist.

Limitations in Current Research Include

- Sample size and demographics: Many studies examining age-related changes in the female urethra suffer from limitations in sample size and demographic diversity. A larger and more diverse pool of participants is needed to draw comprehensive conclusions about how aging affects the female urethra across various populations.
- Longitudinal studies: Longitudinal studies tracking the same individuals over time are essential to capture the dynamic nature of age-related changes in the female urethra. Existing research often relies on cross-sectional data, offering only a static snapshot of urethral changes. Long-term studies are vital for

understanding the progression and variance in aging-related alterations.

Complex Interplay of Factors Involved

- Genetic predisposition: Genetic factors contribute to an individual's susceptibility to UI and urethral changes with aging. Uncovering these genetic predispositions is a challenging but crucial avenue for further research.
- Hormonal changes: Hormonal fluctuations during menopause have known effects on the female urogenital system, but the exact role of hormonal changes in urethral aging remains complex and not fully elucidated. Understanding the interplay between hormones and the urethra is critical.
- Lifestyle and behavioral factors: Lifestyle choices, such as diet, physical activity, and smoking, can affect the female urethra. The interaction of these factors with aging-related changes is not yet fully understood and requires more investigation.

Future Directions for Research Would Include

- Advancements in imaging technologies: Cutting-edge imaging technologies, such as high-resolution MRI and real-time ultrasound, hold great promise for providing more detailed insights into the female urethra. Advancements in imaging will allow for a more nuanced understanding of age-related changes in the anatomic and functional characteristics of the urethra.
- Targeted therapeutic approaches: Future research should focus on developing targeted therapeutic approaches tailored to address specific age-related urethral changes. Customized interventions will provide better outcomes for aging women with UI.
- Public health implications: Future research should focus on developing targeted therapeutic approaches tailored to address specific age-related urethral changes. Customized interventions will provide better outcomes for aging women with UI.

SUMMARY

Urethral function is an important contributor to stress and UI pathogenesis. Because urethral function declines by 15% each decade,[7] even in the absence of childbirth, understanding the role of urethral failure in the aging population is important. Neurovascular, smooth muscle, striated muscle, and connective tissue changes collectively influence urethral function, leading to a greater susceptibility to UI as women age. Striated muscle loss and a higher connective-tissue proportion are evident among the older female urethras compared to younger female urethras. Aging decreases the quantity and overall distribution of intramuscular nerves within the striated urethral sphincter, decreasing the number of striated muscle cells over time. Understanding these age-related alterations is essential for developing effective prevention and treatment strategies to improve the quality of life for aging women. Imaging technologies, including MRI and ultrasound, have been crucial in advancing our understanding of age-related changes in the female urethra. MRI offers detailed structural insights, such as the decrease in striated muscle signal intensity, while ultrasound provides real-time dynamic observations, such as age-related changes in urethral mobility and vascularity factors, both contributing to our knowledge of UI in aging women.

In summary, while we have made significant strides in understanding the female urethra's changes with aging, substantial gaps in knowledge persist. Addressing these gaps will enhance our understanding of age-related alterations and pave the way for more effective prevention and treatment strategies, ultimately improving the quality of life for aging women.

CLINICS CARE POINTS

- Aging typically leads to a decline in urethral function, and individuals with poor urethral function are more likely to fail operations for stress incontinence that focus on urethral support.
- The fact that urethral weakness also plays a role in urge incontinence suggests that interventions such as pelvic muscle training may play a role in treatment.
- Advanced imaging technologies such as MRI and ultrasound provide valuable insights into the physiologic changes that occur in the aging female urethra. MRI offers structural information, while ultrasound allows for real-time dynamic observations, both contributing to our understanding of UI in aging women. Further research in this area is essential to enhance our knowledge and improve prevention and treatment strategies.
- To date, interventions that can be demonstrated to increase urethral function have not been developed but, when they are, they will target this unaddressed impairment in incontinence.

DISCLOSURE

The authors declare no conflict of interest. This study was supported by departmental funding provided to Dr Z. Sadeghi, by the Department of Urology at the University of California, United States, Irvine. Dr J. DeLancey and Dr U.G.J. Balis had their effort supported by RC2 DK122379, and NIH, United States.-NIAMS, United States R01NS120060 grant.

REFERENCES

1. DeLancey JOL. Structural support of the urethra as it relates to stress urinary incontinence: the hammock hypothesis. Am J Obstet Gynecol 1994;170: 1713–23.
2. DeLancey JOL. Anatomy and physiology of urinary continence. Clin Obstet Gynecol 1990;33:298–307.
3. Shah AP, Mevcha A, Wilby D, et al. Continence and micturition: An anatomical basis. Clin Anat 2014;27: 1275–83.
4. Falah-Hassani K, Reeves J, Shiri R, et al. The pathophysiology of stress urinary incontinence: a systematic review and meta-analysis. Int Urogynecol J 2021;32:501–52.
5. Lukacz ES, Whitcomb EL, Lawrence JM, et al. Urinary frequency in community-dwelling women: what is normal? Am J Obstet Gynecol 2009;200:552.e1–7.
6. Pipitone F, Sadeghi Z, DeLancey JOL. Urethral function and failure: A review of current knowledge of urethral closure mechanisms, how they vary, and how they are affected by life events. Neurourol Urodyn 2021;40:1869–79.
7. Trowbridge ER, Wei JT, Fenner DE, et al. Effects of aging on lower urinary tract and pelvic floor function in nulliparous women. Obstet Gynecol 2007;109: 715–20.
8. Minassian VA, Drutz HP, Al-Badr A. Urinary incontinence as a worldwide problem. Int J Gynecol Obstet 2003;82:327–38.
9. Lukacz ES, Santiago-Lastra Y, Albo ME, et al. Urinary Incontinence in Women: A Review. JAMA 2017;318:1592–604.
10. Wu JM, Vaughan CP, Goode PS, et al. Prevalence and trends of symptomatic pelvic floor disorders in U.S. women. Obstet Gynecol 2014;123:141–8.
11. Baczewska B, Wiśniewska K, Muraczyńska B, et al. Assessment by women on selected aspects of quality of life and on disease acceptance after undergoing urogynecological procedures for urinary incontinence. J Clin Med 2023;12:4894.
12. Gibson W, Hunter KF, Camicioli R, et al. The association between lower urinary tract symptoms and falls: Forming a theoretical model for a research agenda. Neurourol Urodyn 2018;37:501–9.
13. Steibliene V, Aniuliene R, Aniulis P, et al. Affective Symptoms and Health-Related Quality of Life Among Women with Stress Urinary Incontinence: Cross-Sectional Study. Neuropsychiatric Dis Treat 2020;16:535–44.
14. Gümüşsoy S, Kavlak O, Dönmez S. Investigation of body image, self-esteem, and quality of life in women with urinary incontinence. Int J Nurs Pract 2019;25:e12762.
15. Schreiber Pedersen L, Lose G, Høybye MT, et al. Predictors and reasons for help-seeking behavior among women with urinary incontinence. Int Urogynecol J 2018;29:521–30.
16. Agarwala N, Liu CY. Minimally invasive management of urinary incontinence. Curr Opin Obstet Gynecol 2002;14:429–33.
17. Oelrich TM. The urethral sphincter muscle in the male. Am J Anat 1980;158:229–46.
18. Rud T, Andersson KE, Asmussen M, et al. Factors maintaining the intraurethral pressure in women. Invest Urol 1980;17:343–7.
19. DeLancey JO. Structural aspects of the extrinsic continence mechanism. Obstet Gynecol 1988;72: 296–301.
20. Gosling JA. The structure of the female lower urinary tract and pelvic floor. Urol Clin North Am 1985;12: 207–14.
21. Gosling JA, Dixon JS, Critchley HOD, et al. A comparative study of the human external sphincter and periurethral levator ani muscles. Br J Urol 1981;53:35–41.
22. Carlile A, Davies I, Rigby A, et al. Age changes in the human female urethra: a morphometric study. J Urol 1988;139:532–5.
23. Clobes A, DeLancey JOL, Morgan DM. Urethral circular smooth muscle in young and old women. Am J Obstet Gynecol 2008;198:587.e1–5.
24. Perucchini D, DeLancey JOL, Ashton-Miller JA, et al. Age effects on urethral striated muscle: I. Changes in number and diameter of striated muscle fibers in the ventral urethra. Am J Obstet Gynecol 2002; 186:351–5.
25. Perucchini D, DeLancey JOL, Ashton-Miller JA, et al. Age effects on urethral striated muscle: II. Anatomic location of muscle loss. Am J Obstet Gynecol 2002; 186:356–60.
26. Tanagho EA, Meyers FH, Smith DR. Urethral resistance: its components and implications. I. Smooth muscle component. Invest Urol 1969;7:136–49.
27. Semmelink HJF, de Wilde PCM, van Houwelingen JC, et al. Histomorphometric study of the lower urogenital tract in pre- and postmenopausal women. Cytometry 1990;11:700–7.
28. van Geelen H, Sand PK. The female urethra: urethral function throughout a woman's lifetime. International Urogynecology Journal 2023;34(6):1175–86.
29. Zinner NR, Sterling AM, Ritter RC. Role of inner urethral softness in urinary continence. Urology 1980; 16:115–7.

30. Delancey JOL, Ashton-Miller JA. Pathophysiology of adult urinary incontinence. Gastroenterology 2004; 126:S23–32.

31. Huisman AB. Aspects on the anatomy of the female urethra with special relation to urinary continence. Contrib Gynecol Obstet 1983;10:1–31.

32. Berkow SG, Amboy P. The corpus spongeosum of the urethra: its possible role in urinary control and stress incontinence in women. Am J Obstet Gynecol 1953;65:346–51.

33. PANDIT M, et al, DeLancey JO, Ashton-Miller JA, et al. Quantification of intramuscular nerves within the female striated urogenital sphincter muscle. Obstet Gynecol 2000;95:797–800.

34. Ulmsten U, Falconer C. Connective tissue in female urinary incontinence. Curr Opin Obstet Gynecol 1999;11:509–15.

35. Falconer C, Ekman-Ordeberg G, Blomgren B, et al. Paraurethral connective tissue in stress-incontinent women after menopause. Acta Obstet Gynecol Scand 1998;77:95–100.

36. Petros PEP, Ulmsten UI. An integral theory of female urinary incontinence. Acta Obstet Gynecol Scand 1990;69:7–31.

37. Kwon J, Lee E, Park H, et al. Overactive bladder medication, how long should it be sustained?: Mirabegron interferes with the central sensitization induced by the mice model of overactive bladder. Neurourol Urodyn 2022;41:S7–256.

38. Hipp JD, Cheng JY, Toner M, et al. Spatially Invariant Vector Quantization: A pattern matching algorithm for multiple classes of image subject matter including pathology. J Pathol Inform 2011; 2:13.

39. Jackson SR, Avery NC, Tarlton JF, et al. Changes in metabolism of collagen in genitourinary prolapse. Lancet 1996;347:1658–61.

40. Keane DP, Sims TJ, Abrams P, et al. Analysis of collagen status in premenopausal nulliparous women with genuine stress incontinence. Br J Obstet Gynaecol 1997;104:994–8.

41. Falconer C, Blomgren B, Johansson O, et al. Different organization of collagen fibrils in stress-incontinent women of fertile age. Acta Obstet Gynecol Scand 1998;77:87–94.

42. Chen B, Yeh J. Alterations in connective tissue metabolism in stress incontinence and prolapse. J Urol 2011;186:1768–72.

43. Francis WJA. The onset of stress incontinence. BJOG 1960;67:899–903.

44. Nager CW, Schulz JA, Stanton SL, et al. Correlation of urethral closure pressure, leak-point pressure and incontinence severity measures. Int Urogynecol J 2001;12:395–400.

45. Schick E, Dupont C, Bertrand PE, et al. Predictive value of maximum urethral closure pressure, urethral hypermobility and urethral incompetence in the diagnosis of clinically significant female genuine stress incontinence. J Urol 2004;171:1871–5.

46. DeLancey JOL, Trowbridge ER, Miller JM, et al. Stress urinary incontinence: relative importance of urethral support and urethral closure pressure. J Urol 2008;179:2286–90.

47. HILTON P, STANTON SL. Urethral pressure measurement by microtransducer: the results in symptom-free women and in those with genuine stress incontinence. Br J Obstet Gynaecol 1983; 90:919–33.

48. Rud T. Urethral pressure profile in continent women from childhood to old age. Acta Obstet Gynecol Scand 1980;59:331–5.

49. Fleischmann N, Flisser AJ, Blaivas JG, et al. Sphincteric urinary incontinence: relationship of vesical leak point pressure, urethral mobility and severity of incontinence. J Urol 2003;169:999–1002.

50. McGuire EJ, Fitzpatrick CC, Wan J, et al. Clinical assessment of urethral sphincter function. J Urol 1993;150:1452–4.

51. Han JY, Park J, Choo MS. Long-term durability, functional outcomes, and factors associated with surgical failure of tension-free vaginal tape procedure. Int Urol Nephrol 2014;46:1921–7.

52. Schick E, Tessier J, Bertrand PE, et al. Observations on the Function of the Female Urethra: I: Relation Between Maximum Urethral Closure Pressure at Rest and Urethral Hypermobility. Neurourol Urodyn 2003;22:643–7.

53. Burden H, Warren K, Abrams P. Leak point pressures: how useful are they? Curr Opin Urol 2015; 25:317–22.

54. Kobayashi S, Shinno Y, Kakizaki H, et al. Relevance of detrusor hyperreflexia, vesical compliance and urethral pressure to the occurrence of vesicoureteral reflux in myelodysplastic patients. J Urol 1992;147:413–5.

55. Sidi AA, Dykstra DD, Gonzalez R. The value of urodynamic testing in the management of neonates with myelodysplasia: A prospective study. J Urol 1986;135:90–3.

56. McGuire EJ, Woodside JR, Borden TA, et al. Prognostic value of urodynamic testing in myelodysplastic patients. J Urol 1981;126:205–9.

57. Sinha D, Nallaswamy V, Arunkalaivanan AS. Value of Leak Point Pressure Study in Women With Incontinence. J Urol 2006;176:186–8.

58. Bump RC, Elser DM, Theofrastous JP, et al. Valsalva leak point pressures in women with genuine stress incontinence: reproducibility, effect of catheter caliber, and correlations with other measures of urethral resistance. Continence Program for Women Research Group. Am J Obstet Gynecol 1995;173:551–7.

59. Nager CW, Brubaker L, Litman HJ, et al. A randomized trial of urodynamic testing before stress-incontinence surgery. N Engl J Med 2012; 366:1987–97.

60. Swift SE, Utrie JW. The need for standardization of the Valsalva leak-point pressure. Int Urogynecol J 1996;7:227–30.

61. Roy C, Ohana M, Labani A, et al. Evaluation of the female bladder neck and urethra using MRI with fiber tractography: Prospective study on a large cohort of continent women. Neurourol Urodyn 2021;40:1441–9.

62. Itani M, Kielar A, Menias CO, et al. MRI of female urethra and periurethral pathologies. Int Urogynecol J 2016;27:195–204.

63. Macura KJ, Genadry RR, Bluemke DA. MR imaging of the female urethra and supporting ligaments in assessment of urinary incontinence: spectrum of abnormalities. Radiographics 2006;26:1135–49.

64. Macura KJ, Genadry RR. Female urinary incontinence: pathophysiology, methods of evaluation and role of MR imaging. Abdom Imag 2008;33:371–80.

65. Masteling M, Chen L, DeLancey J, et al. Quantification of aging effects on urethral morphology using MRI. Philadelphia: ICS; 2018.

66. Pregazzi R, Sartore A, Bortoli P, et al. Perineal ultrasound evaluation of urethral angle and bladder neck mobility in women with stress urinary incontinence. BJOG 2002;109:821–7.

67. Zhao B, Wen L, Liu D, et al. Urethral configuration and mobility during urine leaking described using real-time transperineal ultrasonography. Ultrasonography 2022;41:171.

68. Lone F, Sultan AH, Stankiewicz A, et al. Vascularity of the urethra in continent women using colour doppler high-frequency endovaginal ultrasonography. Springerplus 2014;3:619.

69. Liang CC, Chang SD, Chang YL, et al. Three-dimensional power Doppler measurement of perfusion of the periurethral tissue in incontinent women – a preliminary report. Acta Obstet Gynecol Scand 2006; 85:608–13.

70. Larsson L, Degens H, Li M, et al. Sarcopenia: Aging-Related Loss of Muscle Mass and Function. Physiol Rev 2019;99:427.

Urinary Catheters
Materials, Coatings, and Recommendations for Selection

John T. Stoffel, MD[a],*, Lisa Yu, RN[b]

KEYWORDS

- Urinary catheter • Clean intermittent catheterization • Urinary retention • Catheter material

KEY POINTS

- Urinary catheters have been used to treat urinary retention for more than 3000 years and have evolved with advances in technology.
- The introduction of galvanized rubber materials is the foundation for the modern urinary catheter.
- Hydrophilic coating on catheters may reduce urethral trauma and incidence of catheter-acquired urinary tract infections.
- Comparing the efficacy and safety of types of urinary catheters is challenging due to short follow-up, lack of standardized end points, and heterogenous study cohorts.
- The selection of a catheter type for a person requires education and evaluation of multiple variables to determine proper safety and quality of life goals.

INTRODUCTION

Catheters have long played a key role in the management of both acute and chronic urinary symptoms. They can be either indwelling or intermittently placed and are commonly used to treat urinary retention, manage incontinence, and protect the kidneys. Catheters can also have a much broader role in medical systems and are used to provide data for medical care; for example, intensive care units and anesthetists rely on urinary catheters to provide accurate measurements of a person's fluid balance, physicians use them to get an uncontaminated specimen for assessment of urinary infections, and catheters can be an integral part of end of life care plans, providing dignity and solace for patients and families. Indeed, catheters are used as a versatile tool in maintaining both patient safety and a stable quality of life.

There can be considerable morbidity related to catheter usage. In a study of national data from 2001 to 2010, indwelling urinary catheters were associated with 3.8 million preventable urinary tract infections (UTIs).[1] UTI also remains a common problem for people performing clean intermittent catheterization (CIC). The Neurogenic Bladder Research Group (NBRG) spinal cord injury registry of 1479 spinal cord injured people showed that CIC users had a three to four times greater odds of having a UTI or visiting an emergency room (ER) compared those voiding spontaneously.[2,3] It is well-known that indwelling and intermittent catheters have also been associated with urethral/bladder injury and hematuria.[4,5]

Catheter usage and care plans are also tied to quality of life for people. For example, the NBRG registry demonstrated that people with indwelling catheters reported a higher urinary quality of life compared with people performing intermittent catheterization, independent of level of injury.[6] There is also a considerable time burden associated with managing a bladder with a catheter. People with spinal cord injuries can spend up to

[a] Department of Urology, University of Michigan, 3875 Taubman Center, 1500 East Medical Center Drive, Ann Arbor, MI 48109, USA; [b] Neurourology/Incontinence/Reconstruction, University of Michigan/Michigan Medicine, 1500 East Medical Center Drive, Ann Arbor, MI 48109, USA
* Corresponding author.
E-mail address: jstoffel@med.umich.edu

Urol Clin N Am 51 (2024) 253–262
https://doi.org/10.1016/j.ucl.2024.01.003
0094-0143/24/© 2024 Elsevier Inc. All rights reserved.

53 minutes per day performing intermittent catheterization, compared with the 7 minutes per day neurologically intact people spend voiding.[7] The time spent managing a catheter can significantly impact how a person interacts with others and society in general, so the choice of other catheter type is an important medical decision.

However, little is known about how to match patient phenotype with catheter type to maximize safety and quality of life. There have been some small forays into examining psychosocial difference between people who use indwelling versus intermittent catheters,[8] but there is less information examining how the catheter selection process occurs. This lack of information partly stems from poor education on the different types of catheters available for use and the data surrounding their efficacies. The purpose of this review is to compare the physical aspects of urinary catheters such as material, coating, and insertion techniques and to propose an educational strategy for incorporating these variables into a tangible educational process.

History of the Urinary Catheter

The word catheter is derived from the ancient Greek kathiénai, "to let down" which aptly describes its primary purpose.[9] Reviewing the history of the urinary catheter over time is helpful in understanding how catheter selection evolves in lock step with technological changes.

Rigid catheters

Catheterization has likely existed as a medical treatment for thousands of years and one of the earliest documentations of catheter usage comes from *The Sushruta Samhita,* an early Indian medical text from 1000 BCE. Here, catheters, which were made out of wood and covered with ghee, were used to drain the bladders of people with urinary retention.[10] Other early reports of catheters note rolled onion leaves covered with lacquer from China and straight twigs soaked and bundled together from Persia. By the fifth century BCE, Hippocrates discussed drainage of urine and the harm that can occur with bladder injuries. *It has been reported that Erasistratus of Alexandria invented an S-shaped catheter in 300 BCE,* and this model persisted for another 400 years as evidenced by catheters that have been recovered from a surgeon's house in Pompeii, Italy (c 79 ACE)[11] **(Fig. 1)**.

Flexible catheters

An advancement in catheter technology occurred in the middle ages when malleable catheters began to be produced which reduced urethral trauma

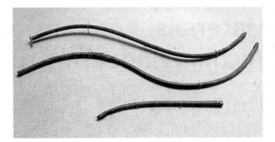

Fig. 1. Example of S-shaped catheters found in House of the Surgeon, Pompeii, Italy.

during passage. Silver was the metal of choice because it was durable, held its shape when bent, and was thought to have some antiseptic properties. *Ambroise Pare, considered by some to be the father of modern surgery and surgeon/barber to the 16th century French kings Henry II and Charles II, created curved catheters of different diameters to facilitate a less traumatic passage into the bladder.*[11,12] The solid metal design ultimately gave way to a woven silver variety (seventeenth–eighteenth centuries) that was easier to manufacture. Once they were more readily available, catheters became a widely accepted tool to treat urinary retention and there are reports of men's hats in eighteenth-century England created with brims wide enough to hide a catheter within.[13] *The modern Coudé catheter (French "elbow") was first introduced in the early nineteenth century, and although still made of a malleable metal, it had the characteristic curved nose that is known to contemporary urologists.* This design for navigating an enlarged prostate continues to be used today.[9]

The next major evolution of urinary catheters came with the discovery of rubber and the vulcanization process invented by Goodyear in the mid-nineteenth century. Rubber catheters had been available since the 1700s, but the rubber was brittle and prone to fracturing with temperature changes. One of the first vulcanized, shaped rubber catheters was created by Auguste Nelaton of St Louis Hospital in Paris.[10] It was created out of a firm vulcanized red rubber, the echoes of which continue today as the classic "red rubber catheter." Once catheters could be mass produced, sizing became standardized and the French measuring scale of 3 mm = 1 Fr was adopted, reflecting the French physicians work in pioneering urinary catheterization.

Self-retaining catheters

Self-retaining catheters for prolonged urinary drainage continued to evolve. Some earlier designs included areas where the catheter could be sewn to the male glans or female labia to keep it from inadvertently being removed. The limitations of these were obvious and were later replaced with elaborate bandages and taping techniques. In the early to mid-nineteenth century, Malecot and de Pezzar created winged and mushroom-tipped catheters, respectively, that were designed to be self-retaining. These designs have survived into today, although they have limited use today in urinary catheterization. *The modern catheter design is attributed to Frederick Foley, who described a self-retaining catheter with an inflatable balloon in 1929 as a way to improve hemostasis after transurethral prostate surgery.*[14] He applied for the patent in 1935, but it was ultimately awarded to Paul Raiche of the Davol Rubber Company of Providence, Rhode Island in 1936[15] and the C.R. Bard company ultimately began manufacturing self-retaining catheters of Foley's design. Today, the design remains similar to Foley's original description, although Bard modified the materials by changing to a latex balloon in 1960s and a silicone-coated elastomer over latex (**Fig. 2**).

Intermittent catheterization

World War II brought in changes in catheterization. *Sir Ludwig Guttman, a German born neurosurgeon, developed a sterile intermittent catheterization technique at the National Spinal Injuries Center at Stoke Mandeville Hospital in Buckinghamshire in the 1940*s to treat injured Royal Air Force pilots. His goal was to reduce the dependence on indwelling catheters because he observed that many people arriving at the hospital had chronically obstructed catheters and were frequently ill from pyelonephritis.[16] His catheterization technique required sterile conditions and was performed by trained medical professionals. Using a technique of no-touch catheterization every 6 hours, upper tract UTIs markedly decreased. Catheterization continued until spinal shock had resolved and patients could void per urethra. Most men were managed with a condom catheter at this point.

The next revolution in catheterization came in the 1970s when Jack Lapides of the University of Michigan began advocating for intermittent catheterization as a long-term management strategy, with the important advancement of being performed by the patient themselves. Instead of Guttman's no-touch technique, Lapides described a clean technique to be performed at regular intervals.[17] The guiding principle was that bladder volume, rather than bacterial presence, was the greatest driver of morbidity associated with urinary retention. Dr Lapides reasoned that catheterization could be performed by anyone if clean technique minimized urethral and bladder trauma. Although initially derided, his philosophy transformed the concept of intermittent catheterization from a medical procedure performed only by professions into a routine, patient-controlled intervention.

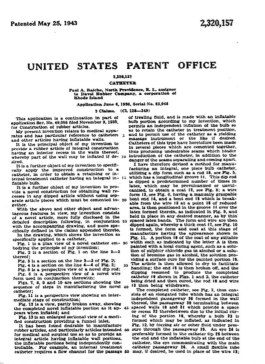

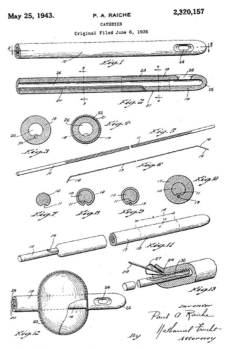

Fig. 2. US patent of self-retaining urinary catheter. Patent issued to Paul Raiche and eventually produced by C.R. Bard.

Table 1
Key figures in urinary catheter development

Person	Timeframe	Advancement
Erasistratus	500 BCE	S shaped curved metal catheter
Ambroise Pare	1500s	Malleable silver metal catheter
Auguste Nelaton	1850s	Rubber Catheter
Frederick Foley	1930s	Self-Retaining catheter balloon
Ludwig Guttman	1940s	Sterile Intermittent catheterization
Jack Lapides	1970s	Clean intermittent catheterization

Table 1 summarizes some of the key figures in catheter development.

Modern Modifications to Urinary Catheters

Catheter material: plastic, silicone, latex, and polyvinyl chloride

Today, catheters can be made of plastic, silicone, rubber/latex, or polyvinyl chloride (PVC). *There are little data examining how catheter material composition reduces urethral or bladder morbidity or improves urinary quality of life.* Starting with animal model data, Hosseinpour and colleagues performed a study comparing morbidity of latex catheter to silicone catheters in a rabbit model and did not note a difference when comparing the incidence of UTIs or cystitis.[18] However, a similar study comparing latex and Nelatone (a soft and flexible plastic) in a different rabbit model by the same group of researchers showed that subjects with Nelatone catheters had fewer UTIs (20% UTI incidence Nelatone, 60% Latex; $P<.01$).[19] In one of the few human trials, Erickison and colleagues compared the morbidity of silicone catheters to a hydrogel-coated latex catheter in a prospective, randomized trial for 85 post-urethroplasty male patients. At a mean follow-up of 20 months, they found no difference in stricture recurrence or postoperative complications between the two groups.[20]

In comparative studies comparing catheters in people performing intermittent catheterization, Witjes and colleagues randomized 98 neurologically impaired people to PVC catheters for self-catheterization and they were compared with 97 people who were randomized to non-PVC catheters. The tested catheters were single-use PVC catheters (LoFric Primo) and had a hydrophilic layer of polyvinyl pyrrolidone and sodium chloride. After 4 weeks, there was no statistical difference in

patient-reported handling of catheter or satisfaction. Both groups reported similar adverse events (8% PVC vs 10% non-PVC). UTI was more commonly reported in the PVC group (seven in PVC group, three in non-PVC), although this was not statistically significant.[21] It should be noted, however, that 4 weeks may be too short of a time interval to detect differences. A 2011 literature review by Chartier-Kastler and colleagues identified 19 studies that compared PVC catheters with standard gel lubricant to other catheter materials and coating. The review suggested that PVC catheters in general caused more urethral inflammation and microscopic hematuria than other catheter materials. However, the review does not use a standardized methodology for comparison so it is difficult to separate the impact of coating on catheters from underlying catheter material.[22]

The choice of catheter material may be subject to regional practice patterns. More PVC catheters are used in the United States and more silicone catheters are used in Europe. Given the limited number of patients and lack of standardized comparisons, it is difficult to extrapolate existing data to recommend a specific catheter material at this time.

Catheter coatings

Hydrophilic It has been postulated that urethral trauma is a mechanism by which catheters can cause UTIs and inflammation. An approach to reducing catheter-related morbidity is to lower the resistance of the catheter as it is passed through the urethra into the bladder. Hydrophilic catheters are designed to do this via a precoating with a polymer material which binds with water (or saline) and creates a slippery layer that reduces tissue resistance in the urethral lumen (**Fig. 3**). *There are data that suggest a hydrophilic catheter decreases the incidence of UTIs for people performing intermittent catheterization.* Cardenas and colleagues performed a prospective, randomized trial of 114 spinal cord injured people (224 recruited) in 15 United States centers comparing single-use hydrophilic-coated (Speedi-Cath) or PVC uncoated catheters. They found that the time to a first, symptomatic UTI was significantly delayed ($P = .038$) and corresponded to a 33% decrease in the daily risk of developing the first symptomatic UTI in the hydrophilic group.[4] A limitation of this study was that the participants were not blinded and thus introduced a potential bias for UTI evaluation.

Studies comparing hydrophilic and non-hydrophilic catheters have been combined and studied in systematic reviews and meta-analysis. Rognoni and Tarricone performed a systematic review comparing morbidity and quality of life

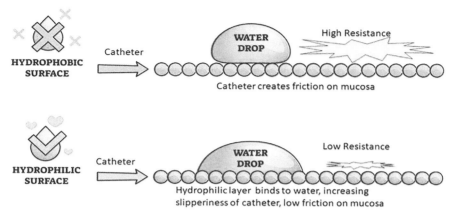

Fig. 3. Hydrophilic catheters bind water to lower resistance when passing along urethral tissue.

between single-use hydrophilic catheters and non-hydrophilic catheters in a population performing intermittent catheterization. They identified 695 patients across 9 studies and found a statistically significant decreased risk of UTIs in hydrophilic catheter users compared with non-hydrophilic catheter users (RR = 0.84; 95% CI, 0.75–0.94; P = .003).[23] A more recent meta-analysis and systematic review by Plata and colleagues (seven randominzed controlled trial [RCTs], two cross over studies) also found that hydrophilic catheter users had a lower risk of UTIs compared with non-hydrophilic catheter users (RR = 0.78; 95% CI 0.62–0.97.).[24] Overall, these systematic reviews provide strong enough evidence to suggest that there is some protective benefit of a hydrophilic coating on a catheter against the development of UTI.

The impact of hydrophilic catheters on urethral trauma during intermittent catheterization is less clear. In Rognoni and Tarricone's study, there were three trials that reported hematuria or urethral bleeding; hydrophilic catheter users reported more hematuria compared with non-hydrophilic users 31% versus 22%.[23] The investigators speculate that this may reflect the lack of education regarding intermittent catheterization rather than morbidity related to material. Hedlund and colleagues performed as systematic literature review comparing hydrophilic and PVC catheters. They found that up to 25% of patients using PVC catheters had urethral strictures in one study, compared with zero new strictures with hydrophilic catheters, and most of the strictures developed after more than 5 years of CIC.[25]

In principle, it stands to reason that a less traumatic insertion of a catheter will result in better patient comfort but *comparative studies are also inconclusive on whether hydrophilic catheters improve quality of life during when used during for*

intermittent catheterization. Evidence showed lower or neutral quality of life (QoL) when using a hydrophilic catheter in some studies[26,27] and less discomfort in others.[28] It is challenging to separate the lack of education regarding catheter use, pre-existing expectations, and neurologic functioning from these studies and extrapolate to a generalized population. Furthermore, no specific type of hydrophilic coating has been found to be definitively superior in reducing morbidity or maximizing quality of life. Shamout and colleagues all performed a systematic review (2188 patients, 31 studies total) which did not detect any difference in effectiveness between the types of hydrophilic coating when three types of catheters were compared.[29] It should be noted that the Shamout and colleagues' review was not conducted with the same methodology as the Rognoni[23] and Plata's[24] studies.

Antimicrobial *Another approach to reducing the morbidity of catheter-related infections is to coat the catheter surface with antimicrobial material to reduce biofilm accumulation. Substances used as coating include silver alloy, other noble metal alloy, and nitrofurazone.*

Sun and colleagues performed a meta-analysis of the efficacy of silver alloy catheters and noble metal catheters in preventing bacteria for short-term indwelling urethral catheterization of less than 14 days. Thirteen studies were included in the analysis and the investigators found that both catheters reduced the risk of bacteriuria (silver RR 0.63, 95% CI 0.44–0.90, P = .01 and noble metal catheters RR 0.58, 95%CI 0.41–0.81, P = .001). The data also suggested that silver alloy catheters delay bacteria growth for greater than 1 week. The risk of symptomatic catheter aquired urinary tract infection (CAUTI) was not well assessed in this analysis and the investigators noted that the data are difficult to combine due to differing methodology, selection criteria, and end points.[30] A larger meta-analysis with different inclusion criteria focused on prevention of CAUTI. Lam and colleagues evaluated 26 randomized controlled trials comparing silver or antiseptic-coated catheters to standard catheters in an inpatient population. This included 12,422 hospitalized adults in 25 parallel group trials, and 27,878 adults in one large cluster-randomized cross-over trial. They concluded that comparisons between silver alloy-coated catheter and standard catheter yielded no significant difference in symptomatic CAUTI (RR 0.99, 95% CI 0.85–1.16) in the meta-analysis.[31]

Several silver-coated catheters are available for use commercially but remain expensive. In addition, there is a theoretic concern that noble metals could cause toxicity through absorption into the blood stream. Other researchers have investigated using silver nanoparticles to impregnate catheters because nanoparticles use a smaller amount of silver spread over a larger surface area. This reduces the overall amount of heavy metal on the catheter and its potential toxicity. Rugaie and colleagues demonstrated the feasibility of this in an in vitro study and showed that a silver nanoparticle catheter reduced *Escherichia coli* biofilm by 50% to 60% compared with uncoated controls with limited slough of the silver particles.[32] Silver nanoparticle catheters are not readily available for use outside of investigative research studies at this point. *Overall, it is not clear if silver and noble metal catheters reduce catheter-acquired UTI, but caution should be used before extrapolating the data due to the limited data surrounding extended dwell time.*

There are less data available on the efficacy of a nitrofurazone catheter. Nitrofurazone is similar structurally to nitrofurantoin, a broad-spectrum antibiotic against both gram-positive and gram-negative bacteria (with the exception of pseudomonas). A nitrofurazone catheter theoretically reduces UTI through a continued time release of nitrofurazone into the bladder which would reduce colonization and biofilm formation. Lee and colleagues all performed an observational study comparing nitrofurazone catheters against standard silicone catheters in a 177 patient cohort using indwelling catheters. They found no statistical difference in CAUTI incidence between the two groups overall, but a lower incidence of CAUTI developing after 5 to 7 days in the nitrofurazone group (13% vs 19%, P = .03).[33] Menezes and colleagues randomized renal transplant recipients into receiving nitrofurazone-coated or regular silicone catheters. In the 176 patient cohort, there were no differences in incidence of bacteriuria (12% vs 11%, P = .99) or CAUTI (8% vs 7%,

P = .99). However, more catheter-related complications occurred in nitrofurazone group (47% vs 26%, P = .007).[34]

Vopni and colleagues[35] performed a meta-analysis of 15 studies which pooled data from both silver/noble metal and nitrofurazone-coated catheters, which included several of the above-noted studies. Catheter dwell time for each study ranged from 0 to 30 days. Five of the fifteen studies showed a protective effect against CAUTI and analysis of the pooled data in this study showed coated catheters were protective against CAUTI, yielding a conditional odds ratio of 0.80 and a 95% confidence interval of 0.74 to 0.88.[35] However, caution must still be taken in extrapolating these findings to a broader recommendation and new coatings are still being introduced which must be rigorously evaluated. *Given these limited data and cost associated with antiseptic catheters, there is no strong argument to use these catheters primarily as a prophylaxis against CAUTI at this time.*

Catheterization technique

Another factor to consider is how the catheter is inserted into the bladder. Because the urethral meatus is generally colonized with bacterial flora, from the perineal region in men and vaginal/perineal region in women, there has been an emphasis on reducing introduction of these organisms into the urethra or bladder during insertion of the catheter. The Health Infection Control Practices Care Advisory Committee from the Center for Disease Control published guidelines for preventing CAUTI in 2009. These included using sterile technique for insertion of indwelling catheters in a hospital setting and reinforcing Lapides recommendation of a clean technique for self-intermittent catheterization.[36]

Aseptic technique Research has examined whether an aseptic, or "No Touch", approach to intermittent catheterization decreased CAUTI risk or improved quality of life. These techniques include wrappers or sleeves that prevent a person from directly touching the catheter during insertion into the urethra. Hudson and Murahata performed an in vitro study in which they seeded gloves with *Staphylococcus aureus* and *E coli* bacteria and then compared colonization of bacteria between hydrophilic and no touch catheters. They reported a difference in colony counts, although the differences were somewhat modest: 5 CFU on no touch catheters compared with 210 to 440 CFU in hydrophilic catheters.[37] There are few human trials comparing aseptic to clean technique for intermittent catheterization. *Getliffe and colleagues did a systematic review of 13 trials comparing single-use and multiple-use catheters. They found a study* with a nonsignificant difference between positive cultures in the sterile (51%) and clean groups (63%) after a short 3-week trial.[38]

Reusable It is more common to reuse catheters for intermittent self-catheterization in the United States compared with Europe. This may reflect different personal costs associated with the difference systems of health care delivery. In Plata and colleagues' meta-analysis, single-use catheters had no advantage in UTI risk reduction (RR = 0.77; 95% CI 0.59–1.00) when single-use catheters are compared with hydrophilic catheter (HC).[24] Prieto and colleagues performed a similar meta-analysis of 23 studies, many of which overlapped with Plata and also could not quantitate a risk advantage for single-use catheters reducing symptomatic UTIs.[39] Other literature notes a quality of life advantage of using a single-use catheter in that it reduces the amount of time needing to clean and care for a re-useable catheter.[40] *Given these limited data, arguments can be made where either single use or a reusable catheter may have an advantage for a specific situation or treatment goal.*

Selection of Urinary Catheter for Use

There does not seem to be an industry-wide consensus on choosing catheters or providing catheterization education and anecdotal evidence supports that patients may receive different information both between different care facilities and even between different clinics within the same organization.

The selection of an indwelling catheter may be determined by resources available in a hospital system, modified somewhat by the selection of an insertion tip or allergy to catheter material. However, *selecting a urinary catheter for starting intermittent catheterization should be thought of as a simultaneous assessment of multiple variables based on patient's needs, body habitus, physiology, and treatment goals.* Helping the patient choose a catheter is a multistep process that begins during the education phase and continues throughout the continuum of care. Multiple education sessions may be required because the patient may request family or caregivers receive education as well at a later date.

Patients need to find the most appropriate catheter for their needs. With continued support by their treatment team, all patients with bladder dysfunction can benefit from intermittent catheterization.

Before reviewing the below variables, medical providers will usually assess education level and any barriers to learning. The following is a proposed approach for catheter selection for intermittent catheterization via a "cloud" assessment (**Fig. 4**).

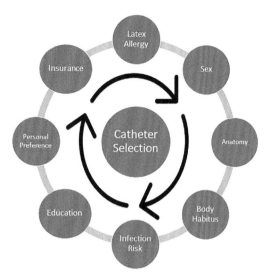

Fig. 4. Simultaneous cloud assessment of patient variables performed when prescribing a urinary catheter for a patient.

Latex allergy

Latex allergy can range from anaphylaxis to irritation. Any reported latex sensitivity defaults a patient to latex catheter category. Patients may develop a latex sensitivity at any point after starting intermittent catheterization and may need to change catheters. There is usually a cost differential with latex-free catheters being more expensive, particularly for specialty catheters.

Sex

Male patients must use a unisex 16″ catheter, however, female patients may use a shorter catheter (6″ female catheter) or unisex 16″ catheter because women have a shorter average urethral length (4–5 cm) versus males (20 cm). Women may prefer using shorter catheter because it is easier to position for the female urethra given its shorter length and position within the vagina. Smaller catheters are also easier to conceal and preferable to some women. All males typically use a standard 16″ catheter. There are no additional catheter length options for men.

Anatomy consideration

Patient should be assessed for possible prostatic enlargement, known urethral strictures and false passages, and prior urethral reconstruction. People with a continent urinary stoma also require special consideration.

An enlarged prostate causes proximal urethral angulation and frequently requires both a larger catheter (16−18 Fr) and a curve catheter tip (eg, Coudé) to successfully access the bladder. Transgendered women may have a prostate and may require a larger catheter with a Coudé tip. In contrast, a urethral stricture will require a small catheter (12 Fr or smaller) and a more rigid catheter. Special care is needed to make sure a person learns proper catheterization technique to avoid causing injury to the urethra. Hydrophilic catheters may be preferred to reduce trauma to stricture. Similarly, people with false passages commonly use Coudé catheters to angle the tip of catheter away from a false passage during catheterization. Hydrophilic catheters may also be preferred so there is less chance of injury.

A continent stoma is a channel between abdominal wall and bladder made out of bladder, appendix, or intestine. Continent stomas generally require smaller catheters (12–14Fr) that are 16″ in length. They may need a curved tip (Coudé) or increased rigidity based on anatomy. People with continent stoma may need to change to a smaller catheter as stoma matures or if scar tissue forms.

Body habitus/body limitations

A person's ability of access the urethra may be altered by body habitus/limitations. With an increased body mass index (BMI), curve tip (Coudé) catheters may be used to access a retracted urethra in both men and women. Catheters with positional aids (grippers, pre-lubrication) may also reduce need for assistance with catheter passage. Fine motor skills or upper extremity limitations also deserve special assessment on hand function. A more rigid catheter, possibly with positional aids, is frequently selected to make it easier for person to pass catheter into urethral meatus and to minimize the impact of loss of dexterity.

People who are generally wheelchair bound and may have physical limitations that do not allow for standard catheterization practices that include draining the urine into a urinal or toilet. Self-contained catheter systems can significantly reduce time to complete catheterization.

Urinary tract infections/bacterial colonization

People with a history of UTIs or those who develop UTIs while on intermittent catheterization may require hydrophilic catheters or self-contained systems if contamination or urethral/bladder injury is a potential source for UTIs. Because bladder irrigation is a common treatment for UTIs in people performing CIC, people performing bladder irrigations will need a catheter that an irrigating syringe can be attached to. People performing bladder irrigation generally cannot use pre-made self-contained catheter kits or compact catheters because an irrigating syringe can not be attached to these systems. Consequently, some people may need an additional catheter type than regularly used to perform irrigation.

Education/cultural/social support

Catheters are selected based on how people are best able to perform the procedure in their everyday life, not just in a medical provider's office. Variables that impact type of catheter and where catheterization is performed include social norms and availability of support. Examples are small easily concealable catheters or self-contained systems for people performing CIC in areas with limited privacy or access to hygiene.

Patient's preference: "the feel of it" Confidence and acceptance of the intermittent catheterization process is important in reducing incidence of urethral injury and in promoting quality of life. Catheter type selection can reduce time needed to catheterization and the need for assistance. Standard practice is to describe several types/brands of catheters. It is important to have options available in the clinic for the patients to touch and to explore differences between pre-lubricated, unlubricated catheters, and tip shape and rigidity. Many patients need to try different catheter types to find the right fit.

Insurance

Currently, insurance status greatly influences the catheter that a patient receives. At the time of teaching, it is frequently unknown by prescribing providers what catheter types are approved by insurance plan and what the cost of catheters will be to the patients. There are hundreds of types of policies that have individual requirements surrounding catheterization documentation and requirements. An out-of-pocket expanse can be significant for specialty catheters (self-lubricated catheters can cost up to and above $2/catheter, self-contained kits can cost in excess of $4/kit).

CLINICS CARE POINTS

- There is directional evidence to suggest hydrophilic catheters are associated with fewer urinary tract infections compared to PVC catheters when performing intermittent catheterization

- Silver and nobel metal catheters may reduce catheter aquired urinary tract infections when used as an indwelling catheter, but data is difficult to extrapolate.

- Single use catheters used for intermittent catheterization, compared to reusable, did not show a definitive reduction in urinary tract infections in several pooled data studies.

- An assessment of multiple patient variables, performed with shared decision making with the patient, can help select the proper catheter for intermittent catheterization.

DISCLOSURE

J.T. Stoffel: Flume Catheter (scientific consultant), Spine X (scientific consultant), and Neurogenic Bladder Research Group (member).

REFERENCES

1. Umscheid CA, Mitchell, Doshi, et al. Estimating the proportion of healthcare-associated infections that are reasonably preventable and the related mortality and costs. Infect Control Hosp Epidemiol 2011; 32(2):101–14.
2. Roth JD, Pariser, Stoffel, et al. Patient subjective assessment of urinary tract infection frequency and severity is associated with bladder management method in spinal cord injury. Spinal Cord 2019; 57(8):700–7.
3. Crescenze IM, Lenherr, Myers, et al. Self-Reported Urological Hospitalizations or Emergency Room Visits in a Contemporary Spinal Cord Injury Cohort. J Urol 2020. https://doi.org/10.1097/JU.0000000000 001386.
4. Cardenas DD, Moore, Dannels-McClure, et al. Intermittent catheterization with a hydrophilic-coated catheter delays urinary tract infections in acute spinal cord injury: a prospective, randomized, multicenter trial. Pharm Manag PM R 2011;3(5):408–17.
5. Feng D, Cheng, Bai, et al. Outcomes comparison of hydrophilic and non-hydrophilic catheters for patients with intermittent catheterization: An updated meta-analysis. Asian J Surg 2020;43(5):633–5.
6. Myers JB, Lenherr, Stoffel, et al. Patient Reported Bladder Related Symptoms and Quality of Life after Spinal Cord Injury with Different Bladder Management Strategies. J Urol 2019;202(3):574–84.
7. Velaer KN, Welk, Ginsberg, et al. Time Burden of Bladder Management in Individuals With Spinal Cord Injury. Top Spinal Cord Inj Rehabil 2021; 27(3):83–91.
8. Welk B, Myers, Kennelly, et al. Using conjoint analysis to measure the importance of psychosocial traits in the choices of bladder management after spinal cord injury. Neurourol Urodyn 2021;40(6): 1643–50.
9. Feneley RC, Hopley IB, Wells PN. Urinary catheters: history, current status, adverse events and research agenda. J Med Eng Technol 2015;39(8):459–70.
10. Bloom DA, McGuire EJ, Lapides J. A brief history of urethral catheterization. J Urol 1994;151(2):317–25.
11. Mattelaer JJ, Billiet I. Catheters and sounds: the history of bladder catheterisation. Paraplegia 1995; 33(8):429–33.
12. Hernigou P. Ambroise Paré III: Paré's contributions to surgical instruments and surgical instruments at the time of Ambroise Paré. Int Orthop 2013;37(5): 975–80.
13. Stoffel JT. Intermittent catheterization: from medical procedure to patient-controlled process. Urology Times; 2022.
14. Foley FEB. Cystoscopic Prostatectomy A New Procedure and Instrument; Preliminary Report. J Urol 1929;21(3):289–306.
15. McClure J., Minnesotan invented life-saving catheter, In: Access press - Minnesota's disability newspaper, 2011, Acess Press: Industrial Station; Minneapolis (MN). www.partnersinpolicymaking.co.
16. Frankel HL. The Sir Ludwig Guttmann lecture 2012: the contribution of Stoke Mandeville Hospital to spinal cord injuries. Spinal Cord 2012;50(11): 790–6.
17. Lapides J, Diokno, Silber, et al. Clean, intermittent self-catheterization in the treatment of urinary tract disease. J Urol 1972;107(3):458–61.
18. Hosseinpour M, Noori, Amir-Beigi, et al. Safety of latex urinary catheters for the short time drainage. Urol Ann 2014;6(3):198–201.
19. Nouri S, Sharif, Hosseinpour, et al. A comparison between foley and nelatone urinary catheters in causing urinary tract infection in animal models. Nurs Midwifery Stud 2015;4(1):e24363.
20. Erickson BA, Navai, Patil, et al. A prospective, randomized trial evaluating the use of hydrogel coated latex versus all silicone urethral catheters after urethral reconstructive surgery. J Urol 2008;179(1): 203–6.
21. Witjes JA, Del Popolo, Marberger, et al. A multicenter, double-blind, randomized, parallel group study comparing polyvinyl chloride and polyvinyl chloride-free catheter materials. J Urol 2009; 182(6):2794–8.
22. Chartier-Kastler E, Denys P. Intermittent catheterization with hydrophilic catheters as a treatment of chronic neurogenic urinary retention. Neurourol Urodyn 2011;30(1):21–31.
23. Rognoni C, Tarricone R. Intermittent catheterisation with hydrophilic and non-hydrophilic urinary catheters: systematic literature review and meta-analyses. BMC Urol 2017;17(1):4.
24. Plata M, Santander, Zuluaga, et al. Hydrophilic versus non-hydrophilic catheters for clean intermittent catheterization: a meta-analysis to determine their capacity in reducing urinary tract infections. World J Urol 2023;41(2):491–9.
25. Hedlund H, Hjelmås, Jonsson, et al. Hydrophilic versus non-coated catheters for intermittent catheterization. Scand J Urol Nephrol 2001;35(1):49–53.

26. Kiddoo D, Sawatzky, Bascu, et al. Randomized Crossover Trial of Single Use Hydrophilic Coated vs Multiple Use Polyvinylchloride Catheters for Intermittent Catheterization to Determine Incidence of Urinary Infection. J Urol 2015;194(1):174–9.

27. Lucas EJ, Baxter, Singh, et al. Comparison of the microbiological milieu of patients randomized to either hydrophilic or conventional PVC catheters for clean intermittent catheterization. J Pediatr Urol 2016;12(3):172–8.

28. Johansson K, Greis, Johansson, et al. Evaluation of a new PVC-free catheter material for intermittent catheterization: a prospective, randomized, crossover study. Scand J Urol 2013;47(1):33–7.

29. Shamout S, Biardeau, Corcos, et al. Outcome comparison of different approaches to self-intermittent catheterization in neurogenic patients: a systematic review. Spinal Cord 2017;55(7):629–43.

30. Sun Y, Ren P, Long X. Role of noble metal-coated catheters for short-term urinary catheterization of adults: a meta-analysis. PLoS One 2020;15(6): e0233215.

31. Lam TB, Omar, Fisher, et al. Types of indwelling urethral catheters for short-term catheterisation in hospitalised adults. Cochrane Database Syst Rev 2014;(9):CD004013.

32. Rugaie OA, Abdellatif, El-Mokhtar, et al. Retardation of Bacterial Biofilm Formation by Coating Urinary Catheters with Metal Nanoparticle-Stabilized Polymers. Microorganisms 2022;10(7).

33. Lee SJ, Kim, Cho, et al. A comparative multicentre study on the incidence of catheter-associated urinary tract infection between nitrofurazone-coated and silicone catheters. Int J Antimicrob Agents 2004;24(Suppl 1):S65–9.

34. Menezes FG, Corrêa, Medina-Pestana, et al. A randomized clinical trial comparing Nitrofurazone-coated and uncoated urinary catheters in kidney transplant recipients: Results from a pilot study. Transpl Infect Dis 2019;21(2):e13031.

35. Vopni R, Voice, de Riese, et al. Use of Antimicrobial-Coated Catheters in Preventing Catheter-Associated Urinary Tract Infections and Bacteriuria: A Meta-Analysis for Clinicians. Urol Pract 2021;8(6):705–12.

36. Gould CV, U.C.A.R.K.G., Pegues DA, and the and H.I.C.P.A.C.H. 4, GUIDELINE FOR PREVENTION OF CATHETERASSOCIATED URINARY TRACT INFECTIONS 2009, CDC, Editor. 2009, Available at: https://www.cdc.gov/infectioncontrol/guidelines/cauti/. p. 1-61.

37. Hudson E, Murahata RI. The 'no-touch' method of intermittent urinary catheter insertion: can it reduce the risk of bacteria entering the bladder? Spinal Cord 2005;43(10):611–4.

38. Getliffe K, Fader, Allen, et al. Current evidence on intermittent catheterization: sterile single-use catheters or clean reused catheters and the incidence of UTI. J Wound Ostomy Continence Nurs 2007; 34(3):289–96.

39. Prieto JA, Murphy, Stewart, et al. Intermittent catheter techniques, strategies and designs for managing long-term bladder conditions. Cochrane Database Syst Rev 2021;10(10):CD006008.

40. Newman DK, New, Heriseanu, et al. Intermittent catheterization with single- or multiple-reuse catheters: clinical study on safety and impact on quality of life. Int Urol Nephrol 2020;52(8):1443–51.

The Role of Upper Extremity Motor Function in the Choice of Bladder Management in Those Unable to Volitionally Void due to Neurologic Dysfunction

Michael Juszczak, MD[a], Kazuko Shem, MD[b],
Christopher S. Elliott, MD, PhD[c],*

KEYWORDS

• Neurogenic bladder • Upper extremity motor function • Epidemiology

KEY POINTS

- It is estimated that 425,000 individuals with neurologic bladder dysfunction (spinal cord injury, spina bifida and multiple sclerosis) are unable to volitionally void and must rely on catheter drainage.
- Upper extremity (UE) motor function is one of the most important factors in determining the type of bladder management chosen in individuals who cannot volitionally void.
- Those with poor UE motor function more often choose an indwelling catheter, while those with normal UE motor function more often choose clean intermittent catheterization (CIC).
- After spinal cord injury, up to 40% of persons have an increase in their functional upper motor function as it relates to the predicted ability to perform CIC of their bladder.
- UE motor function can be improved with non-surgical (tenodesis splints, functional electrical stimulation) and surgical procedures (tendon transfer, nerve transfer, catheterizable channels).
- Novel bladder management solutions for those with impaired UE motor function and concurrent impairments in volitional voiding continue to be an area of need.

INTRODUCTION

Epidemiology of Neurogenic Bladder Requiring Catheterization

Neurogenic bladder (NGB) dysfunction in the form of an inability to empty the bladder is a common problem for those who have neurologic disease with the most common being those with spinal cord injury (SCI), spina bifida (SB), and multiple sclerosis (MS). In the United States, it is estimated that there are 203,000 persons with SCI, 141,000 with SB, and 80,000 with MS, who are unable to volitionally void.[1] Together, these three groups account for ~425,000 persons who are reliant on catheter drainage of the bladder.[1–6] Compared with the general population, those with neurologic disease face many challenges, which include bladder management difficulties that significantly reduce the quality of life (QoL) and increase the rate of medical complications.[7–9]

a Department of Physical Medicine and Rehabilitation, Tower Health, Reading Hospital Rehabilitation at Wyomissing, Reading, PA 19610, USA; b Department of Physical Medicine and Rehabilitation, Santa Clara Valley Medical Center, San Jose, CA 95128, USA; c Division of Urology, Department of Urology, Stanford University Medical Center, Santa Clara Valley Medical Center, Valley Specialties Center-Division of Urology, 4th Floor, 751 South Bascom Avenue, San Jose, CA 95128, USA
* Corresponding author.
E-mail address: christopher.elliott@hhs.sccgov.org

Urol Clin N Am 51 (2024) 263–275
https://doi.org/10.1016/j.ucl.2024.01.002
0094-0143/24/© 2024 Elsevier Inc. All rights reserved.

For those with NGB who are unable to volitionally void, clean intermittent catheterization (CIC), the act of passing a catheter through the urethra into the bladder every 4 to 6 hours, is recommended as the gold standard approach to bladder management because it reduces long-term morbidity.[10,11] Unfortunately, for many who are unable to void due to neurologic disease, upper extremity (UE) motor function limitations make the task of independently performing CIC difficult if not impossible. Patients with poor UE function face multiple challenges when performing CIC which can include removing the catheter from a sealed package; removing ones' clothing to access the urethra; guiding the catheter through the urethra into the bladder; holding a urine receptacle during bladder drainage; disposing urine and catheterization materials after bladder drainage; and then getting redressed. Consequently, for many, CIC can only be performed with the aid of an around-the-clock caregiver[12] which is often either not fully covered by insurance and/or beyond the capabilities of assisting family. This review serves to highlight how UE limitations affect bladder management choices and the current options to improve UE motor impairment.

Among the three main groups with neurologic disease resulting in an inability to volitionally void, UE motor function is most often affected in those with SCI, specifically those with injuries to the cervical spinal segment from which UE motor function signaling originates. Conversely, those with SB are thought to rarely have UE function limitations based on their lumbosacral spinal cord malformations that spare the cervical segments.[13] In those with MS, certain sections of the population have UE functional limitation based on the affected portion of the nervous system; however, epidemiologic study in this area is limited.[14] As a result, studies of the effects of UE motor limitations on bladder management have mainly focused on those with SCI; however, these can be applied to any individual, whether a neurologic disease is present or not.

ASSESSING UPPER EXTREMITY STRENGTH AND MOTOR FUNCTION TO PERFORM CLEAN INTERMITTENT CATHETERIZATION

Accurately assessing UE motor strength and function and its potential recovery following neurologic injury can be challenging as there are few suitable outcome measures to assess UE functional status from a research standpoint.[15] Adequate outcome measures need to have increased responsiveness (ie, a measure's ability to capture clinically meaningful changes with respect to a given variable) to predict functionality and changes in overall functional status that can influence bladder management selection over time due to evolving UE motor function.[16] Two standardized tools to assess muscle strength of the UE in SCI are the International Standards for Neurologic Classification of Spinal Cord Injury (ISNCSCI) and the International Classification for Surgery of the Hand in Tetraplegia (ICSHT), which was developed specifically for surgical planning of the UE in tetraplegia.[17] Although ISNCSI measures UE strengths only in five key muscles, the ICSHT measures strength of nine muscles and it also tests two-point discrimination on the thumb and index fingers. However, information about changes in UE function in addition to strength testing may aid clinicians in developing more personalized treatment plans and in setting more realistic outcome expectations.[18,19] Some of the UE functional measures that have been validated in SCI are the Spinal Cord Injury-Functional Index (SCI-FI), Capabilities of Upper Extremity Instrument, Jebsen Hand Function Test, Sollerman Hand Function Test, Tetraplegia Hand Activity Questionnaire, Van Lieshout Test, Grasp and Release Test, and Graded and Redefined Assessment of Strength, Sensibility and Prehension (GRASSP).[17] The authors highlight a few of these existing tools as follows.

Spinal Cord Injury-Functional Index

The SCI-FI is a psychometrically robust set of instruments developed to improve the measurement of physical functioning in those living with SCI.[20,21] It consists of item banks measuring activity limitations including self-care, basic mobility, and fine motor capability among others.[20–22] For measuring UE function, the SCI-FI fine motor domain has been shown to be responsive to UE motor change for individuals with tetraplegia and incomplete paraplegia.[23]

Tulsky and colleagues used growth mixture modeling to explore[24] the trajectories of recovery with tasks specifically related to dressing, eating, grooming, bathing, and toileting. In all, several distinct patterns of motor recovery have been found ranging from no recovery to gradual recovery to those improvements that are rapid and substantial in nature. This information may be used to assist in the timing of surgical procedures such as tendon transfers and the creation of a catheterizable channel if there is not expected to be significant motor recovery to allow for independent CIC.

Graded and Redefined Assessment of Strength, Sensibility, and Prehension

The GRASSP measures UE sensorimotor function and is designed to capture changes in neurologic recovery of UE function. The GRASSP measure differs from other assessments of UE function in that it was developed for use in those with neurologic impairment based on concepts related to functional status. Repeated use over time provides a recovery profile for multiple domains of function and importantly captures changes in neurologic status rather than changes in functional status alone (which may improve due to learned compensation strategies as opposed to actual neurologic recovery). Specifically, the battery of tests in the GRASSP are used to assess all domains of UE function which include hand strength (the motor force generated that allows for hand dexterity and object manipulation), sensibility (the ability of the hand to discriminate between different forms of tactile sensation), and prehension (the act of co-ordinated reaching and grasping)[25]

Kalsi-Ryan and colleagues administered the GRASSP to individuals with SCI and validated its use as a standardized UE impairment measure to detect changes in UE function.[26] In a prospective analysis of 127 patients with tetraplegia, they found that improvements in the GRASSP subdomain of strength were most sensitive in detecting clinically meaningful change with respect to physical functioning.[27] The GRASSPs unique ability to capture information related to UE function may allow for more informed decision-making for targeted interventions such as functional electrical stimulation (FES) to generate more motor force in weakened muscles. To our knowledge, its use to predict bladder management capabilities has not been performed but remains an interesting potential application.

An Algorithm for the Ability to Self-Catheterize Based on Upper Extremity Motor Strength Scores

As the National Spinal Cord Injury Database (NSCID) data set (which houses information on more than 36,000 persons with SCI) does not use formal measures of UE motor function such as SCI-FI or GRASSP, Zlatev and colleagues proposed an algorithm for a person's ability to self-catheterize based solely on UE motor scores collected at the time of acute rehabilitation discharge (which are part of the NSCID data set).[28] Included in this algorithm are portions of the neurologic examination that assess bilateral motor strength at the C5–C8 levels based on the ISNCSCI. In the ISNCSCI, motor scores are individually graded from 0 to 5 (0 = total paralysis; 1 = palpable or visible contraction; 2 = active movement, full range of motion with gravity eliminated; 3 = active movement, full range of motion

against gravity; 4 = active movement, full range of motion against moderate resistance; and 5 = active movement, full range of motion against full resistance). As trying to characterize one of six possible motor scores at four motor levels bilaterally results in more than 1.6 million possible combinations, a simplification of the motor data was performed where the scores at C5–C8 levels were instead transformed into a binary variable consisting of the ability or inability to achieve active motion against moderate or full resistance, reclassified as "strong" (manual muscle test grade 4 or 5) or "weak" (manual muscle test grade 0, 1, 2, or 3). With this modification, a total of 257 combinations result, allowing for meaningful patient grouping based on expert opinion as either (A) able to catheterize; (B) possibly able to catheterize; (C) able to catheterize only with reconstructive surgical assistance; or (D) unable to catheterize with 99% of patients successfully categorized, and less than 1% of patients being classified as outliers (**Fig. 1**).[28]

Although this study was the first to propose an algorithm to classify the UE motor strength required to perform the discrete act of self-catheterization, a potential limitation is that the authors rely on expert opinion, extrapolating from experience and prior literature what motor score might result in what degree of function. In addition, the authors were unable to directly test their algorithm against a gold standard. Hence, the UE motor function findings of this group, which comprise a large degree of the UE motor function/bladder management literature, can be questioned to a certain degree. It is reassuring however that in a subsequent manuscript examining bladder management and measures of the SCI-Fine Motor Index described above, similar trends in UE motor function and bladder management choice were found, suggesting that the algorithm to predict the ability to self-catheterize proposed by Zlatev and colleagues likely capture much of its intended meaning.

THE ROLE OF UPPER EXTREMITY MOTOR FUNCTION ON BLADDER MANAGEMENT CHOICE IN THOSE UNABLE TO VOLITIONALLY VOID

Those with a neurologic impairment sparing the cervical spinal segments are typically able to independently perform CIC as the nerves to the UE muscles are usually intact, resulting in preserved UE function. However, those with cervical SCI experience varying levels of UE weakness, which can make performing CIC a challenge as independently performing CIC is a multistep process consisting of potentially needing to (1) remove the

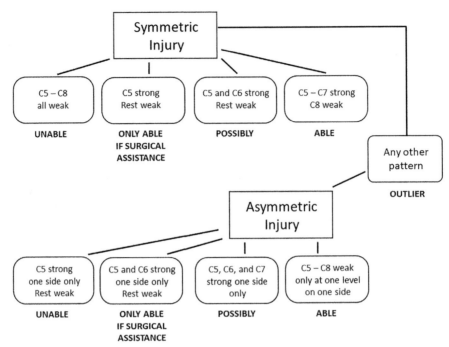

Fig. 1. Algorithm for the predicted ability to self-catheterize based on UE motor strength scores. (*From* Zlatev DV, Shem K, Elliott CS. How many spinal cord injury patients can catheterize their own bladder? The epidemiology of upper extremity function as it affects bladder management. *Spinal Cord*. 2016;54(4):287–291. https://doi.org/10.1038/sc.2015.169, with permission.)

catheter from its packaging; (2) transfer to a toilet/bed or advantageous position in a wheelchair; (3) remove clothing overlying the genitalia; (4) expose the urethra (either putting the penis on stretch or spreading the vaginal labia; (5) guide the catheter through the urethra; (6) dispose of drained urine; (7) replace ones clothing; and (8) potentially needing to transfer back to a wheelchair.

As a result, the degree of UE motor impairment has been thought by many to be the characteristic most significantly associated with the method of bladder management chosen/prescribed at discharge from acute inpatient rehabilitation in those with SCI. Yilmaz and colleagues examined barriers to performing CIC in 269 patients with traumatic SCI who had been performing CIC for at least 3 months. Of those unable to independently perform CIC long term, insufficient hand function (56.1%) was cited as the primary barrier, whereas being unable to appropriately position (35.4%) and spasticity (8.5%) were other commonly cited obstacles.[29] Along these lines, another study of neurologic level of injury and bladder management suggested that CIC rates increase as neurologic level increased (C4 = 0%, C5 = 36.4%, C6 = 66.7%, C7 = 85.7%)[30]

To study the effects of UE motor function on bladder management in a more robust and

statistically significant manner, Zlatev and colleagues examined data on 4,481 individuals in the NSCID at the time of acute rehabilitation discharge using the algorithm described in **Fig. 1**.[28] They found that in the general SCI population, 59% of patients were categorized as "able to catheterize," 12.9% as "possibly able to catheterize," 4% as "able to catheterize with surgical assistance, and 23% as "unable to catheterize." This correlated well with the type of bladder management chosen at rehabilitation discharge with those deemed "able to catheterize" more likely to be discharged performing CIC (73%) than an indwelling catheter (18%) and those deemed "unable to catheterize" more likely to be discharged with an indwelling catheter (58%) compared with CIC (36%). However, although UE motor function was found to be an important factor in dictating bladder management, it was not wholly predictive of discharge bladder management outcomes with 33% of those discharged home with an indwelling catheter deemed "able to self-catheterize" and 14% of patients discharged home with CIC deemed "unable to self-catheterize."[28]

To follow-up this basic epidemiologic study capturing trends at the time of rehabilitation discharge, Zlatev and colleagues further analyzed the relationship between UE motor strength and bladder management in 5112 individuals 1 year after SCI (a time where long-term bladder management choices have typically been made), again using the NSCID. Using multivariate logistic regression models, the authors specifically examined variables affecting (A) a lack of CIC adoption at discharge from acute rehabilitation; (B) CIC discontinuation within the first year after discharge from acute rehabilitation; and (C) continuation of an indwelling catheter rather than converting to CIC at 1 year follow-up after discharge from acute rehabilitation. Using the same previously published algorithm on UE strength (see **Fig. 1**) to predict the ability to self-catheterize, they examined the impact of UE strength, age, gender, BMI, and the American Spinal Injury Association Impairment Scale (AIS) classification. For all three modeled scenarios, UE strength was the most significant predictor for lack of CIC adoption and adherence in people with SCI 1 year after rehabilitation discharge with age and sex also playing more minor roles that also achieved statistical significance (**Table 1**).[31]

UPPER EXTREMITY MOTOR RECOVERY AFTER SPINAL CORD INJURY

Based on prior research demonstrating that individuals with SCI generally experience at least one motor level of improvement following initial injury, Elliott and colleagues followed up their existing UE motor function research by examining the chance of improvement in the ability to self-catheterize during the recovery phase after SCI.[32–34] This was thought to be important as understanding changes in UE strength would theoretically guide realistic discussions about performing independent CIC during acute rehabilitation and additionally to help guide the timing of reconstructive surgeries to facilitate CIC, as there are no established clinical guidelines that speak to their appropriate timing.

Examining a cohort of persons from the NSCID data set with cervical SCI ($n = 1428$) and available motor examinations both at the time of rehabilitation discharge AND at 1 year follow-up, they found that using their algorithm, 40% of patients with SCI will experience an improvement in categorization of UE motor function level over the first year after injury. Overall, an improvement from "possibly able to catheterize," "able to catheterize with surgical assistance," or "unable to catheterize" improved to being "able to catheterize" in 39%, 11%, and 9% of persons, respectively (**Fig. 2**).[35] The degree of improvement, while noted in all groups, was most influenced by AIS class, with more incomplete injuries more likely to improve.[35]

IMPACT OF UPPER EXTREMITY MOTOR RECOVERY ON BLADDER MANAGEMENT AFTER SPINAL CORD INJURY

Given that UE motor function is a key component of individuals adopting and adhering to CIC, one would expect that the improvements in UE motor function during the first year after SCI noted above would be associated with an increase in CIC utilization. However, in a follow-up study of the same model systems SCI cohort ($n = 1428$) at 1 year follow-up, Elliott and colleagues found that those with improvements in UE motor function did not have significant increases in the uptake of CIC.[36] In fact, despite increases in UE function that would predict the ability to perform self-catheterization, CIC dropout (ie, transitioning from CIC to an indwelling catheter) was more common in the first year after rehabilitation discharge than CIC adoption, even when stratifying the data to account for differing UE motor function capability. Specifically, CIC dropout rates among those in the cohort initially deemed "less than able to independently catheterize (a group consisting of "possibly able to catheterize," "only able to catheterize with surgical assistance," or "unable to catheterize") were not significantly altered by whether there was UE motor improvement to be "able to independently catheterize" (34.3% CIC dropout) compared with those who remained "less than able to independently catheterize" (30.0% CIC dropout). In addition, the adoption of CIC did not significantly increase in those with a UE motor transition from "less than able to catheterize" to "able to catheterize" (12.7%) when compared with those "less than able to catheterize" who did not have significant UE improvement (9.2%). Overall, significantly increased rates of CIC adoption were only observed in those that were initially classified as "able to independently catheterize" who had been discharged from rehabilitation with a non-CIC method of bladder management. This was tempered however by the fact that despite individuals in this group having stable motor function at 1 year follow-up, they were still more likely to discontinue CIC ($n = 43$) than adopt CIC ($n = 22$), as illustrated in **Fig. 3**.[36]

On the whole, these findings reinforce the notion that although UE motor function significantly matters (especially when decisions are being made during acute rehabilitation), there are other variables impacting long-term bladder management choices. Based on the studies of CIC discontinuation, the most common sources of patient dissatisfaction are the *4 I's* (urinary *Incontinence*, urinary tract *Infection*, bladder management *Independence*, and bladder management *Inconvenience*) with

Table 1
Logistic regression modeling of: (A) a lack of CIC adoption at discharge from acute rehabilitation; (B) CIC discontinuation within the first year after discharge from acute rehabilitation; and (C) continuation of an indwelling catheter rather than converting to CIC at 1 y follow-up after discharge from acute rehabilitation

		Choice of an Indwelling Catheter over CIC at Time of Rehabilitation Discharge	P-Value	Conversion to an Indwelling Catheter from CIC During the First Year after Rehabilitation Discharge	P-Value	Continuing with an Indwelling Catheter over Converting to CIC During the First Year after Rehabilitation Discharge	P-Value
Age		1.02 (1.02–1.03)	<.001	1.02 (1.01–1.03)	<.001	1.02 (1.01–1.03)	<.001
Gender	Male	Reference	—	Reference	—	Reference	—
	Female	1.73 (1.50–2.00)	<.001	1.13 (0.86–1.47)	.379	2.49 (1.68–3.69)	<.001
AIS Class	A	Reference	—	Reference	—	Reference	—
	B	0.89 (0.76–1.06)	.196	0.87 (0.66–1.13)	.299	0.76 (0.50–1.16)	.200
	C	0.79 (0.66–0.94)	.008	0.62 (0.44–0.85)	.003	0.49 (0.31–0.78)	.003
	D	0.81 (0.68–0.98)	.028	0.55 (0.36–0.86)	.008	0.45 (0.24–0.82)	.009
UE motor function to self-catheterize	Able	Reference	—	Reference	—	Reference	—
	Possibly Able	3.22 (2.70–3.83)	<.001	2.41 (1.75–3.31)	<.001	5.50 (3.30–9.20)	<.001
	Only with surgical assistance	3.44 (2.61–4.53)	<.001	2.32 (1.36–3.93)	.002	4.01 (2.00–8.02)	<.001
	Unable	5.20 (4.52–5.98)	<.001	2.78 (2.16–3.56)	<.001	6.33 (4.33–9.25)	<.001

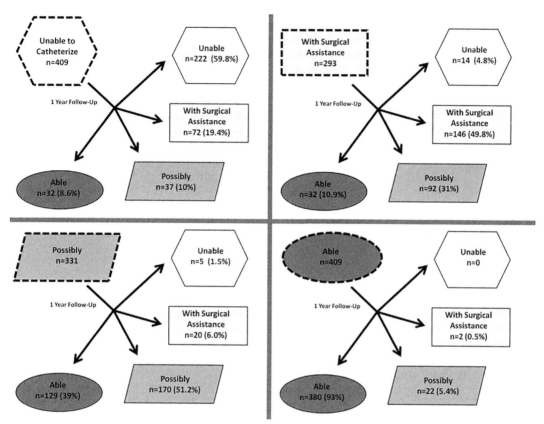

Fig. 2. Changes observed in UE motor function as it pertains to the predicted ability to independently self-catheterize from the time of discharge from acute rehabilitation to 1-year follow-up. (*Data from* Elliott CS, Zlatev D, Crew J, Shem K. Do appreciable changes in the upper extremity motor capability to perform clean intermittent catheterization come about with time after traumatic spinal cord injury?. *Neurourol Urodyn.* 2019;38(3):975–980. https://doi.org/10.1002/nau.23943.)

important modifiers such as increasing age, female gender (a group with more difficulty accessing the urethra), the time it takes to perform CIC (with overweight/obese females requiring significantly more time to catheterize), lack of caregiver assistance, and a lack of appropriate public facilities to perform CIC when away from home also playing a role.[37–40]

IMPROVING UPPER EXTREMITY MOTOR FUNCTION BEYOND INITIAL RECOVERY

Although UE motor function may improve in a significant proportion of the SCI population as noted above, the improvements are often limited for many. The authors describe both nonsurgical (tenodesis aids) and surgical measures (UE reconstruction, neural transfer) that can be considered to further improve UE function to increase functional independence with respect to feeding, grooming, hygiene, performing body weight transfers and performance of CIC.[41]

Tenodesis Effect and Aids

Tenodesis grasp is a normal function of the hand where active wrist flexion allows for passive finger extension and active wrist extension allows for passive finger flexion, as depicted in **Fig. 4**.[42] Tenodesis allows those with impaired UE motor function to grasp and release objects by changing the positioning of their wrists. The ability to grasp objects can lead to increased functional independence including the act of performing CIC.[43] The tenodesis can be augmented using an external orthotic (tenodesis splint). Briefly, the tenodesis splint is worn over an individual's forearm to further promote active wrist extension to bring about passive finger flexion and facilitate pinching and grasping movements of the hand. Tenodesis splints are commonly used in people living with C6 tetraplegia with intact extensor carpe radialis muscle to help provide prehension (grasp) and to assist with performing CIC independently (see **Fig. 4**).[44,45]

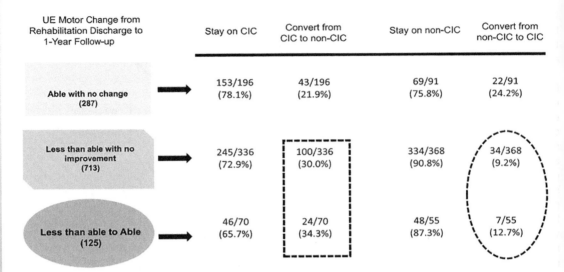

UE Motor Change from Rehabilitation Discharge to 1-Year Follow-up	Stay on CIC	Convert from CIC to non-CIC	Stay on non-CIC	Convert from non-CIC to CIC
Able with no change (287)	153/196 (78.1%)	43/196 (21.9%)	69/91 (75.8%)	22/91 (24.2%)
Less than able with no improvement (713)	245/336 (72.9%)	100/336 (30.0%)	334/368 (90.8%)	34/368 (9.2%)
Less than able to Able (125)	46/70 (65.7%)	24/70 (34.3%)	48/55 (87.3%)	7/55 (12.7%)

Fig. 3. Changes in bladder management from rehabilitation discharge to 1-year follow-up stratified by changes in the predicted ability to self-catheterize. (*Data from* Elliott CS, Seufert C, Zlatev D, Kreydin E, Crew J, Shem K. Do improvements in upper extremity motor function affect changes in bladder management after cervical spinal cord injury? [published online ahead of print, 2021 Nov 18]. *J Spinal Cord Med.* 2021;1–7). https://doi.org/10.1080/10790268.2021.1999715. Does not require permission.)

Upper Extremity Reconstruction/Tendon Transfers

A tendon transfer is a procedure where a tendon of a functional muscle is moved from its normal anatomic insertion and transplanted to the tendon of a new target muscle.[46] When individuals with tetraplegia do not have tenodesis, the goal of UE reconstruction is to restore active elbow extension and/or wrist extension and/or pinch/grasp to perform activities of daily livings (ADLs) with or without the need for adaptive equipment. In addition to tendon transfers, thumb carpometacarpal joint arthrodesis is used to establish better positioning of the thumb to restore key grip which is critical for self-CIC.[46,47] UE reconstruction procedures may be appropriate for individuals with neurologic impairment between C4 and C8 to help foster independent self-catheterization.

Generally, tendon transfer procedures are only performed in muscles with intact sensation and strength. Appropriate sensation is tested using the Weber two-point discrimination test and defined as the ability to distinguish between 1 and 2 points on the thumb greater than 10 mm apart, whereas adequate strength is defined as manual muscle

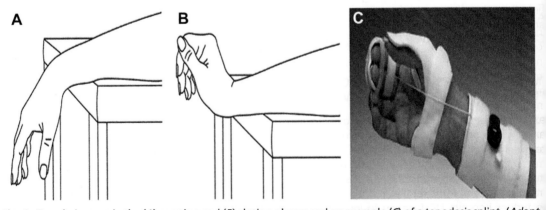

Fig. 4. Tenodesis grasp in the (*A*) opening and (*B*) closing phases and an example (*C*) of a tenodesis splint. (*Adapted from* Jung HY, Lee J, Shin HI. The natural course of passive tenodesis grip in individuals with spinal cord injury with preserved wrist extension power but paralyzed fingers and thumbs. *Spinal Cord.* 2018;56(9):900–906. https://doi.org/10.1038/s41393-018-0137-4. Permission Pending.)

testing scores of at least 4 out of 5 (4 = active movement, full range of motion against moderate resistance, 5 = active movement, full range of motion against full resistance).[48,49]

Before UE reconstruction surgery, a comprehensive multidisciplinary assessment by physiatrists, surgeons, and occupational therapists is essential to ensure that the patient might functionally benefit from the procedure. Psychological assessments are also routinely incorporated to assess a patient's motivation and commitment to continue rehabilitation following the UE reconstruction and to help set realistic postoperative expectations and goals. Practically, one can expect to gain one level of improvement in motor function with a successful tendon transfer procedure (ie, moving from C6 to C7). When successful, UE reconstruction procedures have been associated with improved psychological well-being and an improved QoL.[50,51]

Three prior studies have shown an improvement in bladder management ability after reconstructive UE surgery using tendon transfer techniques.[47,52,53] In one study, all eight individuals with C5–C6 SCI underwent tendon transfers who could not self-catheterize at baseline were able to catheterize after UE surgery[53] However, in another study, only 51% of people with C6 SCI and 86% of people with C7 or C8 SCI were able to perform CIC independently after UE reconstruction surgery.[52] More recently, Bermuz and colleagues reported on 20 individuals with C5–C7 tetraplegia who underwent UE surgery and noted that improvement in the key-grip strength was associated with the ability to independently perform CIC with global satisfaction and QoL measures higher in individuals who were able to perform CIC.[47]

Nerve Transfers

A nerve transfer procedure entails severing an intact motor fascicle and nerve branch from a major peripheral nerve and reimplanting it into a non-innervated muscle below the neurologic level of injury.[54] In contrast to tendon transfers, nerve transfers offer the possibility of axonal sprouting in the newly re-innervated muscle, allowing for axonal regeneration of up to five local motor axons, which may further facilitate neuromuscular recovery.

Historically, the optimal timing, patient selection, indication, and functional outcomes following nerve transfers have been thought to only extend to those who are within 12 months of neurologic injury.[55,56] However, work by Javeed and colleagues evaluating the clinical utility of nerve transfers in restoring UE motor function demonstrates that independent of the timing of the procedure (median time of 21 months after SCI, range 6–142 months after SCI), UE nerve transfer recipients have statistically significant improvements in (A) elbow extension, with 70% of participants achieving greater than 3 out of 5 manual motor testing (MMT) scores, (B) finger extension, with 79% of participants achieving greater than 3 out of 5 MMT scores, and (C) finger flexion, with 52% of participants achieving greater than 3 out of 5 MMT scores. In addition, they demonstrate continued neurologic recovery for up to 48 months after the nerve transfer, supporting the notion of ongoing nerve regeneration and neuroplasticity that may further aid UE motor recovery. To date, no specific data on nerve transfer outcomes as it relates to bladder management have been performed.[57]

Electrical Stimulation

One other therapy with potential long-term promise is FES therapy to improve UE function in SCI.[58] The protocols for transcutaneous FES have been developed with the intent to be used primarily as short-term training therapy to achieve more voluntary function. FES can also be implanted as a neuroprostheses with one system being able to stimulate 12 muscles in the UE.[59] Of note, however, implantable neuroprostheses have not been widely available in the US and their potential effect on bladder management has not been studied.

Surgical Creation of Catheterizable Channels for Catheterization

Although the above procedures can improve one's ability to independently perform CIC through improvements in UE function, the fact is that most individuals require two functioning UEs to perform CIC (one hand to grasp the penis/spread the labia, and the other to insert the catheter). Hence, for individuals with only one functional UE, independent CIC can be extremely problematic if not impossible to perform. To aid in these circumstances or when urethral access is difficult for other reasons (urethral stricture, female gender, lower extremity spasticity), surgical procedures that create a catheterizable channel can be performed to promote CIC use. During catheterizable channel procedures, a section of tubularized intestine (appendix, ileum) is used to create a connection from the bladder to the skin of an accessible location on the lower abdomen (typically umbilical or periumbilical) in order to facilitate CIC when in a seated position. The optimal catheterizable channel stoma site is often patient-specific and requires a multidisciplinary approach with those that are

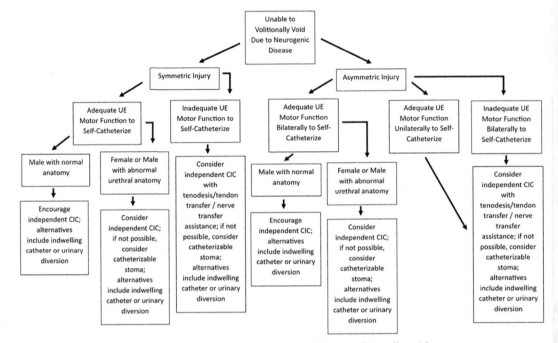

Fig. 5. proposed bladder management algorithm for those unable to volitionally void.

wheelchair bound often requiring higher placement of the stomal location.[60] Catheterizable channel use to facilitate CIC has been associated with higher levels of self-esteem, QoL, and in reducing the time and effort needed to perform catheterization.[61,62] Specifically in a cohort of female patients with tetraplegia who underwent surgical creation of a catheterizable stoma, Walsh and colleagues found that mean catheterization time decreased from 27 minutes per episode of catheterization to 8 minutes.[63]

Although catheterizable channel procedures are often successful, there are unique long-term considerations. Patients undergoing channel creation via an ileocecocystoplasty procedure, which uses the distal ileum and ileocecal valve, are at risk vitamin B12 deficiency and diarrhea due to malabsorption of bile salts.[64] Other commonly reported complications can include urethral or stomal incontinence, stomal stenosis, and bladder calculi.

In a retrospective chart analysis by the Neurogenic Bladder Research Group of 114 individuals who underwent catheterizable stoma procedures, 20% were found to require a revision of the channel (for stenosis or incontinence) and 10% were noted to abandon the use of the channel long term.[65] Hence, although excellent outcomes can be achieved, ideal outcomes are not always achieved and improvements in this area are needed.

SUMMARY

Although CIC is considered a gold standard for bladder management in those unable to volitionally void due to neurologic injury, the adoption and adherence to CIC is less than ideal. This likely speaks to a need to address barriers to CIC such as urinary incontinence (which can be treated pharmacologically or with botulinum toxin injections) and UTI (which can be treated with bladder management alterations and antibiotics), though a significant driving force behind opting for non-CIC bladder management options is impaired UE motor function in a large segment of the neurogenic population. To date, although certain interventions such as UE reconstruction, nerve transfer, tenodesis aids, catheterizable stoma creation, and time after injury may result in improved UE motor function and an improved ability to self-catheterize, the fact is that a large proportion of the neurogenic population does not adopt these measures which often require specialized surgery. Whether failure to adopt these measures is due to lack of medical support or patient choice is unclear, though it speaks to the need for novel bladder management systems, beyond CIC or indwelling catheters with a specific focus on those with limited UE function. Until that time, the authors offer our bladder management algorithm based on our 30+ years' experience with the neurogenic population in the hopes that it aids others and encourage future research on this understudied area of urology (**Fig. 5**).

CLINICS CARE POINTS

- After spinal cord injury, up to 40% of persons have an increase in their functional upper motor function as it relates to the predicted ability to perform CIC of their bladder. The degree of UE motor function return is predicated on the degree of the initial injury andthe completeness of injury.

- Despite the importance of UE motor function in choosing a bladder management, individuals who are discharged from spinal cord injury rehabilitation with abnormal UE motor function are no more likely to adopt CIC practices when their UE motor function significantly improves over time, compared to individuals without significant upper extremity improvement. This suggests that other factors also affect long-term bladder management choices.

DISCLOSURE

The authors have nothing to disclose.

REFERENCES

1. Sun AJ, Comiter CV, Elliott CS. The cost of a catheter: An environmental perspective on single use clean intermittent catheterization. Neurourol Urodyn 2018;37(7):2204–8.
2. Wallin MT, Culpepper WJ, Campbell JD, et al. The prevalence of MS in the United States. Neurology 2019;92(10):e1029–40.
3. Mahajan S, Frasure HE, Ruth Ann M. The prevalence of urinary catheterization in women and men with multiple sclerosis. Journal of Spinal Cord Medicine 2013;36(6):632–7.
4. Bowman RM, McLone DG, Grant JA, et al. Spina Bifida Outcome: A 25-Year Prospective. Pediatr Neurosurg 2001;34(3):114–20.
5. Faleiros F, Pelosi G, Warschausky S, et al. Factors influencing the use of intermittent bladder catheterization by individuals with spina bifida in Brazil and Germany. Rehabil Nurs 2018;43(1):46–51.
6. Spinal cord injury (SCI) 2016 facts and figures at a glance. Journal of Spinal Cord Medicine 2016; 39(4):493–4.
7. Oh SJ, Hyeon Ku J, Gyun Jeon H, et al. Health-related quality of life of patients using clean intermittent catheterization for neurogenic bladder secondary to spinal cord injury. Urology 2005;65(2):306–10.
8. Westgren N, Levi R. Quality of life and traumatic spinal cord injury. Arch Phys Med Rehabil 1998;79(11): 1433–9.
9. Skelton F, Salemi JL, Akpati L, et al. Genitourinary complications are a leading and expensive cause of emergency department and inpatient encounters for persons with spinal cord injury. Arch Phys Med Rehabil 2019;100(9):1614–21.
10. Kennelly M, Thiruchelvam N, Averbeck MA, et al. Adult neurogenic lower urinary tract dysfunction and intermittent catheterisation in a community setting: risk factors model for urinary tract infections. Advances in Urology 2019;2019:1–13.
11. Weld KJ, Dmochowski RR. Effect of bladder management on urological complications in spinal cord injured patients. J Urol 2000;163(3):768–72.
12. Seth JH, Haslam C, Panicker JN. Ensuring patient adherence to clean intermittent self-catheterization. Patient Prefer Adherence 2014;8:191–8. https://doi.org/10.2147/PPA.S49060. Published 2014 Feb 12.
13. Sager C, Barroso U Jr, Bastos JM, et al. Management of neurogenic bladder dysfunction in children update and recommendations on medical treatment. Int Braz J Urol 2022;48(1):31–51. https://doi.org/10.1590/S1677-5538.IBJU.2020.0989.
14. Stoffel JT, Dray EV. Urological care for patients with progressive neurological conditions. Switzerland: Springer Nature; 2019.
15. Dunn JA, Sinnott KA, Bryden AM, et al. Measurement issues related to upper limb interventions in persons who have tetraplegia. Hand Clin 2008; 24(2):161. https://doi.org/10.1016/j.hcl.2008.01.005.
16. Revicki DA, Cella D, Hays RD, et al. Responsiveness and minimal important differences for patient reported outcomes. Health Qual Life Outcomes 2006;4(70). https://doi.org/10.1186/1477-7525-4-70.
17. Mulcahey MJ, Hutchinson D, Kozin S. Assessment of upper limb in tetraplegia: considerations in evaluation and outcomes research. J Rehabil Res Dev 2007;44(1):91–102. https://doi.org/10.1682/jrrd.2005.10.0167.
18. Pretz CR, Kozlowski AJ, Charlifue S, et al. Using Rasch motor FIM individual growth curves to inform clinical decisions for persons with paraplegia. Spinal Cord 2014;52(9):671–6. https://doi.org/10.1038/sc.2014.94.
19. Kozlowski AJ, Pretz CR, Dams-O'Connor K, et al. An introduction to applying individual growth curve models to evaluate change in rehabilitation: a national institute on disability and rehabilitation research traumatic brain injury model systems report. Arch Phys Med Rehabil 2013;94(3):589–96. https://doi.org/10.1016/j.apmr.2012.08.199.
20. Jette AM, Tulsky DS, Ni P, et al. Development and initial evaluation of the spinal cord injury-functional

index. Arch Phys Med Rehabil 2012;93(10):1733–50. https://doi.org/10.1016/j.apmr.2012.05.008.

21. Tulsky DS, Jette AM, Kisala PA, et al. Spinal cord injury-functional index: item banks to measure physical functioning in individuals with spinal cord injury. Arch Phys Med Rehabil 2012;93(10):1722–32. https://doi.org/10.1016/j.apmr.2012.05.007.

22. World Health Organization. International Classification of Functioning, Disability and Health (ICF). www.who.int. Published 2001. https://www.who.int/standards/classifications/international-classification-of-functioning-disability-and-health.

23. Kisala PA, Boulton AJ, Slavin MD, et al. Spinal cord injury-functional index/capacity: responsiveness to change over time. Arch Phys Med Rehabil 2022; 103(2):199–206. https://doi.org/10.1016/j.apmr.2021.10.005.

24. Tulsky DS, Boulton AJ, Kisala PA, et al. Physical function recovery trajectories after spinal cord injury. Arch Phys Med Rehabil 2022;103(2):215–23. https://doi.org/10.1016/j.apmr.2021.09.012.

25. Kalsi-Ryan S, Curt A, Fehlings M, et al. Assessment of the Hand in tetraplegia using the graded redefined assessment of strength, sensibility and prehension (GRASSP). Top Spinal Cord Inj Rehabil 2009;14(4):34–46.

26. Kalsi-Ryan S, Beaton D, Curt A, et al. The graded redefined assessment of strength sensibility and prehension: reliability and validity. J Neurotrauma 2012; 29(5):905–14. https://doi.org/10.1089/neu.2010.1504.

27. Kalsi-Ryan S, Balbinot G, Wang JZ, et al. Minimal clinically important difference of graded redefined assessment of strength, sensibility, and prehension version 1 in acute cervical traumatic spinal cord injury. J Neurotrauma 2022;39(23–24):1645–53. https://doi.org/10.1089/neu.2021.0500.

28. Zlatev DV, Shem K, Elliott CS. How many spinal cord injury patients can catheterize their own bladder? The epidemiology of upper extremity function as it affects bladder management. Spinal Cord 2016; 54(4):287–91. https://doi.org/10.1038/sc.2015.169.

29. Yılmaz B, Akkoç Y, Alaca R, et al. Intermittent catheterization in patients with traumatic spinal cord injury: obstacles, worries, level of satisfaction. Spinal Cord 2014;52(11):826–30. https://doi.org/10.1038/sc.2014.134.

30. Kriz J, Relichova Z. Intermittent self-catheterization in tetraplegic patients: a 6-year experience gained in the spinal cord unit in Prague. Spinal Cord 2014; 52(2):163–6. https://doi.org/10.1038/sc.2013.154.

31. Zlatev DV, Shem K, Elliott CS. Predictors of long-term bladder management in spinal cord injury patients-Upper extremity function may matter most. Neurourol Urodyn 2018;37(3):1106–12. https://doi.org/10.1002/nau.23430.

32. Marino RJ, Ditunno JF Jr, Donovan WH, et al. Neurologic recovery after traumatic spinal cord injury:

data from the Model Spinal Cord Injury Systems. Arch Phys Med Rehabil 1999;80(11):1391–6. https://doi.org/10.1016/s0003-9993(99)90249-6.

33. Kirshblum SC, O'Connor KC. Predicting neurologic recovery in traumatic cervical spinal cord injury. Arch Phys Med Rehabil 1998;79(11):1456–66. https://doi.org/10.1016/s0003-9993(98)90244-1.

34. Kirshblum S, Millis S, McKinley W, et al. Late neurologic recovery after traumatic spinal cord injury. Arch Phys Med Rehabil 2004;85(11):1811–7. https://doi.org/10.1016/j.apmr.2004.03.015.

35. Elliott CS, Zlatev D, Crew J, et al. Do appreciable changes in the upper extremity motor capability to perform clean intermittent catheterization come about with time after traumatic spinal cord injury? Neurourol Urodyn 2019;38(3):975–80. https://doi.org/10.1002/nau.23943.

36. Elliott CS, Seufert C, Zlatev D, et al. Do improvements in upper extremity motor function affect changes in bladder management after cervical spinal cord injury? [published online ahead of print, 2021 Nov 18]. J Spinal Cord Med 2021;1–7. https://doi.org/10.1080/10790268.2021.1999715.

37. Herbert AS, Welk B, Elliott CS. Internal and external barriers to bladder management in persons with neurologic disease performing intermittent catheterization. Int J Environ Res Public Health 2023;20(12): 6079. https://doi.org/10.3390/ijerph20126079.

38. Patel DP, Herrick JS, Stoffel JT, et al. Reasons for cessation of clean intermittent catheterization after spinal cord injury: Results from the Neurogenic Bladder Research Group spinal cord injury registry. Neurourol Urodyn 2020;39(1):211–9. https://doi.org/10.1002/nau.24172.

39. Lane GI, Driscoll A, Tawfik K, et al. A cross-sectional study of the catheter management of neurogenic bladder after traumatic spinal cord injury. Neurourol Urodyn 2018;37(1):360–7. https://doi.org/10.1002/nau.23306.

40. Velaer KN, Welk B, Ginsberg D, et al. Time Burden of Bladder Management in Individuals With Spinal Cord Injury. Top Spinal Cord Inj Rehabil 2021; 27(3):83–91. https://doi.org/10.46292/sci20-00007.

41. Meiners T, Abel R, Lindel K, et al. Improvements in activities of daily living following functional hand surgery for treatment of lesions to the cervical spinal cord: self-assessment by patients [published correction appears in Spinal Cord. 2003 Mar;41(3): 204.]. Spinal Cord 2002;40(11):574–80. https://doi.org/10.1038/sj.sc.3101384.

42. Jung HY, Lee J, Shin HI. The natural course of passive tenodesis grip in individuals with spinal cord injury with preserved wrist extension power but paralyzed fingers and thumbs. Spinal Cord 2018;56(9):900–6. https://doi.org/10.1038/s41393-018-0137-4.

43. Pripotnev S, Bruce J, Novak CB, et al. Quantifying Tenodesis Hand Function in Cervical Spinal Cord

Injury: Implications for Function. J Hand Surg Am 2023;48(7):700–10. https://doi.org/10.1016/j.jhsa.2023.04.004.

44. Tenodesis Thermoplastic Splint Kit Indications. https://www.ncmedical.com/wp-content/uploads/2011/07/Tenodesis-Splint-Kit_11_web.pdf.

45. Cuccurullo S, Lee J. Physical medicine and rehabilitation board review. New York, NY: Demos Medical; 2015.

46. Liew SK, Shim BJ, Gong HS. Upper limb reconstruction in tetraplegic patients: a primer for spinal cord injury specialists. Korean J Nutr 2020;16(2):126–37. https://doi.org/10.13004/kjnt.2020.16.e48.

47. Bernuz B, Guinet A, Rech C, et al. Self-catheterization acquisition after hand reanimation protocols in C5-C7 tetraplegic patients. Spinal Cord 2011;49(2):313–7. https://doi.org/10.1038/sc.2010.120.

48. A report from the international federation of societies for surgery of hand: from the committee on spinal cord injuries 1980. Paraplegia 1981;19(6):386–8. https://doi.org/10.1038/sc.1981.72.

49. MOBERG E. Criticism and study of methods for examining sensibility in the hand. Neurology 1962;12:8–19. https://doi.org/10.1212/wnl.12.1.8.

50. Sinnott A, Brander P, Siegert R, et al. Life impacts following reconstructive hand surgery for tetraplegia. Top Spinal Cord Inj Rehabil 2009;15(2):90–7.

51. Dunn JA, Sinnott KA, Rothwell AG, et al. Tendon transfer surgery for people with tetraplegia: an overview. Arch Phys Med Rehabil 2016;97(6 Suppl):S75–80. https://doi.org/10.1016/j.apmr.2016.01.034.

52. Kiyono Y, Hashizume C, Ohtsuka K, et al. Improvement of urological-management abilities in individuals with tetraplegia by reconstructive hand surgery. Spinal Cord 2000;38(9):541–5. https://doi.org/10.1038/sj.sc.3101046.

53. Hashizume C, Fukui J. Improvement of upper limb function with respect to urination techniques in quadriplegia. Paraplegia 1994;32(5):354–7. https://doi.org/10.1038/sc.1994.60.

54. Fox IK, Miller AK, Curtin CM. Nerve and tendon transfer surgery in cervical spinal cord injury: individualized choices to optimize function. Top Spinal Cord Inj Rehabil 2018;24(3):275–87. https://doi.org/10.1310/sci2403-275.

55. Gordon T, Yang JF, Ayer K, et al. Recovery potential of muscle after partial denervation: a comparison between rats and humans. Brain Res Bull 1993;30(3–4):477–82. https://doi.org/10.1016/0361-9230(93)90281-f.

56. Anastakis DJ, Malessy MJ, Chen R, et al. Cortical plasticity following nerve transfer in the upper extremity. Hand Clin 2008;24(4):425–vii. https://doi.org/10.1016/j.hcl.2008.04.005.

57. Javeed S, Dibble CF, Greenberg JK, et al. Upper limb nerve transfer surgery in patients with tetraplegia. JAMA Netw Open 2022;5(11):e2243890.

58. Kapadia N, Moineau B, Popovic MR. Functional electrical stimulation therapy for retraining reaching and grasping after spinal cord injury and stroke. Front Neurosci 2020;14:718. https://doi.org/10.3389/fnins.2020.00718.

59. Bryden A, Peljovich A, Hoyen H, et al. Surgical restoration of arm and hand function in people with tetraplegia. Top Spinal Cord Inj Rehabil 2012;18(1):43–9.

60. Karsenty G, Chartier-Kastler E, Mozer P, et al. A novel technique to achieve cutaneous continent urinary diversion in spinal cord-injured patients unable to catheterize through native urethra. Spinal Cord 2008;46(4):305–10. https://doi.org/10.1038/sj.sc.3102104.

61. Zommick JN, Simoneau AR, Skinner DG, et al. Continent lower urinary tract reconstruction in the cervical spinal cord injured population. J Urol 2003;169(6):2184–7. https://doi.org/10.1097/01.ju.0000061761.24504.47.

62. Chulamorkodt NN, Estrada CR, Chaviano AH. Continent urinary diversion: 10-year experience of Shriners hospitals for children in Chicago. J Spinal Cord Med 2004;27(Suppl 1):S84–7. https://doi.org/10.1080/10790268.2004.11753447.

63. Walsh K, Troxel SA, Stone AR. An assessment of the use of a continent catheterizable stoma in female tetraplegics. BJU Int 2004;94(4):595–7. https://doi.org/10.1111/j.1464-410X.2004.05007.x.

64. Roth JD, Koch MO. Metabolic and nutritional consequences of urinary diversion using intestinal segments to reconstruct the urinary tract. Urologic Clinics of North America 2018;45(1):19–24.

65. Cheng PJ, Sorena K, Roth JD, et al. Contemporary multicenter outcomes of continent cutaneous ileocecocystoplasty in the adult population over a 10-year period: a neurogenic bladder research group study. Neurourol Urodyn 2020;39(6):1771–80.

Integrating Patient Preferences with Guideline-Based Care in Neurogenic Lower Urinary Tract Dysfunction After Spinal Cord Injury

Vivian Wong, MD[a],*, Giulia M. Ippolito, MD, MS[b], Irene Crescenze, MD[c]

KEYWORDS

- Neurogenic bladder • SCI • Care path • Shared decision-making

KEY POINTS

- There are several options for the management of neurogenic bladder that can be broadly classified into voiding, clean intermittent catheterization, indwelling catheterization, or surgical reconstruction.
- A shared decision-making approach can be used to elicit patient preferences and discuss clinically appropriate bladder management options with consideration to potential harms and benefits.
- Follow-up for patients with neurogenic bladder is dependent not only on clinical risk profile but also on social and community considerations, such as social infrastructure and caregiver availability.

INTRODUCTION

The management of neurogenic lower urinary tract dysfunction (NLUTD) among patients with spinal cord injury (SCI) has evolved significantly over the last century. The advances have been aimed at preventing renal damage and minimizing infectious complications. There has been a shift in improved urologic clinical outcomes after the introduction of clean intermittent self-catheterization (CIC) by Lapdes in 1972.[1] Since then, the rates of renal disease-associated mortality have significantly declined in SCI population, and now, the primary cause of mortality is respiratory complications.[2] Despite initial improvement in outcomes, the urologic-related hospitalization rates that have stayed relatively flat over the last 30 years.[3] One explanation is that

further improvement in outcomes is limited by nonclinical barriers. Studies show that despite CIC being considered the best medical management option for NLUTD, many individuals transition back to indwelling catheters over time.[4–6] Presumably, individual and social factors often drive the change of management for many people with NLUTD as resources and support systems change, and personal goals evolve. There is a growing need for the medical community to understand social and personal factors that influence bladder management choices among people with neurogenic bladder (**Fig. 1**).

One framework to better understand patient preferences and values is with shared decision-making (SDM). SDM is a collaborative process

a Department of Urology, Ohio State University, 915 Olentangy River Road, Suite 3100, Room 3105, Columbus, OH 43212, USA; b Department of Urology, University of Michigan, 1733 Monterey Court, Ann Arbor, MI 48108, USA; c Department of Urology, Ohio State University, 915 Olentangy River Road, 2nd Floor Suite 2000, Columbus, OH 43212, USA
* Corresponding author.
E-mail address: Vivian.Wong@osumc.edu

Urol Clin N Am 51 (2024) 277–284
https://doi.org/10.1016/j.ucl.2024.02.002
0094-0143/24/© 2024 Elsevier Inc. All rights reserved.

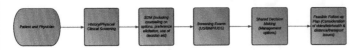

Fig. 1. Patient and physician clinical flow

between patients and clinicians to choose between clinically acceptable options by balancing patient preferences and values with potential harms and benefits.[7] SDM is best suited for situations where there is clinical equipoise, meaning the clinical outcomes are similar among various options, making the decision preference sensitive. The decision for bladder management style after SCI may be a preference-sensitive decision. For the purposes of this article, we review the role of SDM in a setting of guideline-based care pathways for NLUTD care in the SCI population.

DISCUSSION
Guideline-Based Care

Several clinical guidelines have been published to date to summarize the current best practices in NLUTD.[8–10] Neurourologic evaluation should include history, physical examination, validated questionnaires, voiding diary, renal function laboratories, and upper tract imaging.[8,10,11] Urodynamics should be performed at baseline to evaluate lower urinary tract function.[12] Bladder management goals within the first year of an SCI include addressing safe and efficient storage and emptying of urine, continence, and urologic complications.[12] Bladder management options can include CIC, indwelling catheter, voiding, and surgery for bladder augment or diversion; the recommended modality is based on results of baseline testing and evaluation.[13] Currently, CIC is considered the gold standard for the management of urinary retention after SCI, and a 2003 survey showed that 84% of the urologists recommend this as the primary bladder management strategy.[13]

Guidelines also outline the follow-up recommended for NLUTD. This may vary based on etiology of neurologic disease and severity of bladder dysfunction. Per the American Urologic Association (AUA) guidelines, patients should get an annual focused history, physical examination, and symptom assessment.[11] The AUA stratifies patients into low-risk, moderate-risk, or high-risk. Patients with low-risk NLUTD are those who spontaneously void with low PVRs with normal renal function.[11] Moderate-risk patients are those who have urinary retention and elevated PVR with normal renal function.[11] High-risk are those with abnormal renal function and abnormal upper tract imaging.[11] For those with moderate-risk NLUTD, it

is recommended to get annual renal function assessment and upper tract imaging every 1 to 2 years.[11] In high-risk NLUTD, upper tract imaging should be annually and urodynamics should be repeated when clinically appropriate.[11]

In practice, follow-up and management of patients with SCI can be challenging, and many people with SCI are not receiving minimum recommended urologic surveillance.[14] A retrospective review of 7162 patients showed that only 35.7% saw a urologist during a 2 year period while only 48.6% had upper tract evaluation.[14] Patient preferences may diverge from clinical recommendations, making implementation of guideline recommendations complex. For example, clinical guidelines have listed CIC as the gold standard for NLUTD.[15–17] This is because CIC has less risk of urinary tract infections, kidney and bladder stones, urethral fistulas and strictures, and bladder cancer as compared to indwelling catheter.[18–23] While CIC is considered a standard of care for individuals with urinary retention and NLUTD, only 20% of SCI individuals utilizing CIC initially remained on CIC at 30 year follow-up.[14] There is a paucity of data to help understand rates of CIC utilization. Common reasons reported by patients on reasons to stop CIC include inconvenience and dislike of intermittent catheterization.[4,24–27] For instance, a survey of patients with SCI showed that those with indwelling catheters spent 68% less time with bladder management than individuals who used CIC.[12] CIC can be time consuming, as this survey showed each catheterization episode averaged around 8.5 minutes, and this must be repeated every 3 to 4 hours while awake.[12] In addition, there are not always toileting facilities that can accommodate CIC.[28]

There is a need for a better and more individually tailored approach to evaluation, management, and follow-up of NLUTD that would allow people to intergrade personal and support system values and preferences with recommended clinical algorithms. To do this effectively, it is necessary to understand the patient's opinions and preferences, deliver appropriate education, and to create a treatment plan that is a feasible and durable version of guidelines.

Patient Care Preferences in Rehabilitation

The field of urology plays a large role in the recovery and rehabilitation of people with SCI. Bladder dysfunction is a common cause of significant co-morbidity. In a large cohort of individuals with NLUTD due to SCI during the 1 year follow-up period from diagnosis, 39.0% had a urology visit and 33.3% were hospitalized. Urinary tract infections were the largest culprit of hospitalizations.[29] People with SCI feel that bladder and bowel dysfunction negatively impact social interactions, relationships, and quality of life.[30,31] Social plans are limited by the accessibility of bathrooms, and lack of understanding from friends and family causes stress and anxiety.[30,31] Better bladder and bowel control is associated with greater independence, positive affect, and well-being. Common themes that affect choices of bladder management include anxiety regarding bladder management in public, risks of urinary tract infections and embarrassment from incontinence.[32] Choices are typically influenced by their own physical abilities, social and familial support, and health professionals' opinion.[33]

Navigating urologic care decisions can be central to return into community; understanding factors that influence decision-making in this population is important to promoting patient-centered care. The degree of control people feel they have over their life is one key factor to adjustment back into community life.[34–36] Lindberg and colleagues found there were 5 main themes that were important for patients in the rehabilitation process: respect and integrity, planning and decision-making, information and knowledge, motivation and encouragement, and involvement of family.[37] Some people with SCI have reported feeling disempowered and disillusioned with the health care system, many times due to lack of SCI education and communication between care team and patients.[38] A shared decision-making approach with emphasis on patient preference elicitation and understanding of decisional needs and control can help build a collaborative clinical team. For example, in one study, people with SCI felt respected when the treatment team took time to get to know them, to listen, an integral part of SDM.[37] Furthermore, the opportunity to join in on the discussion of their own care and rehabilitation and be able to collaboratively guide their treatment plan was integral to their success.[37] Patients look to their treatment team to encourage them to push forward with their recovery as well as motivate them in new goals.[37] As such, clinician opinions can significantly influence patient decision-making on treatment options, significantly impacting their decision.[33] In addition to clinicians, patients' social support is integral in decision-making. A strong social support system positively impacts the performance status of patients and their quality of life,[7] and some patients find it important to involve family in their medical care.[37]

It is clear that patient partnership in the development of the care plan is important for successful rehabilitation including bladder and bowel management. The participation may benefit from being tailored to each individual, and the treatment team should be ready and willing to be flexible in the rehabilitation plans. One method to promote patient-centered, individualized care is through the use of SDM and decision aids.

Understanding preferences and shared decision-making

The Institute of Medicine's definition of patient-centered care is "care that is respectful of and responsive to individual patient preferences, needs and values."[39] It highlights "that patient values guide all clinical decisions."[39] Decision aids were created in response to increased patient-centered care and to encourage patients to have more autonomy in their own medical decision-making. The purpose of decision aids is to supplement the physician–patient counseling about choices in their treatment options.

Decision aids vary by specialty and topic matter but generally include information about the decision in consideration of evidence-based facts about the condition, treatment options, risks and benefits, and uncertainties. These focus on providing specific and personalized information to patients to aid them in decision-making for their own care—help identify patient's values and guide patients to the health care decision that aligns with those values.[40] Decision aids decrease indecision about patient's values and decisional conflicts related to feeling uninformed. The length of consultation using decision aids was only 2.6 minutes longer than consultation without using decision aids.[40] Patients who utilized decision aids were more satisfied with their decision and the process.[40] Subgroup analysis also show that there were not any differences of knowledge or risk perception when decision aids were given prior to consultation versus during the consultation with provider.[40] Overall, decision aids facilitate patient-driven decision-making while having a positive effect on patient–clinician communication and patient satisfaction. The International Patient Decision Aids Standards Collaboration has worked to standardize the quality and validity of patient decision aids, and in collaboration in 2016, the Washington State Health Authority created a program to certify decision aids.[41]

In the field of urology, there have been multiple studies studying the effects of decision aids on prostate-specific antigen (PSA) screening. A

Cochrane review evaluated 13 studies and showed that in many of those cases, decision aids decrease the number of patients choosing to undergo PSA testing.[40] Another study in 2011 surveyed urologists in the United States and found that among 711 urologists, 33.7% used decision aids with their patients for the discussion of localized prostate cancer.[42] However, a 2019 survey of 2219 respondents to the AUA Annual Census showed that a majority reported using SDM regularly.[43] When polled about specific aspects of SDM, most urologists provide important information about the patient's treatment options but significantly fewer ask for patient values and preferences.[43] In addition, only half of the urologists in the study gave decision aids regularly on various urologic clinical scenarios.[43]

There is a paucity of decision aids available for functional urologic conditions, including NLUTD. There are no validated decision aids on the management of NLUTD at this time, but a publicly available decision aid detailing "Bladder Management After Spinal Cord Injury" is available on the NBRG.org developed by Crescenze.[44] This interactive decision aid, based on the decision aid based on the Ottawa Decision Support Framework, guides patients with NLUTD through decision on bladder management modality by clarifying their choices, comparing options, identifying decisional needs, and planning care. While outcomes of this decision aid have not yet been studied, decision aids in other functional conditions like overactive bladder have been met positively by patients. These decision aids have been shown to decrease patient's uncertainty in decision-making and reduced patients' conflict about treatment.[45,46]

Care of Neurogenic Lower Urinary Tract Dysfunction

Delivering education

Informed patients are central to patient-centered care and SDM.[47] Traditionally, education during SDM is initiated by the clinician team. In NLUTD due to SCI, bladder management education may begin during acute inpatient and rehabilitation admissions. However, the delivery of education on bladder management in this population is variable across the different health care settings. Patients' readiness, learning, style, and relevance to current health priorities must be considered when educational information is delivered, and appropriate timing may not align with the duration of rehabilitation stay.[48]

Recently, with the growth of the model systems organization, as well as several national advocacy groups such as Craig Nielsen Foundation,[49] Paralyzed Veterans of America,[50] and Christopher and Dana Reeve Foundation,[51] there has been an expansion of online resources accessible to patients for education. There has been increased funding for patient-centered care through organizations such as the Patient-Centered Outcomes Research Institute.[52] Also, the expansion of social media platforms has led to a remarkable increase in peer-to-peer communication and education venues. Social media has been shown to be effective at implementing health behavioral change.[53] Unfortunately, not all information that is being shared via social media outlets is validated or accurate as there are no quality assessments, monitoring, or oversight. Additionally, when turning to social media for information, there is generation, racial and income-based discrepancies in the use of these resources that need to be considered.[54]

Upon discharge from the rehabilitation, NLUTD care can be led by urologists and comanaged with physical medicine and rehabilitation and primary care physicians. Individuals with SCI continue to rank subspecialty providers input as the most valuable source of information, despite limitations on clinician time with patients.[48] In accordance with guidelines, the urology team is charged with providing education on NLUTD management options and follow-up plans based on risk stratification.[11] Patient pamphlets and instructions have been used in a clinical setting and may be provided to patients for education purposes, but there is a need for a more effective, succinct, and reliable mode of information delivery in the clinical setting. Electronic health records and patient interface materials, like virtual care navigation, is a promising alternative for delivering patient education.

Care navigation is partnership between patient and navigator where navigators identify patients' needs and provide education and guidance in relation to their care.[55] It has been shown to be effective in oncology[56] and primary care,[57] but due to limited resources, this often is not an option. Several vendors offer virtual care navigation options. Epic Inc., which provides software for electronic medical records for a large portion of American hospitals, has developed and integrated a virtual care companion called MyChart Care Companion.[58,59] This has been utilized in fields such as pregnancy and heart failure.[58,59] These virtual care navigation platforms may be used to create and implement a bladder care pathway to provide NLUTD education, collect surveillance and follow-up information, and administer shared decision-making tools. The benefits of virtual platforms are minimal resource requirement, targeted education, and patient-related outcomes monitoring, which can trigger medical intervention and follow-up.

Funded by grant from the Craig Neilson Foundation, Crescenze and colleagues have developed an NLUTD MyChart care companion called *Virtual Bladder Care Pathway*[60] to help guide individuals with SCI through the early stages of bladder education and management that is currently being evaluated in a clinical setting *Virtual Bladder Care Pathway*[60] incorporates a decision aid to elicit patients' values and preferences and includes monitoring and safety surveillance questionnaires to identify patients at risk for adverse events. Future iterations could facilitate guideline-based follow-up recommendations beyond the acute phase of SCI.

In addition to virtual care navigation, telemedicine can be instrumental to improve follow-up for individuals with SCI. Telemedicine can minimize transportation and caregiver burden and maximize convenience and cost-effectiveness of follow-up.[61,62] Historically, urology has been slow to adopt telehealth technology but long-standing barriers to the adoption of this technology have been decreasing in recent years with the coronavirus disease 2019 pandemic.[63] Telehealth may decrease barriers and offer financial savings associated with travel and improved access to care for patients with limited mobility and those in rural areas with otherwise limited access to subspecialty care.[64,65]

People with SCI need close urologic follow-up after injury to evaluate and provide NLUTD care, which can help minimize long-term morbidity. Future areas that may improve connection between providers and patients with SCI are virtual care pathways and the use of telehealth. Patients with SCI would also benefit from coordinated multidisciplinary care. There is literature in the pediatric urology realm that describes multidisciplinary care clinics that treat patients with NLUTD.[61,62] Teams within these clinics include neurology, urology, nephrology, psychiatry, physical therapist, occupational therapists, nutritionists, social workers, and many others.[61,62] Coordination of care is a major obstacle to maintaining multidisciplinary care for these patients but can be mitigated with the use of telemedicine. For those medical systems that do not have a multidisciplinary care clinic, primary care providers and nursing coordinators can potentially act as a hub for information and referrals with clear communication between the specialists and the primary team.

Neurogenic Lower Urinary Tract Dysfunction Considerations Beyond Spinal Cord Injury

While a robust rehabilitation program is often the key to success for individuals with SCI, those who suffered stroke or have a developing neurodegenerative disorder are sometimes at a disadvantage. The burden of education on bowel and bladder management in an outpatient setting falls on the primary care physicians and neurologists who have limited time and resources to support yet another complex aspect of care. The rehabilitation team that is supporting these individuals through their functional decline is often not trained in addressing options for bowel and bladder management. Referral to urology may be placed late in patient's disease. There is a need to optimize bladder care early in these populations and early referral to urology as well as subspecialty Physical Medicine and Rehabilitation or PT/OT physical therapy/occupational therapy services is well warranted. Implementation of telehealth care pathways for these populations can offer patients education and resources on bladder management, link to the health care team, and minimize the burden on the rehabilitation system.

SUMMARY

The care of patients with NLUTD due to SCI is complex. Traditional approaches to care of patients with NLUTD due to SCI did not incorporate patient preferences and values, which are central to the success of any bladder management routine. Despite the recognized importance of SDM and decision aids on patient-centered care, there is a paucity of research on patient values and preferences within the SCI population. We describe virtual resources to facilitate education, care, and follow up including decision aids and virtual care navigators that are currently available for use and, through this, identify a critical need for creation and validation of these tools within this population.

CLINICS CARE POINTS

- Patients value independence most after SCI. They rely on family support and health care opinion to guide them in their decisions for bladder management.

- Engaging in SDM is a patient-centered approach to selecting an individualized bladder management strategy after SCI.

- SDM should incorporate both education about management options (including potential harms and benefits) as well as elicitation of patient values and preferences.

- Follow-up for NLUTD should consider patient's individualized circumstances, and management may need to be adjusted not only based on clinical risks that arise but also on social and community circumstances.

DISCLOSURE

Giulia Ippolito, MD: None. I. Crescenze: Investigator for Medtronic Inc.

REFERENCES

1. Lapides J, Diokno AC, Silber SJ, et al. Clean, intermittent self-catheterization in the treatment of urinary tract disease. J Urol 1972;107(3):458–61.

2. van den Berg ME, Castellote JM, de Pedro-Cuesta J, et al. Survival after spinal cord injury: a systematic review. J Neurotrauma 2010;27(8):1517–28.

3. Crescenze IM, Lenherr SM, Myers JB, et al. Self-reported urological hospitalizations or emergency room visits in a contemporary spinal cord injury cohort. J Urol 2021;205(2):477–82.

4. Lane GI, Driscoll A, Tawfik K, et al. A cross-sectional study of the catheter management of neurogenic bladder after traumatic spinal cord injury. Neurourol Urodyn 2018;37:360–7.

5. Sekar P, Wallace DD, Waites KB, et al. Comparison of long-term renal function after spinal cord injury using different urinary management methods. Arch Phys Med Rehabil 1997;78(9):992–7.

6. Cameron AP, Lai J, Saigal CS, et al. NIDDK Urological Diseases in America Project. Urological Surveillance and Medical Complications after Spinal Cord Injury in the United States. Urology 2015;86(3):506–10.

7. Implementation of Shared Decision Making into Urological Practice - American Urological Association. https://www.auanet.org/guidelines-and-quality/quality-and-measurement/quality-improvement/clinical-consensus-statement-and-quality-improvement-issue-brief-(ccs-and-qiib)/shared-decision-making. [Accessed 27 November 2023].

8. Kavanagh A, Baverstock R, Campeau L, et al. Canadian Urological Association guideline: Diagnosis, management, and surveillance of neurogenic lower urinary tract dysfunction - Full text. Can Urol Assoc J 2019;13(6):E157–76.

9. Tate DG, Wheeler T, Lane GI, et al. Recommendations for evaluation of neurogenic bladder and bowel dysfunction after spinal cord injury and/or disease. J Spinal Cord Med 2020;43(2):141–64.

10. EAU Guidelines. edn presented at the EAU Annual Congress Milan 2023. ISBN 978-94-92671-19-6. Available at: https://uroweb.org/eau-guidelines/citing-usage-republication.

11. Ginsberg DA, Boone TB, Cameron AP, et al. The AUA/SUFU Guideline on Adult Neurogenic Lower Urinary Tract Dysfunction: Diagnosis and Evaluation. J Urol 2021;206:1097.

12. Velaer KN, Welk B, Ginsberg D, et al. Time Burden of Bladder Management in Individuals With Spinal Cord Injury. Top Spinal Cord Inj Rehabil 2021; 27(3):83–91.

13. Razdan S, Leboeuf L, Meinbach DS, et al. Current practice patterns in the urologic surveillance and management of patients with spinal cord injury. Urology 2003 May;61(5):893–6.

14. Cameron AP, Wallner LP, Tate DG, et al. Bladder management after spinal cord injury in the United States 1972 to 2005. J Urol 2010;184(1):213–7.

15. Abrams P, Agarwal M, Drake M, et al. A proposed guideline for the urological management of patients with spinal cord injury. BJU Int 2008;101(8):989–94.

16. Consortium for Spinal Cord Medicine. Bladder management for adults with spinal cord injury: a clinical practice guideline for health-care providers. J Spinal Cord Med 2006;29(5):527–73.

17. Stöhrer M, Blok B, Castro-Diaz D, et al. EAU guidelines on neurogenic lower urinary tract dysfunction. Eur Urol 2009;56(1):81–8.

18. Esclarín De Ruz A, García Leoni E, Herruzo Cabrera R. Epidemiology and risk factors for urinary tract infection in patients with spinal cord injury. J Urol 2000;164(4):1285–9.

19. West DA, Cummings JM, Longo WE, et al. Role of chronic catheterization in the development of bladder cancer in patients with spinal cord injury. Urology 1999;53(2):292–7.

20. Weld KJ, Dmochowski RR. Effect of bladder management on urological complications in spinal cord injured patients. J Urol 2000;163(3):768–72.

21. Weld KJ, Graney MJ, Dmochowski RR. Differences in bladder compliance with time and associations of bladder management with compliance in spinal cord injured patients. J Urol 2000;163(4):1228–33.

22. Groah SL, Weitzenkamp DA, Lammertse DP, et al. Excess risk of bladder cancer in spinal cord injury: evidence for an association between indwelling catheter use and bladder cancer. Arch Phys Med Rehabil 2002;83(3):346–51.

23. Chen Y, DeVivo MJ, Roseman JM. Current trend and risk factors for kidney stones in persons with spinal cord injury: a longitudinal study. Spinal Cord 2000; 38(6):346–53.

24. Myers JB, Lenherr SM, Stoffel JT, et al. Patient Reported Bladder Related Symptoms and Quality of Life after Spinal Cord Injury with Different Bladder Management Strategies. J Urol 2019;202(3):574–84.

25. Hearn JH, Selvarajah S, Kennedy P, et al. Stigma and self-management: an Interpretative Phenomenological Analysis of the impact of chronic recurrent urinary tract infections after spinal cord injury. Spinal Cord Ser Cases 2018;4:12.

26. Crescenze IM, Myers JB, Lenherr SM, et al. Predictors of low urinary quality of life in spinal cord injury patients on clean intermittent catheterization. Neurourol Urodyn 2019;38(5):1332–8.

27. Yeh HL, Kuo HC, Tsai CH, et al. Reasons for Altering Bladder Management and Satisfaction with Current Bladder Management in Chronic Spinal Cord Injury Patients. Int J Environ Res Publ Health 2022; 19(24):17032.

28. Joshi AD, Shukla A, Chawathe V, et al. Clean intermittent catheterization in long-term management of neurogenic bladder in spinal cord injury: Patient perspective and experiences. Int J Urol 2022; 29(4):317–23.

29. Manack A, Motsko SP, Haag-Molkenteller C, et al. Epidemiology and healthcare utilization of neurogenic bladder patients in a US claims database. Neurourol Urodyn 2011;30(3):395–401.

30. Braaf S, Lennox A, Nunn A, et al. Social activity and relationship changes experienced by people with bowel and bladder dysfunction following spinal cord injury. Spinal Cord 2017;55(7):679–86.

31. Hicken BL, Putzke JD, Richards JS. Bladder management and quality of life after spinal cord injury. Am J Phys Med Rehabil 2001;80(12): 916–22.

32. Welk B, Myers JB, Kennelly M, et al. A qualitative assessment of psychosocial aspects that play a role in bladder management after spinal cord injury. Spinal Cord 2021;59:978–86.

33. Engkasan J, Ng C, Low W. Factors influencing bladder management in male patients with spinal cord injury: a qualitative study. Spinal Cord 2014; 52:157–62.

34. Boschen KA, Tonack M, Gargaro J. Long-term adjustment and community reintegration following spinal cord injury. Int J Rehabil Res 2003;26(3): 157–64.

35. Wu SY, Kuo HC. Satisfaction with Surgical Procedures and Bladder Management of Chronic Spinal Cord Injured Patients with Voiding Dysfunction Who Desire Spontaneous Voiding. J Personalized Med 2022;12(10):1751.

36. Rivers CS, Fallah N, Noonan VK, et al. Health conditions: effect on function, health-related quality of life, and life satisfaction after traumatic spinal cord injury. a prospective observational registry cohort study. Arch Phys Med Rehabil 2018;99(3):443–51.

37. Lindberg J, Kreuter M, Taft C, et al. Patient participation in care and rehabilitation from the perspective of patients with spinal cord injury. Spinal Cord 2013; 51(11):834–7.

38. Krysa JA, Gregorio MP, Pohar Manhas K, et al. Empowerment, communication, and navigating care: the experience of persons with spinal cord injury from acute hospitalization to inpatient rehabilitation. Front Rehabil Sci 2022;3:904716.

39. National Research Council. Crossing the quality chasm: a new health system for the 21st century. Washington, DC: National Academies Press; 2001.

40. Stacey D, Légaré F, Lewis K, et al. Decision aids for people facing health treatment or screening decisions. Cochrane Database Syst Rev 2017;4(4): CD001431.

41. Washington State Health Authority. Patient decision aid certification criteria 2016. www.hca.wa.gov/hw/ Documents/sdm_cert_criteria.pdf.

42. Wang EH, Gross CP, Tilburt JC, et al. Shared Decision Making and Use of Decision Aids for Localized Prostate Cancer : Perceptions From Radiation Oncologists and Urologists. JAMA Intern Med 2015; 175(5):792–9.

43. Lane GI, Ellimoottil C, Wallner L, et al. Shared Decision-making in Urologic Practice: Results From the 2019 AUA Census. Urology 2020;145:66–72.

44. Lane G, Crescenze I. Decision Aid: Bladder Management After Spinal Cord Injury (SCI). https://www.med.umich.edu/1librr/urology/BladderManagementAfterSpinalCordInjuryDecisionAid.pdf. [Accessed 20 November 2023].

45. Khanijow KD, Leri D, Arya LA, et al. A Mobile Application Patient Decision Aid for Treatment of Overactive Bladder. Female Pelvic Med Reconstr Surg 2021;27(6):365–70.

46. van Til JA, Drossaert CH, Renzenbrink GJ, et al. Feasibility of web-based decision aids in neurological patients. J Telemed Telecare 2010;16(1):48–52.

47. Elwyn G, Frosch D, Thomson R, et al. Shared decision making: a model for clinical practice. J Gen Intern Med 2012;27(10):1361–7.

48. Wolfe DL, Potter PJ, Jutai JW, et al. Long term physical impact of spinal cord injury: the role of rehabilitation in educating consumers to reduce complications over the long-term. Presented at First Joint Scientific Meeting of the American Spinal Injury Association (28th Annual Meeting) and the International Medical Society of Paraplegia (41st Annual Meeting). J Spinal Cord Med 2002;22(suppl 1):S50.

49. Craig H. Home. Neilsen Foundation. https://chnfoundation.org/. [Accessed 11 December 2023].

50. Home. Paralyzed Veterans of America. 2022. https://pva.org/.

51. Christopher & Dana Reeve Foundation. Christopher & Dana Reeve Foundation. Published. 2019. https://www.christopherreeve.org/.

52. About PCORI. About PCORI | PCORI. 2021. https://www.pcori.org/about/about-pcori.

53. Naslund JA, Kim SJ, Aschbrenner KA, et al. Systematic review of social media interventions for smoking cessation. Addict Behav 2017;73:81–93.

54. Chirumamilla S, Gulati M. Patient Education and Engagement through Social Media. Curr Cardiol Rev 2021;17(2):137–43.

55. Dohan D, Schrag D. Using navigators to improve care of underserved patients: current practices and approaches. Cancer 2005;104(4):848–55.

56. Cantril C, Haylock PJ. Patient navigation in the oncology care setting. Semin Oncol Nurs 2013; 29(2):76–90.

57. Carter N, Valaitis RK, Lam A, et al. Navigation delivery models and roles of navigators in primary care: a scoping literature review. BMC Health Serv Res 2018;18(1):96.

58. Madson R. Mayo Clinic Care Plans supporting better outcomes, lower health care costs delivered via Epic. Mayo Clinic News Network. 2018. https://newsnetwork.mayoclinic.org/discussion/mayo-clinic-care-plans-supporting-better-outcomes-lower-health-care-costs-delivered-via-epic/.

59. How Can Epic Care Companion Improve Patient Health? Surety Systems. 2023. https://www.suretysystems.com/insights/how-can-epic-care-companion-improve-patient-health/. [Accessed 28 November 2023].

60. Crescenze I. Virtual Bladder Care Pathway. 2021. https://app.dimensions.ai/details/grant/grant.9881340.

61. Syed ST, Gerber BS, Sharp LK. Traveling towards disease: transportation barriers to health care access. J Community Health 2013;38(5):976–93.

62. Sager C, Barroso U Jr, Bastos JM, et al. Management of neurogenic bladder dysfunction in children update and recommendations on medical treatment. Int Braz J Urol 2022;48(1):31–51.

63. Touchett H, Apodaca C, Siddiqui S, et al. Current Approaches in Telehealth and Telerehabilitation for Spinal Cord Injury (TeleSCI). Curr Phys Med Rehabil Rep 2022;10(2):77–88.

64. Hospitals and health systems implementing EPIC in 2022/2023 | Definitive Healthcare. Available at: www.definitivehc.com https://www.definitivehc.com/resources/healthcare-insights/hospitals-and-health-systems-implementing-epic#:~:text=What%20percentage%20of%20health%20system.

65. Modi PK, Portney D, Hollenbeck BK, et al. Engaging telehealth to drive value-based urology. Curr Opin Urol 2018;28(4):342–7.

A Framework for Addressing Health Disparities in Adult Neurogenic Lower Urinary Tract Dysfunction—Systematic Review and Neurogenic Bladder Research Group Recommendations

Shanice Cox, MS[a], Taiwo Dodo-Williams, BS[b], Brandee Branche, MD[c], Natalia García-Peñaloza, MD[b], Mayra Lucas, MD, MPH[d], Yahir Santiago-Lastra, MD[e],*, Neurogenic Bladder Research Group[1]

KEYWORDS

- Health equity • Neurogenic bladder • Urology • Health disparities • Social determinants of health

KEY POINTS

- Health disparities in neurogenic lower urinary tract dysfunction (NLUTD): The article underscores the existence of significant health disparities in NLUTD, particularly related to the social determinants of health and neighborhood disadvantage.
- Conceptual framework by the Neurogenic Bladder Research Group (NBRG): The NBRG introduces a framework for evaluating and addressing these disparities, integrating literature evidence and stakeholder input to improve clinical care, research, and advocacy.
- Call for inclusive research: The article emphasizes the need for broader, more inclusive research in NLUTD, focusing on diverse patient populations and a range of socio-demographic factors, to address the current limitations in understanding and treating NLUTD disparities.

INTRODUCTION

Over the past several decades, a burgeoning body of evidence has shattered the monolithic view that medical care is the solitary influencer of health, even when that care is preventive. This paradigm shift paints a more nuanced picture, acknowledging that while medical care is crucial, it is not the singular force shaping health outcomes. Social sciences like anthropology, sociology, and social

[a] Burnett School of Medicine at TCU, Fort Worth, TX 76129, USA; [b] University of California – San Diego School of Medicine, La Jolla, CA 92093, USA; [c] University of Michigan Medical School, Ann Arbor, MI 48109, USA; [d] University of California - San Francisco School of Medicine, San Francisco, CA 94143, USA; [e] Division of Uro-gynecology, Neuro-Urology and Reconsructive Pelvic Surgery, Department of Urology, University of California - San Diego, 9400 Campus Point Drive, MC7897, La Jolla, CA 92037, USA
[1] The members of the Neurogenic Bladder Research Group that contributed as coauthors to the writing of various sections throughout this article are listed in the acknowledgment section.
* Corresponding author.
E-mail address: ysantiagolastra@health.ucsd.edu

Urol Clin N Am 51 (2024) 285–295
https://doi.org/10.1016/j.ucl.2024.02.007

urologic.theclinics.com

epidemiology have expanded insights and methodologies for researching health and health care disparities faced by systemically marginalized groups.[1] However, these academic advances are virtually absent from the urologic literature, especially when examining neurogenic lower urinary tract dysfunction (NLUTD). When the social determinants of health (SDOHs) are ignored as influences, the chasm between a disease's biomedical explanation and the societal influences at play result in constrained research designs, ineffective clinical practice, and reductive interpretations of racial, ethnic, and socioeconomic disparities in health outcomes. Assessing health equity for NLUTD patients is challenging due to diverse diagnoses, varying disabilities, life stages, and the significant impact of each patient's unique NLUTD condition, disability, and personal experiences on their health disparities.[2]

To address this significant gap in health equity research and clinical care, the Neurogenic Bladder Research Group (NBRG) has proposed a framework for evaluating disparities in adult NLUTD. Our objective is to underscore several important themes related to health equity in NLUTD populations by first incorporating evidence from the literature and then synthesizing qualitative input from key NBRG stakeholders into a conceptual framework. This serves both as a call to action and a practical guide for researchers and clinicians to integrate considerations of these disparities into their practices, research efforts, and advocacy goals.

METHODS
Systematic Review of the Literature

Using the Preferred Reporting Items for Systematic Reviews (PRISMA) guidelines, we conducted a literature search of MEDLINE, EMBASE, and the Cochrane Review Central Register of Controlled Trials to identify studies specifically looking at health disparities within NLUTD conditions and their specific impact on urologic outcomes. The main objective of the systematic review portion of our study was to examine the current interventions specifically targeting the identification or reduction of urologic health disparities in NLUTD. We hypothesized that the available literature would be sparse and focused singularly on racial and/or ethnic disparities without looking much further into contributing SDOHs. In our literature search, we employed Medical Subject Headings and text words pertaining to NLUTD, neurogenic bladder, urology, health disparities, and specified subpopulations identified as high risk for urologic complications by a

group of key stakeholders convened together at a health equity workshop prepared by the NBRG. The NLUTD subpopulations identified by the key stakeholders included spinal cord injury (SCI), spina bifida, movement disorders, and multiple sclerosis. These were selected due to the underlying clinical sequelae that placed these subpopulations at higher risk for long-term urologic complications. The studies eligible for inclusion were published between 2013 and 2023. We omitted conference abstracts lacking complete text, book chapters, articles pertaining to subjects under the age of 18, case reports involving fewer than 10 patients, and articles originating from countries other than the United States. Two independent reviewers conducted all stages of abstract screening, study selection, and data extraction. Any conflicts were resolved by a third reviewer.

Conceptual Framework

The secondary objective involved assembling a team of key stakeholders, including patients, urologic surgeons, physiatrists, allied health professionals, advanced practice providers, patient advocates, caregivers, and nursing. All the stakeholders participate in the care of NLUTD patients or experience the disability themselves. These participants were divided into various focus groups which addressed several important gaps in clinical care and research using the topical themes outlined in **Fig. 1**. The focus groups were transcribed, and subsequently, using qualitative methodology (ATLAS.ti 23.2.1 for Mac), they produced several themes from the analysis.

RESULTS
Systematic Review

A total of 2217 studies were identified for screening after the exclusion of duplicates. After abstract review, 32 full text articles were evaluated for inclusion and exclusion. After full text review and the resolution of conflicts, only 2 studies met our inclusion and exclusion criteria (**Fig. 2—** PRISMA diagram). An aggregate of 5590 participants were represented.

While many studies investigated health disparities, only 2 specifically met our inclusion criteria of focusing specifically on a high-risk NLUTD population and targeting specific urologic outcomes.

The studies revealed disparities in health care outcomes based on race/ethnicity and insurance status. The Smith and colleagues[3] study found Hispanic/Latino participants with spina bifida more likely to experience incontinence and less likely to undergo bladder or bowel surgery

CONCEPTUAL FRAMEWORK FOR EQUITY IN NLUTD

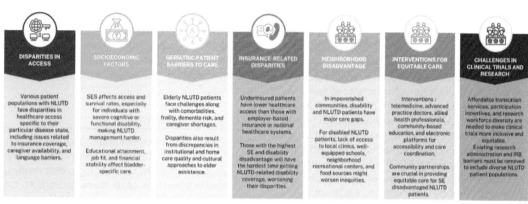

Fig. 1. Workgroup discussions created a conceptual framework for equitable care and research optimization for neurogenic lower urinary tract dysfunction (NLUTD) patients.

compared to non-Hispanic participants. Furthermore, insurance type–influenced health care outcomes were found in the Rude and colleagues[4] study, with participants holding private insurance exhibiting better health indicators, more access to specialized care, and less chronic pain compared to those with public insurance. Both studies highlighted the impact of socioeconomic factors, such as insurance status, education, and employment, beyond racial and ethnic disparities in health care.

Conceptual Framework

The NBRG workgroup comprising diverse stakeholders (identified in acknowledgments) employed

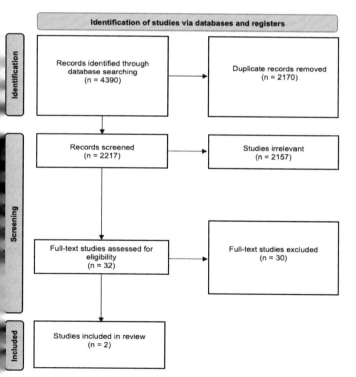

Fig. 2. PRISMA flow diagram for the framework for evaluating health disparities in adult neurogenic lower urinary tract dysfunction.

a mixed-methods approach in 4 focus groups, identifying discussion themes that were then qualitatively assessed using transcription and qualitative software. **Fig. 1** outlines the themes that were identified with a brief synopsis to each theme obtained during the focus group sessions.

DISCUSSION
Systematic Review

Moving forward, future research needs to expand beyond the limitations of current studies by encompassing a more diverse patient population experiencing NLUTD. A comprehensive understanding of disparities demands an exploration of broader sociodemographic factors, beyond race and ethnicity, including SDOHs. The utilization of insurance status, a proxy for health care access, as demonstrated by both studies included in the systematic review, represents a positive step forward.

The NBRG workgroup recognized the need for a more inclusive research approach that incorporates a variety of sociodemographic elements that are currently lacking in the urologic literature. There are stark disparities in health care access and outcomes for individuals with SCIs, especially among systemically marginalized populations. For instance, black patients with SCI have reduced access to essential services like acute inpatient rehabilitation and are less likely to receive surgeries that are crucial for improved health outcomes.[5,6] Moreover, employment status, which is a key determinant of successful community reintegration post-SCI, is significantly lower in systemically marginalized and excluded (SME) groups, further aggravating health care disparities.[6]

There are several important factors that we identified and that are important to highlight. Firstly, the financial aspect of health care post-SCI was a critical area identified by the systematic review, although there are no specific studies correlating this to urologic outcomes. The initial and ongoing health care costs for individuals with SCI and NLUTD are substantial, with a noteworthy proportion lacking private insurance, which imposes a considerable economic burden on the affected individuals and public health care systems.[7] Hospitalization rates are higher among marginalized patients, with urinary tract infections and respiratory complications being the primary causes. However, a few studies identified that Latiné adults with SCI are an exception, potentially due to their stronger social support systems, which correlates with improved outcomes and reduced hospitalization rates.[8] These nuances underscore the need to delve more profoundly into

the effects that community and support structures can have on lifetime health outcomes in NLUTD and in urologic care specifically, as many NLUTD depend on their caregivers and their community for their bladder and bowel management.

Another important observation in the systematic review process was the paucity of prospective studies or community-based participatory research (CBPR). Prospective studies are encouraged to evaluate the impact of various interventions on the disproportionately affected individuals' health outcomes.[9,10]

Conceptual Framework

Herein, we present a closer analysis of the resulting themes from the qualitative analysis. These themes allow us to consider NLUTD urologic outcomes as an integrated function of all these factors so that we can achieve a broader understanding and develop tangible routes for intervention.

THEME 1—DISPARITIES IN HEALTH CARE ACCESS

Various patient populations, including those with spina bifida, cerebral palsy, SCI, and multiple sclerosis, face disparities in health care access specific to their disease state, including issues related to insurance coverage, caregiver availability, geographic location, and language barriers.

The effects of insurance status and health status have been studied across multiple disciplines. Non-private insurance has been shown to be associated with decreased ability to obtain outpatient appointments, surgical care, and increased length of stay.[11–14] Marrie and colleagues[15] reported a higher likelihood of multiple sclerosis patients with private insurance undergoing urologic investigations. Traumatic SCI beneficiaries with non-private insurance have increased morbidity due to the higher prevalence of psychological, cardiac, and metabolic syndromes.[16] Considering the intertwined influence of insurance type and health status, these should be incorporated into practice to improve patient outcomes.

Workgroup Recommendation

Patients with NLUTD are likely to be underinsured. This has specific impacts to the affordability of urologic care, particularly with bladder management. Enhanced care navigation and collaboration with the patient's medical home, especially with Federally Qualified Health Centers, may reduce their need to seek care from health systems that exclude or reduce access to underinsured patients. Federally Qualified Health Centers (FQHCs) and other community-based health care delivery systems will require enhanced education specific to urologic disease and prevention of NLUTD-specific urologic complications.

Specifically with caregiver availability, these issues may be due to complex care needs, continuous care, and physical demands related to high-risk NLUTD conditions. Parents of spina bifida patients are noted to have high levels of parenting stress.[17] Predictive factors for parental stress include being a single parent and need for clean intermittent catheterization (CIC).[18]

Workgroup Recommendation

Some suggested methods to help alleviate caregiver burden include but are not limited to the utilization of support systems/organizations, respite care services, tailored interventions that may reduce stressors, caregiver advocates within the health care team, and the development of uniform protocols for evaluating caregiver educational and resource needs specific to urologic care and bladder management.[18,19]

The presence of language barriers presents challenges in providing superior health care. It has previously been described that language barriers result in more health care costs.[20,21] A systematic review investigating the impact of language barriers in health care reported diminished satisfaction and miscommunication between health providers and patients, ultimately influencing health care outcomes.[21] The presence of an existing chronic condition and the added layer of inadequate language support further complicate access to optimal health care. Addressing these issues involves augmenting the availability of interpreter services, fostering a positive attitude toward their utilization, and raising awareness regarding the availability of such services.[22]

Workgroup Recommendation

Expanding language services, such as interpreters or multilingual staff, can improve health care access for patients facing language barriers. Additionally, community-based partnerships with local sources of language-concordant advocacy, community, and social worker support are essential to further help address the holistic needs of NLUTD patients beyond what can be offered to them at the urologic specialty program.

THEME 2—SOCIOECONOMIC FACTORS

Socioeconomic status plays a critical role in determining health care access and survival rates, particularly among patients with severe cognitive or functional disability and this exacerbates the management of their NLUTD. Issues such as educational attainment, suitability for employment, and financial stability impact the quality of bladder-specific care received by these populations.

The workgroup discussion highlighted the pivotal role of socioeconomic status in shaping health care access and survival rates among individuals grappling with severe cognitive or functional disabilities, notably impacting the management of NLUTD. Emphasizing the role between socioeconomic factors and health care, the discourse underscored how variables like educational attainment, suitability for employment, and financial stability significantly influence the caliber of bladder-specific care received by this population. These observations align with corroborating studies that have consistently demonstrated the profound impact of socioeconomic disparities on health outcomes.[23–26] For instance, a long-term study evaluating the risk factors for cardiovascular disease across different ethnic and racial groups found that participants with low incomes and educational attainment were at a higher risk of adverse health outcomes at 10 years.[27] While physicians cannot directly have an influence on patients' socioeconomic status, some ways in which physicians can help keep costs low for patients include ensuring the use of preventative care, telemedicine services, affordable medication, and collaborating with social workers and other community stakeholders.

Workgroup Recommendation

More enhanced data collection on socioeconomic status of the patients is warranted to truly understand disparities beyond race and ethnicity. Much of the data that currently exists has been obtained from patients who are followed by an established safety net hospital, but many patients with NLUTD experience their disability outside of these sources of health care. In addition to data collection, any research findings obtained from enhanced data collection and CBPR should be integrated into advocacy for policies that address the root causes of the socioeconomic disparities. For example, enhanced data collection on socioeconomic status may help to identify the affordability of bladder management and the socioeconomic factors that drive adherence to bladder management method for individuals who lack access to a health care safety net. These findings can then be used to further public policy changes that address the complex interplay between socioeconomic factors and NLUTD outcomes. Enhanced understanding of socioeconomic variables may also help prepare patients for surgical interventions and prolonged hospitalizations during which employment of the patient and their caregivers may be negatively impacted due to higher acute needs for support.

THEME 3—BARRIERS TO QUALITY CARE FOR GERIATRIC PATIENTS WITH NEUROGENIC LOWER URINARY TRACT DYSFUNCTION

There are more patients with NLUTD reaching elder status than ever before. Geriatric patients with high-risk NLUTD will face multiple challenges, including added comorbidities, frailty, higher risk of dementia, and lack of adequate caregiver availability. Additionally, disparities arise due to differences in the quality of care between institutions and home care, as well as cultural variations in the approach toward support for elders.

While no studies to our knowledge have looked specifically at health care access in geriatric patients with NLUTD, 1 study evaluating facilitators and objective barriers to health care in older Medicare beneficiaries report finance and lack of primary health care provider with decreased likelihood of obtaining recommended medical care.[28]

Workgroup Recommendation

The group participants underscored a need to incorporate the Comprehensive Geriatric Assessment in the routine evaluation of geriatric patients with NLUTD to appropriately address comorbidities, frailty, and cognitive status. Support and education programs for caregivers and respite care facilities in addition to allied health professionals and other multidisciplinary partners can help facilitate day-to-day condition management and emotional support for the geriatric NLUTD patient.

THEME 4—INSURANCE-RELATED DISPARITIES

Access to health care is most heavily influenced by insurance type, with disparities observed between underinsured patients and those with different insurance models, such as employer-based insurance and national health care systems. The workgroup identified that patients with the most socioeconomic and disability-related disadvantage will have the greatest difficulty accessing coverage for their NLUTD-related disability and this can exacerbate inequity.

Lack of equal access to health care can contribute to disparities in health outcomes for individuals with NLUTD. Patients with Medicaid coverage or no insurance may experience more complications, hospitalizations, and have a higher risk of renal insufficiency and downstream complications of NLUTD.[29,30] Patients who rely on subsidized clinics may receive lower quality health care due to a lack of resources such as electronic medical records and emergency departments.

According to the Rude and colleagues study, public insurance has been associated with worse patient outcomes in many disciplines, but the role of insurance has not previously been analyzed regarding high-risk NLUTD. Publicly insured individuals with SCI are more likely to be managed with spontaneous voiding while individuals with private insurance are more likely to be managed with CIC, even when adjusting for variables known to impact bladder management. This may be the result of the insurance status directly influencing management, but further investigation into the etiology of this difference is warranted to uncover potential disparities in outcomes. Additionally, because Medicaid coverage can vary from state to state, NLUTD patients may experience varying degrees of insurance coverage for their chronic conditions based on the state in which they reside.

Workgroup Recommendations

The thematic analysis did not identify a specific recommendation with regards to insurance-related inequity, though legislative advocacy and public policy goals are often centered around insurance coverage and the burden it could potentially create through processes like prior authorization and coverage exclusions.

THEME 5—COMMUNITY VITAL SIGNS, NEIGHBORHOOD DISADVANTAGE

The workgroup identified that patients with disability and NLUTD experience large gaps in care when they live in disadvantaged communities. Inability to access community sources of wellness, like local clinics, well-equipped schools, neighborhood recreational centers, and food sources, can further exacerbate inequity for disabled NLUTD patients.

The patient's neighborhood can significantly impact their health outcomes. Factors such as neighborhood socioeconomic status, neighborhood violence, and lack of access to health care facilities can negatively impact a patient's health.[31,32] To assess SDOHs and the impact of the patient's neighborhood on their health outcomes, community vital signs have been suggested. Community vital signs are measures of social and behavioral aspects that can indicate potential risks to a patient's health based on their environment. These vital signs include factors such as access to healthy food options, public transportation, safe and affordable housing, and community-based resources such as parks, recreation centers, and health clinics.[32]

Workgroup Recommendations

Community vital signs (**Fig. 3**) have the potential to help health care providers understand the environmental factors that may be contributing to a patient's health outcomes and provide tailored care that addresses those factors. However, community vital signs are not yet commonly used in clinical practice, and there is a need for health care providers to be trained in using them effectively. Additionally, community vital signs may require significant data collection and analysis, which may pose challenges to health care providers who do not have access to the necessary resources. The role of the community and of neighborhood disadvantage is an important consideration in establishing future research. Tools such as the Area Deprivation Index may be helpful in quantifying the impacts of the community vital signs on the external stressors experienced by NLUTD patients.

THEME 6—INTERVENTIONS FOR EQUITABLE CARE

Discussions involved implementing various interventions, including telemedicine, the use of advanced practice providers and allied health professionals, community-based education programs, and electronic platforms for improved accessibility and care coordination. Community-based partnerships in clinical care and research

emerged as an important theme in ensuring equitable care for NLUTD patients with socioeconomic disadvantage.

A recent large, prospective study assessing unmet social needs in over 33,000 patients from primary care clinics found a positive cumulative association between the number of social needs and multiple chronic medical conditions. Transportation to health care appointments had the strongest association with multiple medical conditions assessed, which is consistent with other studies. The present study also identified transportation to health care appointments as one of the needs with a strong association to overactive bladder. While these studies from the primary care literature were conducted by a single group at a large, urban medical center, our study represents participants living in a variety of different community types, suggesting transportation affects health care access, care, and outcomes across the country and across multiple different diseases.[33]

Workgroup Recommendation

The group participants emphasized 3 important interventions that can help level inequities, particularly those related to access to care. Firstly, establishing a transportation infrastructure for disabled patients to access clinic buildings, or partnerships with ride-share programs would contribute significantly to enhanced transportation services. While these are available in some health systems, more prevalent availability could considerably improve patient adherence to appointments.

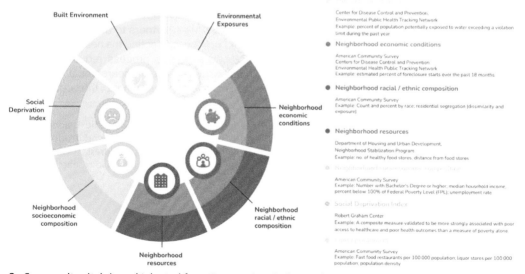

ig. 3. Community vital signs. (*Adapted from* Community Vital Signs (Vital Signs). http://communityvitalsigns.org)

POTENTIAL LEGISLATIVE ADVOCACY AREAS RELEVANT TO HEALTH EQUITY IN NLUTD

Comprehensive Insurance Coverage / Medicaid expansion

Telehealth Accessibility and Expansion of Services

Caregiver Support and Return to Work flexibility

Transportation Equity and Affordability

Disability Inclusion and Accessibility

Physician Workforce Enhancement in Underserved Areas

Reduction of Prior Authorization Burdens

Fig. 4. Potential areas of legislative advocacy and public policy.

For those patients without access to ride-share or public transportation, integration of telehealth services into routine NLUTD care is an essential component of addressing health inequity. The telehealth infrastructure should be available across different platforms and should include audio-only options for patients who do not have the capability to communicate through a video platform. Second, the workgroup also recommended an overhaul of the NLUTD care model to include the patient's neighborhood and community sources of health. Community-based collaborative care models can serve as a powerful resource for the patient to manage their condition effectively without straying far from home. This is essential particularly in rural areas without specialized NLUTD care. Lastly, to drive equity, physicians must themselves become advocates for policy changes that benefit marginalized patients. **Fig. 4** summarizes potential policy positions that are discussed at the local, state, and national levels that are highly relevant to improving equity to NLUTD patients.

The American Urologic Associations Advocacy Summit, held annually in Washington DC, highlights several advocacy goals that advance the specialty and its patients. Included within the advocacy goals are expansion of telehealth flexibilities, addressing workforce issues, and reducing the burdens of prior authorizations. Engagement of the clinician beyond the walls of the clinic has become an important intervention for equitable care.

THEME 7—CHALLENGES IN CLINICAL TRIALS AND RESEARCH

Efforts to make clinical trials more inclusive and drive equity highlight the need for affordable translation services, incentives for participation, and diversification of the research workforce. Barriers in research administration and Institutional Review Board (IRB) processes need to be addressed to ensure the inclusion of diverse NLUTD patient populations.

A growing body of literature supports the role of community engagement in all phases of the research process including hypothesis generation, proposal development, research implementation, and dissemination. Community engagement is the bidirectional, mutually beneficial process of working collaboratively with and through groups of people affiliated by geographic proximity, a health issue, or similar situations. It requires working in partnership with the community in a relationship of transparency and trust to draw on the expertise of all partners to address pressing real-world problems affecting the health of the community partners. This process requires an ongoing relationship between researchers and community representatives throughout the course of the

ADDRESSING CHALLENGES IN NLUTD RESEARCH AND CLINICAL TRIALS

Establish Multilingual Support Systems

Expand Access to Transportation

Integrate Telehealth Services Widely

Use Community Vital Signs in Clinical Assessment

Enhance Community-Based Care Models

Promote Inclusive Clinical Trials

Diversify Research and Clinical Workforce

Streamline Research Administration Processes

Engage in Community-Based Participatory Research (CBPR)

Implement Comprehensive Geriatric Assessments

Fig. 5. Neurogenic Bladder Research Group (NBRG) workgroup recommendations to address the challenges in creating inclusive research.

EXAMPLES OF COMMUNITY BASED PARTICIPATORY RESEARCH IN NLUTD

1. **Transportation and Access to Urological Care:** A study that partners with local transportation services to assess the impact of improved transportation access on appointment adherence and health outcomes for NLUTD patients.

2. **Telehealth Utilization in NLUTD Management:** Research to evaluate the effectiveness of telehealth services in managing NLUTD, focusing on patient satisfaction, health outcomes, and barriers to telehealth use among different communities.

3. **Assessing the Role of Caregiver Support in NLUTD Outcomes:** A study to develop and test caregiver support interventions, including respite care and educational resources, to determine their impact on the well-being of both caregivers and NLUTD patients.

4. **Insurance Navigation and Health Outcomes:** A project that investigates the impact of providing dedicated insurance navigation services on the healthcare utilization patterns and outcomes of NLUTD patients with various insurance types.

5. **Evaluating Community Vital Signs:** Research that maps community vital signs against health outcomes in NLUTD to understand how neighborhood factors like food security and proximity to resourced community clinics affect patient well-being.

6. **Neighborhood Advocacy and NLUTD Management:** A study to create neighborhood advocacy programs that empower NLUTD patients to engage with local health resources and assess the impact of this engagement on their health outcomes.

7. **Socioeconomic Factors and Bladder Management:** Research focused on the correlation between socioeconomic status, bladder management adherence, and the development of urological complications in NLUTD patients.

8. **Cultural Competency Training for Healthcare Providers:** A study that implements cultural competency training for providers and measures the impact on patient-provider communication, trust, and health outcomes in NLUTD care.

9. **Community-Based Health Education Programs:** A study to develop, implement, and assess the effectiveness of community-based health education programs on knowledge, self-management skills, and health outcomes in NLUTD.

10. **Assessing the Efficacy of Multidisciplinary Care Teams:** A pilot study that provides education to "health promoters" – community clinic staff or volunteers that serve as a liaison between the NLUTD patient and their subspecialty clinic.

Fig. 6. Potential community-based participatory research areas of interest. NLUTD, neurogenic lower urinary tract dysfunction.

research and beyond. Communities are best positioned to define the most pressing problems for their members. Engaging community members and centering their lived experiences increases the relevance and cultural rigor of the research and the likelihood of generating meaningful results.[34]

Workgroup Recommendation

In order to move toward equitable research implementation that engages the community directly, the workgroup participants recommended various intervention points to drive inclusive recruitment, engaging idea generation and addressing present challenges in inclusive research. These recommendations are summarized in **Fig. 5**. First, to overcome language barriers and ensure clear communication, the implementation of multilingual support systems and resources is crucial at every stage of both research and clinical care. Additionally, improving patient access to health care facilities through partnerships with transportation and ride-share services is vital, especially for patients with mobility impairments. The expansion of telehealth infrastructures, including both video and audio-only options, can address disparities in technology access and provide flexible care options. Furthermore, integrating 'community vital signs' — key indicators of environmental and social determinants — into clinical assessments allows for more personalized care plans. At the community level, the promotion of collaborative care models can utilize local resources and support systems, enabling patients to effectively manage their conditions within their own neighborhoods or medical homes (for example, the model of the integrated FQHC).

In the realm of clinical research, these strategies include advocating for inclusive clinical trials that reflect the diverse NLUTD populations. This can be achieved by providing affordable translation/interpreter services, offering participation incentives, and ensuring accessible research facilities. To echo the diversity of patients in the workforce, there is a call to diversify the researchers and clinicians themselves. Streamlining administrative processes, such as IRB protocols, is also suggested to speed up the inclusion of varied patient groups in studies. Engaging in CBPR ensures that the research not only involves but is driven by community members, addressing the real-life challenges they face. Lastly, implementing comprehensive geriatric assessments in NLUTD care is essential to cater to the complex needs of the ever-increasing elderly population, considering comorbidities, frailty, and cognitive function. These recommendations are directed toward creating a research and clinical landscape that is inclusive, patient-oriented, and sensitive to the distinct needs of individuals with NLUTD from varied sociodemographic contexts. **Fig. 6** includes potential CBPR research areas of interest for improving NLUTD urologic outcomes.

SUMMARY

This systematic review highlights the disparity in adult NLUTD care, revealing a pattern influenced by racial, ethnic, and economic factors. It calls for a deeper understanding and proactive measures. The conceptual framework, shaped by varied stakeholders, charts a course toward redressing these disparities by recognizing the SDOHs's role in NLUTD. It encourages urologists and researchers to adopt strategies that broaden patient access to crucial services like telemedicine, foster community engagement, and promote collaborative research and advocacy to refine health care delivery. This study serves as a valuable roadmap for mitigating NLUTD disparities through a holistic, fair health care model that weaves in sociodemographic awareness and encourages community participation.

ACKNOWLEDGMENTS

The authors listed here are part of the Neurogenic Bladder Research Group that contributed to the writing of this article: Sara Lenherr, MD; Iryna Crescenze, MD; Guilia Lane, MD; Zhina Sadeghi, MD; Christopher Elliot, MD; Argyrios Stampas, MD; Rose Khavari, MD; Daniel Wood, MD; John T. Stoffel, MD; Michael Albo, MD; Rachel Shapiro, PA-C; Joel Castellanos, MD; Ms. Kassandra Nieves.

DISCLOSURE

The authors have nothing to disclose.

REFERENCES

1. Adler NE, Stewart J. Preface to the biology of disadvantage: socioeconomic status and health. Ann N Y Acad Sci 2010;1186(1):1–4.
2. Wyndaele JJ. The management of neurogenic lower urinary tract dysfunction after spinal cord injury. Nat Rev Urol 2016;13(12):705–14.
3. Smith KA, Liu T, Freeman KA, et al. Differences in continence rates in individuals with spina bifida based on ethnicity. J Pediatr Rehabil Med 2019; 12(4):361–8.
4. Rude T, Moghalu O, Stoffel J, et al. The role of health insurance in patient reported satisfaction with bladder management in neurogenic lower urinary tract dysfunction due to spinal cord injury. J Urol 2021;205(1):213–8.
5. Escalon MX, Houtrow A, Skelton F, et al. Health care disparities add insult to spinal cord injury. Neurol Clin Pract 2021;11(6):e893–5.
6. Meade MA, Lewis A, Jackson MN, et al. Race, employment, and spinal cord injury. Arch Phys Med Rehabil 2004;85(11):1782–92.
7. Skelton F, Salemi JL, Akpati L, et al. Genitourinary complications are a leading and expensive cause of emergency department and inpatient encounters for persons with spinal cord injury. Arch Phys Med Rehabil 2019;100(9):1614–21.
8. Mahmoudi E, Meade MA, Forchheimer MB, et al. Longitudinal analysis of hospitalization after spinal cord injury: variation based on race and ethnicity. Arch Phys Med Rehabil 2014;95(11):2158–66.
9. Jones CP, Jones CY, Perry GS, et al. Addressing the social determinants of children's health: a cliff analogy. J Health Care Poor Underserved 2009;20(4 Suppl):1–12.
10. Jones CP. Levels of racism: a theoretic framework and a gardener's tale. Am J Publ Health 2000; 90(8):1212–5.
11. Ayoade OF, Fowler JR. Effect of insurance type on access to orthopedic care for pediatric trigger thumb. J Hand Surg 2020;45(9):881.e1.
12. Routh JC, Joseph DB, Liu T, et al. Variation in surgical management of neurogenic bowel among centers participating in National Spina Bifida Patient Registry. J Pediatr Rehabil Med 2017;10(3–4): 303–12.
13. Nabi J, Tully KH, Cole AP, et al. Access denied: The relationship between patient insurance status and access to high-volume hospitals. Cancer 2021; 127(4):577–85.
14. Bradley CJ, Dahman B, Bear HD. Insurance and inpatient care: differences in length of stay and costs between surgically treated cancer patients. Cancer 2012;118(20):5084–91.
15. Marrie RA, Cutter G, Tyry T, et al. Disparities in the management of multiple sclerosis-related bladder symptoms. Neurology 2007;68(23):1971–8.
16. Peterson MD, Berri M, Meade MA, et al. Disparities in morbidity after spinal cord injury across insurance types in the United States. Mayo Clin Proc Innov Qual Outcomes 2022;6(3):279–90.
17. Pinquart M. Parenting stress in caregivers of children with chronic physical condition-A meta-analysis. Stress Health J Int Soc Investig Stress 2018; 34(2):197–207.
18. Kanaheswari Y, Razak NNA, Chandran V, et al. Predictors of parenting stress in mothers of children with spina bifida. Spinal Cord 2011;49(3):376–80.
19. Northouse L, Williams AL, Given B, et al. Psychosocial care for family caregivers of patients with cancer. J Clin Oncol 2012;30(11):1227–34.
20. Bischoff A, Denhaerynck K. What do language barriers cost? An exploratory study among asylum seekers in Switzerland. BMC Health Serv Res 2010;10:248.
21. Al Shamsi H, Almutairi AG, Al Mashrafi S, et al. Implications of language barriers for healthcare: a systematic review. Oman Med J 2020;35(2):e122.
22. Vange SS, Nielsen MR, Michaëlis C, et al. Interpreter services for immigrants in European healthcare systems: a systematic review of access barriers and facilitators. Scand J Publ Health 2023. https://doi.org/ 10.1177/14034948231179279. 14034948231179279.
23. Vasileiou ES, Filippatou AG, Pimentel Maldonado D, et al. Socioeconomic disparity is associated with faster retinal neurodegeneration in multiple sclerosis. Brain J Neurol 2021;144(12):3664–73.
24. Calocer F, Ng HS, Zhu F, et al. Low socioeconomic status was associated with a higher mortality risk in multiple sclerosis. Mult Scler Houndmills Basingstoke Engl 2023;29(3):466–70.
25. Vogel TR, Kruse RL, Kim RJ, et al. Racial and socioeconomic disparities after carotid procedures. Vasc Endovasc Surg 2018;52(5):330–4.

26. Pimentel Maldonado DA, Eusebio JR, Amezcua L, et al. The impact of socioeconomic status on mental health and health-seeking behavior across race and ethnicity in a large multiple sclerosis cohort. Mult Scler Relat Disord 2022;58:103451.

27. Shea S, Lima J, Diez-Roux A, et al. Socioeconomic status and poor health outcome at 10 years of follow-up in the multi-ethnic study of atherosclerosis. PLoS One 2016;11(11):e0165651.

28. Kurichi JE, Pezzin L, Streim JE, et al. Perceived barriers to healthcare and receipt of recommended medical care among elderly Medicare beneficiaries. Arch Gerontol Geriatr 2017;72:45–51.

29. Lawrenson R, Wyndaele JJ, Vlachonikolis I, et al. Renal failure in patients with neurogenic lower urinary tract dysfunction. Neuroepidemiology 2001; 20(2):138–43.

30. DeNavas-Walt C., Proctor B.D., Income and Poverty in the United States: 2014; 2015:1-80. Available at: https://www.census.gov/content/dam/Census/library/publications/2015/demo/p60-252.pdf. Accessed December 10, 2023.

31. Neighborhoods and health - Diez Roux. Annals of the New York academy of sciences. Wiley Online Library; 2010. https://nyaspubs.onlinelibrary.wiley.com/doi/10.1111/j.1749-6632.2009.05333.x. [Accessed 10 December 2023].

32. Braveman P, Gottlieb L. The social determinants of health: it's time to consider the causes of the causes. Public Health Rep 2014;129(Suppl 2):19–31.

33. Sebesta EM, Gleicher S, Kaufman MR, et al. Associations between unmet social needs and overactive bladder. J Urol 2022;208(5):1106–15.

34. Klusaritz H, Maki J, Levin E, et al. A community-engaged approach to the design of a population-based prospective cohort study to promote bladder health. Neurourol Urodyn 2023;42(5):1068–78.

The Ideal Neurogenic Bladder Management Team

LaTanya Lofton Hogue, MD[a], Michael Kennelly, MD[b],*

KEYWORDS

- Interdisciplinary team • Neurogenic bladder • Neurogenic lower urinary tract dysfunction
- Neurologic disease

KEY POINTS

- Neurogenic lower urinary tract dysfunction (NLUTD) is prevalent in conditions like spina bifida, spinal cord injury, and MS, causing predictable urinary dysfunction and complications like infections.
- Collaborative care involving neurologists, urologists, physiatrists, and primary care physicians is crucial for NLUTD management to prevent complications.
- Three team models exist: multidisciplinary, interdisciplinary, and transdisciplinary. The interdisciplinary model fosters joint decision-making, enhancing patient outcomes effectively.
- An ideal team comprises professionals from urology, physiatry, nursing, therapy, social work, and gastroenterology, addressing diverse patient needs in NLUTD.
- Telemedicine aids NLUTD management during COVID-19, offering convenience and accessibility. However, challenges like technology literacy and privacy concerns persist.

INTRODUCTION

Neurogenic bladder typically refers to neurogenic lower urinary tract dysfunction (NLUTD) that occurs due to neurologic disease, and it often results in abnormalities of the lower urinary tract, bladder neck, and the urethral sphincters. NLUTD is a widespread problem that affects persons living with neurologic diseases, and because of NLUTD, patients may develop secondary complications, such as recurrent urinary tract infections, renal calculi, urethral strictures, urinary incontinence, and detrusor external sphincter dyssynergia.[1] The secondary complications that may occur are often related to the underlying neurologic condition, and the location of the neurologic disease often causes predictable patterns of symptoms and dysfunction.[2]

Management of NLUTD requires the coordination of a diverse team of professionals operating in conjunction with each other to prevent further complications and achieve the most optimal outcome for the patient throughout the continuum of care for persons living with neurologic diseases. An approach involving various team members including neurologists, urologist, physiatrists, and primary care physicians has been shown to be important for optimizing management of NLUTD.[3]

The goal of this article is to describe the roles of the members of an ideal neurogenic bladder management team, including recommendations for who should comprise members of the team, discussion surrounding when the interdisciplinary team should be implemented, and potential impact of the interdisciplinary team on optimizing patient urologic outcomes and quality of life.

DISCUSSION
Scope of the Problem

NLUTD is a common complication of numerous neurologic conditions, including meningomyelocele

[a] Department of Orthopedic Surgery, Wake Forest School of Medicine, Atrium Health, Carolinas Rehabilitation, 1100 Blythe Boulevard, Charlotte, NC 28203, USA; [b] Department of Urology, Wake Forest School of Medicine, Atrium Health, Carolinas Rehabilitation, 1100 Blythe Boulevard, Charlotte, NC 28203, USA
* Corresponding author. Department of Urology, Wake Forest School of Medicine, Atrium Health, Carolinas Rehabilitation, Charlotte, NC 28203.
E-mail address: Michael.kennelly@atriumhealth.org

Urol Clin N Am 51 (2024) 297–303
https://doi.org/10.1016/j.ucl.2024.02.006

(spina bifida), spinal cord injury, cerebrovascular disease, Parkinson's disease, multiple system atrophy, and multiple sclerosis. Patients may be at high risk of secondary complications of NLUTD due to the underlying neurologic disease. The neurologic disorder often causes specific predictable patterns of lower urinary tract dysfunction.[3] The most common urodynamic pattern of lower urinary tract dysfunction is neurogenic detrusor overactivity (NDO), which often results in urinary incontinence. This pattern is commonly seen in patients with suprapontine lesions, such as Parkinson's disease, multisystem atrophy, dementia, multiple sclerosis, and stroke. These patients may report urinary urgency, frequency, and urinary urge incontinence, and this is often referred to overactive bladder. NDO can also occur in patients with cervical and thoracic spinal cord injury, but patients with suprasacral spinal cord injury typically present with NDO with detrusor sphincter dyssynergia.[4]

Another urodynamic pattern of lower urinary tract dysfunction is detrusor sphincter dyssynergia which is often associated with suprasacral spinal cord injury and diseases of the suprasacral spinal cord. Detrusor sphincter dyssynergia occurs due to discoordinated activity between the detrusor and the urethral sphincters. This results in the detrusor and the urethral sphincter subsequently contracting concurrently leading to urinary symptoms of intermittent obstructive voiding, urinary urgency, and urge incontinence along with incomplete bladder emptying. Sustained high bladder pressures from detrusor sphincter dyssynergia can lead to upper tract changes, including hydroureter, hydronephrosis, and renal deterioration.

Some NLUTD patients develop a noncompliant bladder on urodynamic testing where the bladder loses its ability to accommodate during bladder filling leading to high bladder pressures. In patients with normal or hypoactive urethral sphincter, patients often present with urinary incontinence. However, in NLUTD patients with hypertonic urethral sphincters, poor bladder compliance can be a "silent killer" as the patients are often asymptomatic, but the sustained high bladder pressures often lead to irreversible hydroureter, hydronephrosis, and renal deterioration. Although the exact etiology of poor bladder compliance is unknown, it is thought to be due to the changes in the viscoelastic properties of the bladder leading to fibrosis and loss of elasticity.

In patients with neurologic disease or injury to the cauda equina or sacral roots, including cauda equina syndrome, spina bifida, and diabetic peripheral neuropathy, the most commonly seen form of NLUTD results in bladder hypoactivity that may also be accompanied by impaired sphincter activity. This results in an areflexic bladder or hypotonic bladder with poorly sustained bladder contractions. Thus, these patients frequently report incomplete bladder emptying. Additionally, due to the hypotonic poor urethral function (intrinsic sphincter deficiency), these patients may also present with stress urinary incontinence along with incomplete bladder emptying.[2]

Regardless of the neurologic etiology of the NLUTD, the goals of management are to achieve urinary continence, prevent secondary complications, for example, urinary tract infection, preserve upper urinary function, and improve quality of life for the person with neurogenic bladder.[3,5,6] Thus, at the center of the ideal neurogenic bladder management team is the patient. All treatment recommendations must be specific to the patient and should be made in collaboration with the patient and their caregivers.[7] The benefits of collaborative treatment involving a team approach has been cited as a solution to many concerns facing health care because it is has been shown to correlate with improved patient outcomes, improvement in continuity of care, and decreased costs of providing care.[8]

MODELS FOR TEAM APPROACH TO CARE

Three primary approaches used to describe interactions between team members described in literature include a multidisciplinary team model, an interdisciplinary team model, and a transdisciplinary team model. The multidisciplinary team approach involves each specialty or discipline working independently to treat the patient from their own perspective (**Fig. 1**). The knowledge and skill set of each specialty and discipline is utilized to treat the patient, but there is not frequently a direct plan for communication between team members, and often the members of the multidisciplinary team do not influence the decisions of other members of the team.[9–13]

In the interdisciplinary team model, medical specialists and team members work together in the assessment and treatment of patients by using joint decision-making and goal setting (**Fig. 2**). At the center of the interdisciplinary team model is the premise that each specialty and discipline work in collaboration with each other to treat the patient.[9] Coordination and integration of care between the medical specialists and disciplines result in achieving common goals of patient-centered care, and this has been shown to result in the most optimal patient outcome.[14]

In the transdisciplinary team model, team members do not perform a specific role, but rather each team member can perform any team member role

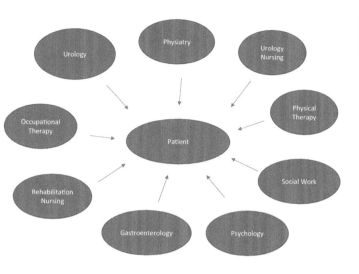

Fig. 1. Components of a multidisciplinary team for neurogenic bladder management.

(Fig. 3). This may result in flexibility in treatment capability, but this often requires that team members be trained in various areas.[15,16] This type of model is rare as multiple boarded providers are needed, which is not practical at most centers.

At the authors' institution, components of both a multidisciplinary approach and an interdisciplinary team approach are used to treat NLUTD depending on the needs of the patients. During the acute care hospitalization prior to transfer to inpatient rehabilitation, the multidisciplinary model of treatment is commonly utilized in the treatment of neurogenic bladder. Initiation of treatment for NLUTD is managed by the admitting physician team, most commonly the acute care hospitalist medicine team or trauma surgery team, depending on the etiology of the patient's neurologic disease. Urology may be consulted for assistance in the management of NLUTD if there is an acute urologic emergency or concern. In the acute setting, initial bladder management often centers on education, training decisions regarding management with a Foley catheter, suprapubic tube, or initiation of intermittent catheterization.

Once the patient's care is transferred to physiatry (either in acute inpatient rehabilitation or in the outpatient clinic), an interdisciplinary team care model is often used. At the authors' institution, patients who are treated for NLUTD are frequently already being comanaged with physiatry. The interdisciplinary management between urology and physiatry frequently begins, while the patient is admitted to inpatient rehabilitation. Urology consultation may be initiated while the patient is admitted to inpatient rehabilitation to assist with bladder management decisions, handle acute urologic interventions if needed or coordinating urodynamic testing.

Components of a transdisciplinary care model are often utilized in the outpatient clinic setting at the authors' institution in the management of NLUTD. Various team members may be used to perform various tasks in managing the patient with NLUTD. For example, nursing staff members may have special certification in rehabilitation nursing, that is, Certified Rehabilitation Registered Nursing, and they may also have undergone training in urology nursing practice, that is, Certification Board

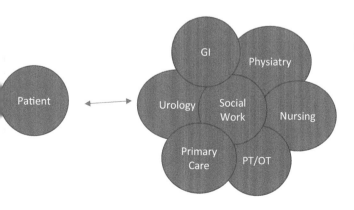

Fig. 2. Components of a transdisciplinary team model for neurogenic bladder management.

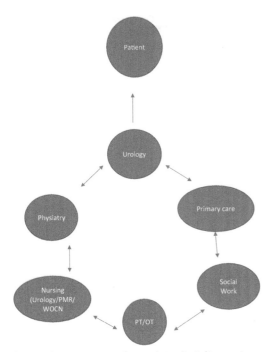

Fig. 3. Components of an interdisciplinary team model for neurogenic bladder management.

for Urologic Nurses and Associates. Additionally, initiation of medications to treat common complications of NLUTD, such as urinary tract infection urinary incontinence, or sexual dysfunction, may be initiated by the physiatrist or urologist. At the author's institution, the certified urology nurse and certified rehabilitation registered nurse are frequently utilized to provide education and training regarding intermittent catheterization techniques, safe techniques for bowel management, answer questions regarding medications utilized for spasticity, and provide education regarding pressure ulcer prevention.

WHO COMPRISES THE IDEAL TEAM?

To achieve the most optimal outcome for the patient, the team will need to include a diverse range of knowledge and professional skills.[10] Many patients who have NLUTD have co-occurring neurologic conditions that often impact other organ systems. Thus, their treatment teams may already include a variety of diverse medical specialists. Medical specialists with expertise in physiatry, urology, nephrology, neurology, gastroenterology, internal medicine, obstetrics, gynecology, physical/occupational therapy, nursing, social work, and pulmonary care may be essential members of the interdisciplinary neurogenic bladder management team.[7] Additionally, other medical professionals

may also be needed depending upon the specific needs and goals of each patient.[10]

The members of the specialized neurogenic bladder management team vary across clinical settings and vary dependent upon the needs of the patient. At the authors' institution, members of the neurogenic bladder management team include urology, physiatry, rehabilitation nursing, urology nursing, social worker, occupational and physical therapy, and the rehabilitation psychologist.

The urologist has specialized training in the prevention and management of acute and long-term complications of NLUTD and in the surgical and nonsurgical management of patients with NLUTD.

The physiatrist is a physician who is specialized in physical medicine and rehabilitation and has specialized training and expertise in the medical and functional assessment of various neurologic conditions that may result in NLUTD. The physiatrist is frequently responsible for coordinating the team approach to care for the patient, and thus frequently, the physiatrist initiates the urology consultation for management of neurogenic bladder.

The gastroenterologist has specialized training and expertise in the medical management of gastrointestinal dysfunction. They have specialized training in the nonsurgical management of patients with neurogenic bowel dysfunction. At the authors' institution, there is a specialized neurogenic bowel clinic to manage unique issues related to patients with GI dysmotility and neurologic disorders that is facilitated by the gastroenterology team.

The rehabilitation nurse is frequently responsible for continence management, while the patient is admitted to the inpatient rehabilitation unit, and often once the patient transitions to outpatient care, the rehabilitation or urology nurses assist in providing ongoing education and support for patients with NLUTD. They may also be responsible for education regarding bladder and function, sexual function, fertility, optimal catheterization techniques, catheter care, and prevention of urinary tract infections and complications.

Occupational and physical therapists assess the functional ability and mobility of the patient with NLUTD. Their primary goal is to optimize the patient's ability to perform activities of daily living, for example, toileting and bladder management care while decreasing risks associated with decreased mobility and decreased functional ability caused by the neurologic condition. Therapists may fabricate custom orthotics or devices that can be used to facilitate increased independence in the management of NLUTD. Additionally, they may also be able to teach patients with NLUTD methods for self-catheterization through the support of orthotic devices to aid in independence of self-catheterization. They also are able to provide instruction regarding methods for improved independence with management of neurogenic bowel dysfunction and neurogenic sexual dysfunction.

The social worker is an important member of the interdisciplinary neurogenic bladder management team as they are utilized to assist with integration into the community. The social worker frequently serves as a case manager and frequently assists with ordering equipment, medications, and supplies needed for management of NLUTD, and they may also be utilized for counseling and guidance regarding navigating insurance and disability benefits.[9,10] At the authors' institution, the social worker provides information regarding patient assistance programs for medication used to treat NLUTD, for example, beta-3 agonists, antimuscarinic medications, and botulinum toxin.

Other medical specialists and professionals may be considered in the interdisciplinary team for management of neurogenic bladder dependent upon the needs of the individual patient.

Examples of Coordination of Care Between Interdisciplinary Team Members

At the authors' institution, coordination of care between interdisciplinary team members has helped to improve patient outcomes and decrease secondary complications for patients with neurogenic bladder.

Patients with neurologic conditions frequently receive botulinum toxin injections for the treatment of upper limb and/or lower limb spasticity. These patients may also require the use of botulinum toxin in the management of detrusor external sphincter dyssynergia and NDO due to NLUTD. Coordination of care between physiatry and urology is imperative in this clinical example in order to decrease the risk of antibody formation that would make the botulinum treatment ineffective. Additionally, coordination of the injection dates is important so that the recommended maximum dose is not exceeded. The maximum dose of onabotulinumtoxin A is 400 units in 3 months, and the only Food and Drug Administration-approved treatment indication for NDO is onabotulinumtoxin A. The goal in this situation is to coordinate injection dates within 24 to 48 hours of each botulinum toxin therapy, and monitoring of the dosing of botulinum toxin is also considered to prevent potential complications. Studies have shown inconsistent results regarding potential for increased incidences of adverse effects in people with neurologic conditions who receive botulinum toxin injections. However, it is recommended that monitoring of the dose of botulinum toxin is warranted in all persons who have neurologic conditions who receive botulinum toxin therapy.[17] This requires the assistance and coordination of care between the patient, urology, physiatry, nursing staff, social work, and ancillary staff.

At the authors' institution, the social work team and urology team are also utilized to coordinate ordering of catheter supplies for patients with NLUTD in both inpatient setting and outpatient setting.

Patients with NLUTD may have issues with urinary and fecal incontinence that may result in pressure ulcer development. In this clinical example, coordination of care with the addition of a wound care team, including the Wound, Ostomy, and Continence Nurses or Certified Wound Specialists, or plastic surgery may be indicated to obtain the most optimal outcome for the patient.

Patients with NLUTD often have co-occurring mobility impairments that impact their overall bladder management. Some of these conditions include mobility deficits, bowel dysfunction, autonomic dysreflexia, pressure ulcers, spasticity, and pressure ulcers that must be comanaged with the interdisciplinary team to achieve the optimal outcome.

Anticholinergic medications are frequently utilized to treat NDO and incontinence, and a frequent side effect of anticholinergic medications is constipation. As a result, patients may have increased difficulty with bowel evacuation. The authors' institution utilizes a gastroenterology motility clinic to provide a comprehensive approach to management of neurogenic bowel.

Role of Telehealth in the Ideal Neurogenic Bladder Management Team

Telemedicine has expanded as an option for health care delivery across the spectrum of medical specialties since the COVID-19 pandemic.[18] Telemedicine is a broad term that involves the use of technology for telecommunications or remote interactions for medical interventions, including the investigation, monitoring, and management of patients and education of patients and staff.[19,20] Options for telemedicine include video visits, eVisits, eConsult (interprofessional consult between a referring provider and a consulting physician), and telesurgery (independent conduction of surgery by a remote surgeon).[21]

Studies have shown that video conferencing can be utilized to incorporate members of the treatment team and patients along with their caregivers as part of team meetings.[20,21] In-person interdisciplinary team meetings are frequently utilized at the authors' institution to discuss patient management and concerns. Telemedicine for the purposes of managing patients with neurogenic bladder who may have limited access to in-person evaluation or limited access to specialty care by the neurogenic bladder management team may offer an alternative treatment strategy.[21–23]

Telemedicine has been shown to offer numerous benefits including convenience, easy access, efficiency, reduced cost of travel, decreased CO_2 emissions to the environment, and high patient satisfaction rates. Additionally, telehealth may also have an impact on reducing health disparities to those patients in underserved populations, for example, patients with physical disabilities. Despite the advantages to telemedicine, there remain limitations to its use as a primary means of medical care. These limitations include lack of acceptance of telemedicine by patients, lack of experience in using technology with both the physician and patient, and concerns regarding privacy and safety.[18,20]

SUMMARY

The ideal neurogenic bladder management team should consist of a diverse team of professionals with unique understanding and expertise in the management of neurogenic lower urinary tract disorder. While there is limited evidence concerning the key components of an ideal neurogenic bladder management team, research shows that collaborative team models can decrease cost of care and improve patient outcomes.[9,10]

CLINICS CARE POINTS

1. Interdisciplinary Collaboration Improves Patient Outcomes:
   a. Pearl: This article emphasizes that an interdisciplinary team approach involving neurologists, urologists, physiatrists, and other specialists is crucial for optimizing the management of neurogenic lower urinary tract dysfunction.
   b. Pitfall: Failing to incorporate interdisciplinary collaboration may result in suboptimal patient outcomes, increased complications, and higher costs of care.

2. Patient-Centered Care is Essential:
   a. Pearl: This article underscores the importance of patient-centered care, emphasizing that all treatment recommendations must be specific to the individual patient and should be made collaboratively with the patient and their caregivers.
   b. Pitfall: Neglecting the patient's unique needs and preferences may lead to ineffective treatments, reduced adherence, and decreased overall quality of life for individuals with neurogenic bladder.

3. Tailored Team Models for Effective Care:
   a. Pearl: This article introduces 3 team models—multidisciplinary, interdisciplinary, and transdisciplinary—highlighting the effectiveness of the interdisciplinary approach in achieving common goals of patient-centered care.
   b. Pitfall: Implementing a team model without considering the specific needs of patients and the clinical setting may lead to inefficiencies and communication gaps among team members, compromising the overall quality of care.

These evidence-based pearls emphasize the importance of collaboration, patient-centered care, and tailored team models in the management of neurogenic bladder, providing a foundation for improved outcomes and enhanced quality of life for patients with neurologic diseases.

DISCLOSURE

The authors have nothing to disclose.

REFERENCES

1. Panicker JN. Neurogenic Bladder: Epidemiology, Diagnosis, and Management. Semin Neurol 2020; 40:569–79.
2. Nseyo U, Santiago-Lastra Y. Long-Term Complications of the Neurogenic Bladder. Urol Clin 2017;44: 355–66.
3. Panicker JN, Fowler CJ, Kessler TM. Lower urinary tract dysfunction in the neurological patient: clinical assessment and management. Lancet Neurol 2015; 14(07):720–32.
4. De Groat WWC. A neurologic basis for the overactive bladder. Urology 1997;50(6A suppl). discussion 53-5363-52.
5. Groen J, Pannek J, Castro Diaz D, et al. Summary of European Association of Urology (EAU) Guidelines on Neuro-Urology. Eur Urol 2016;69(2):324–33.
6. Palma JA, Kaufmann H. Treatment of Autonomic Dysfunction in Parkinson disease and other synoucleinopathies. Mov Disord 2018;33(03):372–90.
7. Agrawal S, Agrawal RR, Wood HM. Establishing a Multidisciplinary Approach to the Management of

Neurologic Disease Affecting the Urinary Tract. Urol Clin 2017;44:377–89.

8. Rice AH. Interdisciplinary collaboration in health care: Education, practice, and research. Natl Acad Pract Forum: Issues Interdiscipl Care 2000;2(1):59–73.

9. Singh R, Kucukdeveci AA, Grabljevec K, et al. The role of interdisciplinary teams in physical medicine and rehabilitation. J Rehabil Med 2018;50:673–8.

10. Neumann V, Gutenbrunner C, Fialka-Moser V, et al. Interdisciplinary team working in physical and rehabilitation medicine. J Rehabil Med 2009;2010(42): 4–8.

11. Ellis g, Sevdalis N. Understanding and improving multidisciplinary team working in geriatric medicine. Age Ageing 2019;48:498–505.

12. Korner M. Interprofessional teamwork in medical rehabilitation: a comparison of multidisciplinary and interdisciplinary team approach. Clin Rehabil 2010;24:745–55.

13. Sheehan D, Robertson L, Ormond T. Comparison of language used and patterns of communication in interprofessional and multidisciplinary teams. J Interprof Care 2007;21:17–30.

14. Baragar B, Schick-Makaroff K, Manns B, et al. "You need a team": perspectives on interdisciplinary symptom management using patient—reported outcome measures in hemodialysis care—a qualitative study. Journal of Patient-Reported Outcomes 2023;7:3–17.

15. Norrefalk JR. How do we define multidisciplinary rehabilitation? J Rehabil Med 2003;35:91–102.

16. Schmitz KH, Bavendam T, Brady SS, et al. Is the juice worth the squeeze? Transdisciplinary team science in bladder health. Neurology and Urodynamics 2020;39:1601–11.

17. Narayanan UG. Botulinum toxin: does the black box warning justify change in practice? Dev Med Child Neurol 2011;53(2):101–2.

18. Gadzinski A, Ellimoottil C. Telehealth in urology after the COVID-19 pandemic. Nat Rev Urol 2020;17:363–4.

19. National Center for Interaction. Telemedicine. Advanced informatics in medicine. 1991. www.telemed.no/omNST/.

20. Ayoub C, El-Asmar J, Abdulfattah S, et al. Telemedicine and Telementoring in Urology: A glimpse of the Past and a Leap into the Future. Frontiers in Surgery 2022;(9):1–9.

21. Irgins I, Rekand T, Arora M, et al. Telehealth for People with spinal cord injury: a narrative review. Spinal Cord 2018;56:643–55.

22. Careau E, Dussault J, Vincent C. Development of interprofessional care plans for spinal cord injury clients through video-conferencing. J Interprof Care 2010;24(1):115–8.

23. Woo C, Seton J, Washington M, et al. Increasing specialty care access through use of an innovative home telehealth-based spinal cord disease management protocol (SCI-DMP). J Spinal Cord Medicine 2016;39:3–12.

A Primer for Primary Care Physicians Managing Neurogenic Bladder Patients

Humphrey O. Atiemo, MD[a],*, John T. Stoffel, MD[b]

KEYWORDS

- Neurogenic bladder • Care coordination • Risk stratification

KEY POINTS

- Neurogenic bladder (NB) patients require a coordinated care team who share common treatment goals.
- NB patients at high or indeterminant risk for renal compromise require close urologic surveillance.
- NB patients at low risk for renal compromise do not require close urologic surveillance and are frequently followed by primary care.
- NB patients with new urinary incontinence, retention, hydronephrosis on imaging, gross hematuria, or more than 3 culture-proven urinary tract infections/year require urologic evaluation.
- NB patients with isolated foul-smelling urine, asymptomatic positive urine dip, or urine culture generally do not require urologic evaluation.

INTRODUCTION

The neurogenic bladder (NB) is a constellation of lower urinary tract symptoms that impact those individuals with underlying neurologic conditions.[1] The prevalence of NB in developed countries is difficult to estimate due to poorly available epidemiologic studies in this patient population. However, due to the prevalence of neurologic diseases that impact the bladder such as stroke, multiple sclerosis, Parkinson's disease, and spinal cord injury, it can be assumed that NB is very common disease entity.[2] The treatment cost of NB in developed countries has been studied with one systematic review reporting annual supportive costs ranging from $2039.69 to $12,219.07 with a lifetime cost of $112,774. These figures represent US dollars from 2022.[3,4] Given the economic burden of NB, the management and prevention of lower urinary tract complications by primary care providers who may encounter these patients is most prudent. This article provides a primer for the management of these patients with a focus on when to escalate care.

NEUROANATOMY AND THE DEVELOPMENT OF NEUROGENIC BLADDER

The bladder has 2 central jobs—to store and empty urine. During storage, the detrusor muscle actively relaxes, and the bladder neck/proximal urethral sphincter tone increases as the bladder volume rises. When a threshold volume is reached, the detrusor muscle contracts in coordination with relaxation of the bladder neck/proximal urethral sphincter complexes and urine is expelled per urethra. The nervous system coordinates the changes between urine storage and bladder emptying. When filling, afferent sensory nerves carry information regarding bladder pressure and wall tension (A fibers) as well as pain and temperature (C fibers) mostly through the pudendal and pelvic nerves

a Department of Urology, Vattikuti Urology Institute, Henry Ford Hospital, Promedica Health System, 2142 North Cove Boulevard, Toledo, OH 43606, USA; b Division of Neurourology and Pelvic Reconstruction, Department of Urology, University of Michigan, 3875 Taubman Center, 1500 East Medical Center Drive, Ann Arbor, MI 48109, USA
* Corresponding author.
E-mail address: Humphrey.Atiemo@promedica.org

Urol Clin N Am 51 (2024) 305–311
https://doi.org/10.1016/j.ucl.2024.02.003
0094-0143/24/© 2024 Elsevier Inc. All rights reserved.

to the sacral spinal cord. The spinal cord carries this information to the midbrain periaqueductal gray region (PAG). Different parts of the cortex then process this information to determine whether the bladder should be storing or it is appropriate to empty. If storing, the PAG inhibits the pontine micturition complex and the sympathetic nervous system is activated to promote bladder relaxation. If emptying, the PAG lifts the inhibition on the pontine micturition complex and the parasympathetic nervous system is activated to start bladder emptying[5] (Fig. 1).

When working properly, the function of the bladder is to store urine at low intravesical pressures and to expel urine efficiently, via relaxation of the urethral sphincter and pelvic floor musculature with the concomitant increase in intravesical pressure due to detrusor contraction.

A NB occurs when there is disruption of this neurologic coordination. Upper motor neuron diseases, suprasacral in location, such as stroke, dementia, and spinal cord injury, often lead to neurogenic detrusor overactivity (DO) with urinary incontinence with loss of coordination from the pontine micturition center. Voiding in this patient population is involuntary and may be associated with detrusor sphincter dyssynergia, which is lack of bladder and sphincteric coordination. Diseases and injury impacting the lower motor neurons and peripheral nerve injury such as cauda equina syndromes and lower lumbar disk herniation most commonly present as delayed bladder sensation voiding impaired voiding. Incontinence in this patient population may be due to incomplete bladder emptying and urinary retention. Prior to the initiation of therapies for incontinence, there should be an assessment of bladder emptying.

Not all neurologic conditions have consistent urologic presentations. Diseases such as multiple sclerosis may impact both upper and motor neuron function and therefore may have a varied presentation of lower urinary tract symptoms.[6] Other conditions, such as spinal cord injury, tend to have more predictable urinary symptoms tied to level of injury (Table 1).

Management Goals

NB should be thought of as a chronic condition and can benefit from the Center for Disease Control's Chronic Care Model to treat it.[7] This strategy, successfully used for management of diabetes, requires 6 elements: (1) an organizing health system; (2) support for self-management such as facilitating patient empowerment; (3) decision support for evidenced base care; (4) coordinating care processes; (5) clinical information systems; and (6) community resources and policies. We proposed that primary care physicians are an integral part of this chronic care model for NB.

A clear definition of treatment goals is needed to best coordinate care. We suggest that clinicians treating patients with NB should be focused on the maintenance of bladder function, urinary continence, reduction of the infectious complications of NB, and the prevention of renal deterioration. These goals can be categorized as addressing a safety issue, a quality-of-life issue, or both.

Safety Issues

Recently, the American Urologic Association Guidelines Panel published a study regarding the management of neurogenic lower urinary tract dysfunction. Patients with NB were stratified as presenting as low risk, unknown risk, and high

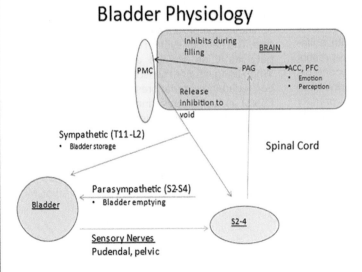

Bladder Physiology

Fig. 1. Neural control of the micturition reflex.

Table 1
Urinary signs and symptom with management options of common neurologic conditions

Neurologic Disease/Injury	Urodynamic Pattern	Clinical Presentation	Risk Stratification	Management Option
Suprapontine: CVA, brain tumor, dementia	Synergic voiding, neurogenic detrusor overactivity, normal bladder compliance	Urinary incontinence	Low	Antimuscarinic/Beta-3 agonist Refer for urodynamic evaluation for persistent symptoms
Suprasacral: MS, spinal cord injury	Synergic/dyssynergic[a] neurogenic detrusor overactivity, normal bladder compliance	Urinary incontinence, urinary retention, poor bladder compliance. autonomic dysreflexia[b]	Indeterminant/ high risk	Refer for urodynamic evaluation with expectant management
Sacral/lower lumbar: Tethered cord, lumbar injury	Chronic nonrelaxing to fixed sphincter, detrusor areflexia, neurogenic detrusor overactivity, normal to reduced bladder compliance	Urine retention, recurrent UTI	Low risk	Intermittent catheterization, suprapubic catheter drainage
Diabetes	Detrusor areflexia, neurogenic detrusor overactivity, impaired bladder contractility, normal bladder compliance, synergic voiding	Poor bladder sensation, urinary retention, urinary incontinence	Low	Check PVR prior to expectant management

Abbreviations: CVA, cerebral vascular accident; UTI, urinary tract infection.
[a] Urinary dyssynergia may manifest in individuals with spinal cord injury above T7.
[b] Autonomic dysreflexia: a syndrome of unopposed sympathetic activity in individuals with spinal cord injury above T6.

Adapted from Kowalik CCG, Wein AJ, Dmochowski RR: Neuromuscular dysfunction of the lower urinary tract, in Partin AW, Peters CA, Kavoussi LR, Dmochowski RR, Wein AJ (eds): CAMPBELL WALSH WEIN UROLOGY, ed 12. Philadelphia, Elsevier, 2020, vol 3, chap 116, p 2600.

risk. "Risk" in this study is geared toward specific safety issues—upper tract deterioration and loss of renal function. High-risk/unknown-risk patients are those at risk of developing urologic complications including renal deterioration. This group includes supraspinal spinal cord lesions (spinal cord injury, multiple sclerosis, transverse myelitis). Low-risk patients are generally those with low risk of developing renal deterioration (ie, stroke, Parkinson's disease, and dementia), empty their bladder well with a low post-void residual (PVR), and do not have recurrent urinary tract infections.[8] High- and indeterminate-risk patients need active urologic surveillance. Many low-risk patients can be followed by primary care. In these cases, primary care physicians should be aware of typical safety issues for NB which include hydronephrosis (with or without change in renal function), chronic urinary tract infections (more than 3/y), and incontinence causing skin break down. Coordination with urologic team can help determine whether a patient with NB is high, indeterminate, or low risk.

Quality-of-Life Issues

Patients with NB benefit from a predictable bladder management regimen that allows them to participate in other daily activities. It is reasonable to assume that patients with NB should be able to hold urine for at least 4 hours during the day, be able to delay urinating 15 minutes when feeling an urge, and have nocturia less than twice per night. Urinary symptoms that impact quality-of-life include urinary incontinence, urinary hesitancy or retention, and bladder pain. Many urinary quality-of-life issues can be discovered during primary care evaluations.

Evaluation

An initial evaluation of the patient with NB should include complete history and physical examination. A pelvic examination is needed, particularly for patients with indwelling urethral catheters, to assess for urethral injury should be performed. Rectal examination in men over the age of 50 years is also important to screen for prostate cancer or to rule out prostatic abscess as source of urinary symptoms. For patients who are spontaneously voiding, a PVR should be assessed. In general, a PVR of less than 25% of total bladder volume is acceptable. A urine analysis can be helpful to assess for a urinary tract infection, but should not be routinely performed in asymptomatic NB patients performing intermittent catheterization or with an indwelling catheter. In these situations, the urinalysis (UA) is frequently falsely positive because of the catheters.

A generalized bladder risk stratification can also be easily performed once the patient has been assessed. In general, risk stratification can be accomplished by identifying the location of the neurologic lesion. Low-risk patients may present with suprapontine lesions such as stroke, Parkinson's disease, brain tumor, and traumatic brain injury will more likely have neurogenic DO with synergistic voiding and low PVRs. Patients with suprasacral spinal cord lesions (spinal cord injury [SCI], multiple sclerosis [MS], transverse myelitis) are at risk for both DO and detrusor-external sphincter dyssynergia and poor bladder compliance. These individuals would be classified as unknown risk and therefore require additional testing for risk stratification by a urologic specialist. These patients require urodynamic evaluation, upper tract imaging, and the assessment of renal function (**Table 2**).

Urinary Incontinence

Neurogenic overactive bladder is common in many neurologic conditions, such as cervical/thoracic spinal cord injury, multiple sclerosis, Parkinson's disease, spina bifida, and cerebral vascular injuries. It is a quality-of-life issue for many people and, in some conditions, may reflect a safety issue such as high bladder storage pressures or can cause skin break down. All patients should be asked if they have urinary incontinence. If positive, it is helpful to differentiate whether the incontinence is an inability to delay urination (overactive bladder) or activity related (stress incontinence).

Prior to urologic referral, it is helpful to have patients perform a voiding diary. People consuming volumes greater than 64 oz/day or high volumes of irritants (coffee, tea, energy drinks, alcohol) can be advised to decrease this intake and see if this mitigates bothersome symptoms. First-line therapy for neurogenic overactive bladder without an elevated PVR usually includes either anticholinergic medications or B3 agonists. However, anticholinergic medications can negatively impact people with slow bowel transit and can precipitate cognitive changes in others. Consequently, beta-3 agonists are generally the preferred oral therapy, although insurance can be a limiting step in prescribing. However, treatment outcomes can be unsatisfactory and may people stop oral overactive bladder (OAB) treatment.[9] It is important to note that addressing urinary symptoms also frequently requires addressing bowel issues. Care should be made to formulate a urinary plan that also includes a sustainable bowel regimen producing a bowel movement every 3 days at the minimum.

Table 2
Key symptoms and signs needing urologic referral in the neurogenic bladder patient

Clinical Symptom	Initial Evaluation	Clinical Sign	Urology Referral
Flank pain	Renal ultrasound/basic metabolic panel	Hydronephrosis/ elevated creatinine	Yes: Urodynamic evaluation needed
Dysuria	Check PVR/urinalysis and culture	Normal PVR, positive cultures	No: Treat expectantly
Hematuria	Urinalysis with microscopy/ renal ultrasound	Renal stone, positive cultures	Yes: Hematuria evaluation needed
Foul-smelling urine	Check PVR/urinalysis	Negative U/A, normal PVR	No: Increase hydration and bladder emptying techniques
Urinary incontinence	Check PVR/urinalysis	Perineal maceration/ yeast dermatitis, normal PVR/ elevated PVR[b]	Yes: Urodynamic evaluation needed if patient refractory to medical management
Urinary frequency[a]	Check PVR/urinalysis	Normal urinalysis, elevated PVR[b]	Yes: Urodynamic evaluation needed

[a] Urinary frequency defined as greater than 8 voids during the awake hours and more than 2 voids after bedtime.
[b] Elevated PVR defined as greater than 250 mL measured immediately after the void.

Urologic assessment for neurogenic overactive bladder can include urodynamics to differentiate between DO and loss of bladder compliance. Treatment may progress to third-line therapy such as intradetrusor onabotulinumtoxin-A injections or fourth-line therapy such as augmentation cystoplasty/urinary diversion if a safety issue persists.

Special attention needs to be given to NB patients, particularly women, reporting urinary leakage around an indwelling catheter. Many NB patients sit in wheelchairs where a significant amount of pressure is placed on the perineum. This pressure, combined with a lack of sensation, can cause soft tissue damage to the urethra and perineum (**Fig. 2**).

Urinary Retention

Urinary retention can be caused by lack of coordination between bladder and sphincters (eg, detrusor sphincter dyssynergia) or loss of bladder contractility. A PVR greater than 300 cc or greater than 25% of bladder capacity can be considered urinary retention. Although alpha blockers may have some benefit in facilitating bladder emptying in MS people,[10] urodynamic evaluation is generally needed and the majority of NB patients will progress to intermittent catheterization, neuromodulation, and/or indwelling catheter to treat this condition. If intermittent catheterization is performed, a schedule of catheterization every 4 to 6 hours during the day is commonly utilized. Ongoing urologic evaluation is usually necessary for these patients.

Hematuria

Hematuria can be differentiated as either microscopic or gross hematuria. For patients without an active urinary tract infection and not using a urinary catheter (intermittent catheterization, urethral catheter, suprapubic tube), we recommend clinicians follow the 2020 American Urologic Association Guidelines on assessing microscopic hematuria.[11] These guidelines recommend that microscopic hematuria is defined as greater than 3 RBC/high-powered field and not assessed via a urine dipstick. However, patients using catheters should not be routinely assessed for microscopic hematuria since a catheter frequently causes urothelial irritation which results in chronic microscopic hematuria.

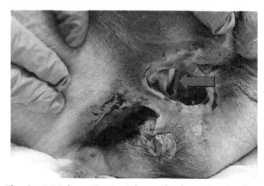

Fig. 2. A Male patient with urethral erosion (*red arrow*) and methylene blue stained fistulous track through decubital ulcer.

Gross hematuria is defined as visible blood in the urine. In general, gross hematuria should be evaluated by a urologist with a CT abdomen/pelvis with and without contrast and with cystoscopy. However, gross hematuria related to indwelling or intermittent catheterization trauma is usually followed conservatively. If bleeding continues, it is subsequently evaluated as earlier. Patients should also be reassured that seeing occasional small blood on the catheter tip during intermittent catheterization does not require a full evaluation.

Hydronephrosis

NB patients with new or worsening hydronephrosis almost universally require urologic evaluation. Some NB patients can develop loss of bladder compliance, which results in high bladder storage pressures. Over time, high bladder pressures cause either urinary reflux or slow drainage of renal from the renal pelvis. This backpressure in the renal collecting system damages the delicate filter mechanisms of the renal parenchyma and can result in loss of renal function. Consequently, any discovery of upper tract changes on imaging necessitates a urodynamic evaluation to measure bladder storage pressures. Treatment of the hydronephrosis in NB patients focuses on bladder interventions such as anticholinergic or B3 agonist oral therapy, intradetrusor botulinum toxin injections, or severely compromised bladders, augmentation cystoplasty, or urinary diversion.

Urinary Calculi

Urinary calculi are relatively common in NB patients and can be classified by location in the urinary tract: renal, ureteral, and bladder. Renal calculi are frequently observed with yearly imaging if patients are not symptomatic or experiencing chronic urinary tract infections. In our cohort of 205 spinal cord injury patients, 17% had radiologic evidence of stones. The median stone size was 4.9 mm. Over 70% of the stones were followed conservatively and only a minority of these required subsequent intervention.[12] In contrast, NB patients with identified ureteral stones should undergo urologic assessment and treatment. Many patients with altered sensorium do not experience symptoms commonly associated with renal obstruction such as flank pain or pressure. Consequently, these patients are at high risk of chronic obstruction or progression to bacteremia. Bladder stones should similarly be assessed and treated by urology. Bladder stones usually represent urine stasis, chronic infection, or debris from catheters. Left untreated, stones can exacerbate urinary

symptoms and urinary tract infections. Some NB patient stones can become truly prodigious in size (**Fig. 3**).

Urinary Tract Infections

Urinary tract infections may present with either typical or atypical symptoms in a neurogenic population. Symptoms and signs of urinary frequency, incontinence, and foul-smelling urine may be present in some, but others may have increased muscular spasticity, sweating, or abdominal pain. We would like to emphasize that foul-smelling urine alone is not always indicative of a urinary tract infection. Many times, urine odor represents dietary choices rather than evidence of an infection.

The standard of care for urinary tract infection in NB patients is to obtain a urine culture. A positive culture is usually defined as greater than 10,000 organisms in combination with urinary-specific symptoms.[11] As mentioned earlier, a positive urine analysis may represent a false positive due to catheter irritation or urinary calculi. Furthermore, a positive urine culture without urinary symptoms in people with catheters does not need to be treated (ISDA). Treatment should be specific for

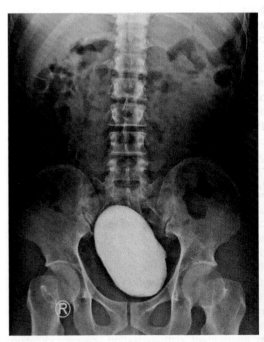

Fig. 3. A male patient with large bladder stone on abdominal plain film. (Eriawan Agung Nugroho et al., Giant bladder stone with history of recurrence urinary tract infections: A rare case, Urology Case Reports, 26, 2019, 100945, https://doi.org/10.1016/j.eucr.2019.100945.)

the cultured organism and limited to a 7 to 10 day course.

NB people with more than 3 culture-proven urinary tract infections in 12 months (or 2 within 6 months) should be referred to urology for evaluation. This usually entails imaging to rule out stones, urodynamic evaluation to assess for bladder pressures, and a PVR to assess for incomplete emptying.

SUMMARY

Managing NB patients requires a team approach. Primary care physicians have significant experience managing populations requiring chronic longitudinal care and are an important part of a NB care team. Urologic issues in these patients can be broadly divided into either safety or quality-of-life issues. Some neurologic conditions, such as spinal cord injury and spina bifida, are associated with high or indeterminate urologic risk for renal complications and should be seen frequently by urologists to mitigate this risk. Other conditions, such as cerebral vascular accidents and Parkinson's disease, have low urologic risk of renal complications and may be followed more frequently by primary care physicians rather than urologists. Care of patients with neurogenic bladder centers around identifying urologic signs and symptoms which may impact either patient safety or quality of life. Some such as new hydronephrosis or ureteral stones require prompt urologic assessment. Others such as positive urine analysis for microscopic hematuria or urinary tract infection may not require urologic assessment. Overall, NB patient care improves when urology and primary care have common goals.

CLINICS CARE POINTS

- Primary care assessment of NB patients should categorize urologic symptoms and signs as either a safety issue or a quality-of-life issue.
- Neurogenic bladder patients with multiple sclerosis or spinal cord injury are at indeterminant or high risk for renal deterioration and should be referred for urological evaluation.

DISCLOSURE

J. Stoffel: Flume catheter (scientific advisor), Spine X (Scientific Advisor).

REFERENCES

1. Panicker JN. Neurogenic Bladder: Epidemiology, Diagnosis, and Management. Semin Neurol 2020;40(5):569–79.
2. Przydacz Mikolaj. Pierre Denys and Jacques Corcos What do we know about neurogenic bladder prevalence and management in developing countries and emerging regions of the world? Annals of Physical and Rehabilitation Medicine 2017;60(5):341–6. Copyright © 2017.
3. Palma-Zamora ID, Atiemo HO. Understanding the Economic Impact of Neurogenic Lower Urinary Tract Dysfunction. Urol Clin North Am 2017;44(3):333–43.
4. Abedi A, Sayegh AS, Ha NT, et al. Health Care Economic Burden of Treatment and Rehabilitation for Neurogenic Lower Urinary Tract Dysfunction: A Systematic Review. J Urol 2022;208(4):773–83.
5. Chai TC, Birder LA. Physiology and pharmacology of the bladder and urethra. In: Partin AW, Peters CA, Kavoussi LR, et al, editors. Campbell WALSH WEIN UROLOGY, vol. 3, 12th edition. Philadelphia: Elsevier; 2020. p. 2461. chap 110.
6. Kowalik CCG, Wein AJ, Dmochowski RR. Neuromuscular dysfunction of the lower urinary tract. In: Partin AW, Peters CA, Kavoussi LR, et al, editors. Campbell WALSH WEIN UROLOGY, vol. 3, 12th edition. Philadelphia: Elsevier; 2020. p. 2600. chap 116.
7. Stellefson M, Dipnarine K, Stopka C. The Chronic Care Model and Diabetes Management in US Primary Care Settings: A Systematic Review. Prev Chronic Dis 2013;10:120180.
8. Ginsberg DA, Boone TB, Cameron AP, et al. The AUA/SUFU Guideline on Adult Neurogenic Lower Urinary Tract Dysfunction: Diagnosis and Evaluation. J Urol 2021;206(5):1097–105.
9. Veenboer PW, Bosch JL. Long-term adherence to antimuscarinic therapy in everyday practice: a systematic review. J Urol 2014;191(4):1003–8.
10. Schneider MP, Tornic J, Sýkora R, et al. Alpha-blockers for treating neurogenic lower urinary tract dysfunction in patients with multiple sclerosis: A systematic review and meta-analysis. A report from the Neuro-Urology Promotion Committee of the International Continence Society (ICS). Neurourol Urodyn 2019;38(6):1482–91.
11. Averch TD, Stoffel J, Goldman HB, et al. AUA White Paper on Catheter Associated Urinary Tract Infections: Definitions and Significance in the Urological Patient. Urol Pract 2015;2(6):321–8.
12. Lane GI, Roberts WW, Mann R, et al. Outcomes of renal calculi in patients with spinal cord injury. Neurourol Urodyn 2019;38(7):1901–6.

Moving?